The Newborn Child

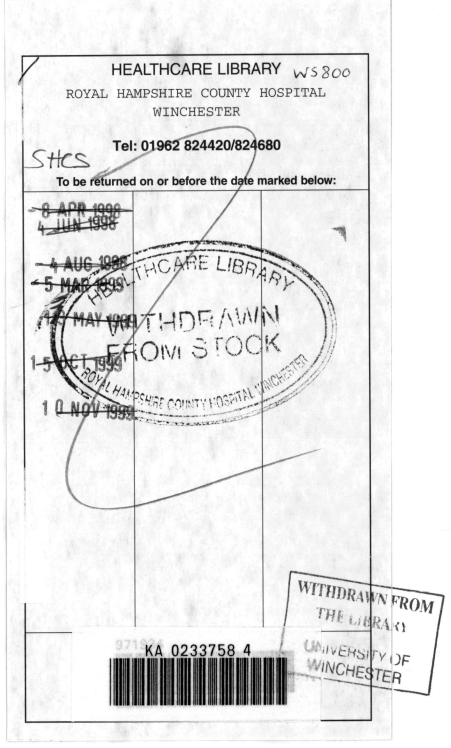

For information on Churchill Livingstone titles, or to place an order, call:

UK: Freephone 0500 566 242
Europe: + 44 131 535 1021
USA/Canada: + 1 201 319 9800
Australia/New Zealand: + 61 3 9699 5400

For Churchill Livingstone

Editorial director: Mary Law
Project manager: Valerie Burgess
Project development editor: Dinah Thom
Design direction: Judith Wright
Project controller: Pat Miller
Copy editor: Adam Campbell
Sales promotion executive: Hilary Brown

The Newborn Child

Peter G B Johnston
MB FRCP FRCPCH
Consultant Paediatrician,
West Dorset General Hospitals NHS Trust, Dorset, UK

EIGHTH EDITION

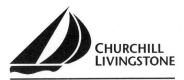

CHURCHILL LIVINGSTONE

NEW YORK EDINBURGH LONDON MADRID MELBOURNE SAN FRANCISCO TOKYO 1998

CHURCHILL LIVINGSTONE
Medical Division of Pearson Professional Limited

Distributed in the United States of America by Churchill
Livingstone, 650 Avenue of the Americas, New York, N.Y.
10011, and by associated companies, branches and
representatives throughout the world.

First edition 1961
Second edition 1967
Third edition 1972
Fourth edition 1977
Fifth edition 1982
Sixth edition 1987
Seventh edition 1994
Eighth edition 1998

ISBN 0 443 05510 6

British Library Cataloguing in Publication Data
A catalogue record for this book is available from the British
Library.

Library of Congress Cataloging in Publication Data
A catalog record for this book is available from the Library of
Congress.

Note
Medical knowledge is constantly changing. As new
information becomes available, changes in treatment,
procedures, equipment and the use of drugs become
necessary. The author and the publishers have, as far as it is
possible, taken care to ensure that the information given in
the text is accurate and up-to-date. However, readers are
strongly advised to confirm that the information, especially
with regard to drug usage, complies with the latest
legislation and standards of practice.

The
publisher's
policy is to use
**paper manufactured
from sustainable forests**

Printed in Singapore

Contents

Preface

From the first edition of this book by Dr David Vulliamy in 1961 through to this eighth revision, the aim has been to give a broad overview encompassing all aspects of care of the baby from the antenatal period through to the end of the first month of life. It is written for midwives and neonatal nurses in training, and for medical students and junior doctors embarking on neonatal care, as an introduction to the subject. I hope that it will not only provide an adequate grounding in good care of the newborn baby, but also stimulate readers to explore individual subjects further in other more detailed texts. This new edition is based on reliable research where it is available and I have provided more suggestions for further reading at the end of each chapter than in previous editions. I have not attempted an exhaustive list of papers on each subject since the whole range of up-to-date publications is readily accessible through computerized nursing and medical literature data bases in medical libraries; readers are advised to consult these if they wish to read the most recent papers on any subject.

In preparing this edition I have tried to keep a proper balance between new innovations in care based on good quality research and the long-established good practices upon which many of the improvements in perinatal care over the last few decades have been based. It is pleasing to see how much research is undertaken by doctors, nurses, midwives, epidemiologists, geneticists and others and to note how the real significance of such papers is increasingly being evaluated by meta-analysis, with the results being published as papers, books and computer data bases. However, such scientific advances must be held in a constructive tension with the personal needs of the parents and child, and on occasions the wider society in which they live.

The areas of greatest change in this edition are aspects of resuscitation of the infant at birth, the rapid advances in genetics, the increased understanding of HIV and other infections, drug abuse and social and ethical matters. However, changes have been made in all sections of the book to incorporate important recent developments. I have also tried to recognise the impact of the increasingly multicultural society in the UK, and although this rarely affects the type of care required, it can have a significant bearing on how it is provided. Mothers and babies have much the same needs wherever they are and whatever their background. I must, however, thank Dr Sadru Jivani from Blackburn particularly for his sound advice about ethnic issues in perinatology which are not commonly encountered in Dorset at the present time.

As with previous editions I have had great help from many of my colleagues at West Dorset Hospital in Dorchester, and to them all I give my thanks. Dr Nick Dennis and the Regional Genetics Service in Salisbury have provided valuable advice and illustrations. Mr Jonathan Scott in Poole helped greatly to enable Louise Phillips to obtain some excellent new photographs. Many others, all acknowledged within the book, provided the illustrations I requested very willingly. Yet others have written the research papers without which this book would not have been possible. Finally my wife Frances and my sons have endured much to see the completion of this edition and without their support it would not have happened. I owe them all a big debt of gratitude.

Dorchester 1997 P.G.B.J.

Introduction

EPIDEMIOLOGY, PERINATAL STATISTICS AND DEFINITIONS

Pregnancy and childbirth are usually natural and normal events, and in Britain in about two-thirds of mothers no intervention other than the help of a midwife is needed to deliver a healthy child who can be cared for with little professional advice. The prospects for the remaining third of mothers and infants have also greatly improved over the years in most developed countries. This has been achieved largely through an increasing understanding by midwives and doctors of the many risks inherent in pregnancy and delivery and of the physiological needs of the infant before, during and after birth, and by learning when and how to intervene in the process. Despite the emphasis placed on it, the influence of expensive and sophisticated technology in improving the overall outcome for mothers and babies has been relatively small, although it has substantially improved the outlook for the minority of infants who are small or premature. Many more babies have benefited from attention to such maternal factors as the nutrition and health of the mother before and during pregnancy; the appropriate management of pregnancy-related disorders; reduction of tobacco and alcohol consumption; prevention and treatment of infections; the active management of prolonged labour; and the promotion of breast feeding. The provision of neonatal resuscitation to minimize the effects of asphyxia, the prevention of hypothermia and hypoglycaemia, and improved nutrition for the newborn infant have had a major impact in reducing the risk of death of babies in the newborn period and improving their health and development for the future. Other factors which influence the outcome for the baby include genetic disorders and the socioeconomic circumstances of the family, which may in some cases be amenable to medical or social intervention.

It has been traditional to measure the effectiveness of perinatal care by improvements in mortality rates year by year, but the quality of life for the surviving children and how it might have been affected by events around this time are equally important, though much more difficult to assess. Although major neurological handicaps such as cerebral palsy or severe developmental delay are often identifiable within a few months of birth, minor impairments in development may not show themselves for several years and are often ill-defined, so it is sometimes impossible to relate them, with certainty, to events around the time of birth.

In Britain, mortality rates have been progressively falling and are low compared with many developing countries, but it should be remembered that even in the mid-1990s some 5800 babies die each year at or around the time of birth, compared with a total of only 1300 in the rest of the first year. Thus even in the relative safety of the current practice of midwifery, obstetrics and neonatology, there is no room for complacency. Concern to preserve the life of a baby rightly has priority, but it is important that nursing and medical care at this critical time of treatment should also aim to prevent permanent disabilities which may be related to events around or during childbirth. If the improvement in results of perinatal care is to continue, all those involved in the care of the child at any stage must be aware of the effects of complications of the pregnancy on the fetus and take an interest in the long-term outcome for the child in order to learn of the effects of their methods of care. Regular local clinical audit meetings and analysis of the annual perinatal statistics, involving clinicians, midwives, pathologists, members of the diagnostic imaging departments and others, are now commonplace and should enable departments to learn together the aspects of care on which they must focus attention to improve clinical practice. These are now supplemented by regional and national initiatives which are attempting to identify factors which adversely influence the outlook for the infant.

Definitions

Before discussing perinatal statistics it is necessary to define the terms used.

Live births and stillbirths

When a baby is born with signs of life, including breathing, beating of the heart and movement of voluntary muscles, it is classified as a *live birth* irrespective of the length of the gestation period or birth weight.

Stillbirth or *late fetal death* has very recently been legally defined in British law as a baby born after 24 weeks of pregnancy who shows no sign of life after delivery from the mother. All babies born before this maturity is reached are regarded as mid-trimester abortions. This recognizes the fact that with modern neonatal intensive care, a small number of infants of only 24 weeks can survive, but that additional advances of care will be needed to save even more immature infants in future.

A *low birth weight baby* weighs 2500 g (5.5 lb) or less at birth. Babies less than 1500 g at birth are often termed 'very low birth weight'.

A *pre-term baby* is born at any time before 37 weeks (259 days) from the first day of the last menstrual period; a *term baby* is born between 37 and 41 completed weeks of gestation (259–293 days); and a *post-term* baby is born after 42 weeks (294 days) or more.

The *newborn or neonatal period* is the first month of life, and *infancy* is the first year.

Mortality statistics

Perinatal deaths include both stillbirths and deaths in the first week, so *perinatal mortality* is a combination of these two groups.

The perinatal mortality rate per 1000 total births has been taken as a general indication of the standard of health care at this time of life and the improving trend in England and Wales over the last 20 years is shown in Figure 1.1. Although stillbirths and first week deaths have differing basic causes, the downward trends in both reflect the continuing improvements in obstetric and neonatal paediatric practice, but it should be remembered that the small number of fetal deaths before 28 weeks of gestation were not included before 1992, and the effect of their inclusion in current mortality figures can clearly be seen as an increase in the perinatal mortality figures.

The decline in perinatal mortality was comparatively disappointing in Britain until the mid-1970s, when it accelerated somewhat to bring it more in line with figures in most other west European countries. This downward trend now appears to be continuing, though at a slower rate than before. Further reductions in the mortality rates will be much harder to achieve in future

because many of the babies dying are too immature to survive with existing methods of care.

The contribution of lethal congenital malformations to perinatal mortality has fallen as more of them are identified prenatally and the pregnancy is subsequently terminated, but if those remaining are excluded, the average perinatal mortality rate drops from approximately 7.5 to about 5.5 per 1000 births. If babies of birth weight below 1000 g, of which about two-thirds will survive, are also excluded the figure comes down to about 4–5 per 1000. There is, however, still a wide variation in different parts of the country, and in some the mortality rate 'adjusted' in this way reaches as low as 3 per 1000.

First-day deaths have fallen considerably over the years, yet even now nearly half of all neonatal deaths occur in the first 24 hours. Although pre-term and low birth weight babies have a much higher risk of dying than larger and more mature babies, studies have shown that around a quarter of neonatal deaths in the UK still occur in babies weighing over 2500 g at birth. Most of

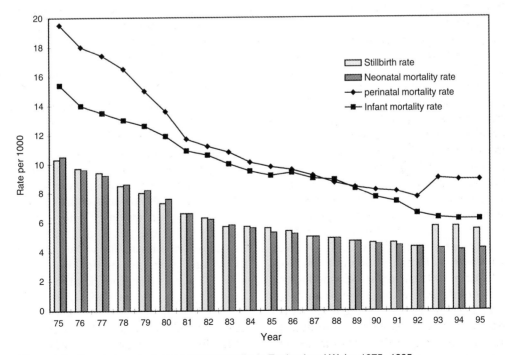

Figure 1.1   Trends in perinatal and infant mortality in England and Wales 1975–1995.

these deaths are caused by factors operating before delivery, especially intrapartum asphyxia or a major congenital malformation.

The death rate in the first month (*neonatal mortality*) is only slightly greater than that of the first week, and its continuing fall is largely the result of improved perinatal care over the years.

Changes in the *infant mortality rate* (deaths in the whole of the first year) are also greatly influenced by neonatal deaths. However, about two-thirds of deaths from the age of 1 month to 1 year (*postneonatal mortality*) are due either to the 'sudden infant death syndrome' or to congenital abnormalities, and although they have fallen recently they are balanced by some extremely immature babies who survive beyond the first month as a result of intensive care but who die later in the first year. This accounts for the fact that the infant mortality was not improving as rapidly as perinatal mortality up to about 1990 (Fig. 1.1). However, the halving of the incidence of cot deaths in Britain which followed the recommendation that babies should sleep supine, reflecting a similar change in New Zealand, has reduced these figures in the last few years (p. 72).

GENERAL FACTORS INFLUENCING PERINATAL HEALTH

The relative impact of different factors on the outcome of pregnancy will vary between one country and another, and between regions of the same country. Where regular antenatal care is not available, such factors as eclampsia, maternal anaemia, sexually transmitted diseases, prenatal infection and prolonged labour have a major impact on the baby's prognosis. By contrast, where antenatal services are well developed these hazards are largely preventable and an adverse outcome for the baby is more likely to be related to low birth weight, maternal smoking, alcohol consumption and socioeconomic factors. In comparing statistics from one country or region with those of another, it is therefore necessary to obtain more detailed information than is offered by the crude mortality rates. Since low birth weight is one major predisposing cause of neonatal death, poor growth in childhood and developmental delay, it is useful to know its prevalence. In Britain the average rate is about 6% of all births, although it varies widely from one region to another. Low birth weight is also directly related to adverse socioeconomic conditions, so these have to be taken into account. The incidence of lethal malformations is another variable factor, and termination of pregnancy after antenatal diagnosis of serious fetal abnormalities also lowers the official perinatal mortality figures.

The causes of perinatal death

The immediate cause of a baby's death is not always easy to establish, and an autopsy carried out by a pathologist with special experience of the newborn is often needed to define it accurately. However, certain maternal and fetal factors are known to predispose the infant to both stillbirth and neonatal death.

A national study in Britain showed that 86% of the causes of stillbirth are complications of the pregnancy or delivery of the infant, such as antepartum haemorrhage, abruption or placenta praevia (41%), hypertension (22%) and complications of the umbilical cord such as knots or prolapse (8%). Approximately 32% of the babies suffered lethal intrauterine hypoxia caused by placental malfunction, 5% were already growth retarded and 8% had congenital malformations. In only 14% of cases was there no definable maternal condition.

In identifying the causes of neonatal death, on the other hand, complications of the pregnancy present a substantial risk in fewer than 50% of cases, and in 35% of deaths the pregnancy and delivery were normal. Very few neonatal deaths relate closely to complications in labour. Congenital malformations were a major factor in 33% of cases, of which nearly half were anomalies affecting the heart and circulation, some 15% were malformations of the respiratory tract and less than 10% were defects in the central nervous system (CNS). This shows a considerable fall in the proportion of CNS abnormalities over the years, which is largely due to identification of these conditions in early pregnancy through screening procedures and subsequent termination of affected infants. A small number of babies die from infections but 45% of deaths before 28 days of age follow complications of immaturity, a high proportion of which are due to respiratory disorders such as hyaline membrane disease. Around 60% of neonatal deaths and 27% of stillbirths occur in babies of less than 1500 g birth weight and the cause in almost all of these is extreme prematurity. The maternal conditions most commonly contributing to neonatal deaths are antepartum haemorrhage, pre-term labour and hypertension acting mostly through premature delivery of the baby, and premature rupture of the membranes. Figure 1.2 shows the recent trends in the causes of neonatal deaths and illustrates that prematurity, congenital abnormalities and asphyxia remain the commonest causes, although the contribution of premature birth is rising as a proportion of the total as the number of babies born with lethal malformations falls.

Even with modern methods of neonatal intensive care, not all such conditions can be successfully treated at the present time and further developments in methods of care will be needed to improve their outlook in future.

The predisposing causes which increase the chances of a baby dying in the neonatal period and which may be amenable to medical or social intervention during the pregnancy or at the time of birth include:

- poor socioeconomic conditions – acting through inappropriate maternal nutrition, a greater amount of general illness and inadequate or late antenatal care
- low birth weight – either from early onset of labour or intrauterine growth failure (especially common in poor social conditions)
- pre-eclampsia
- antepartum haemorrhage
- smoking (more than five cigarettes/day)
- excessive alcohol consumption
- malpresentation (mainly breech)
- disproportion
- post-term birth
- prolonged second stage of labour
- multiple birth
- adverse previous obstetric history (abortion, stillbirth, eclampsia, premature labour, etc.)
- first pregnancy
- maternal disease (diabetes, hypertension, urinary infection, etc.).

Other factors which are not amenable to professional interventions also relate closely to increased perinatal mortality and morbidity. For

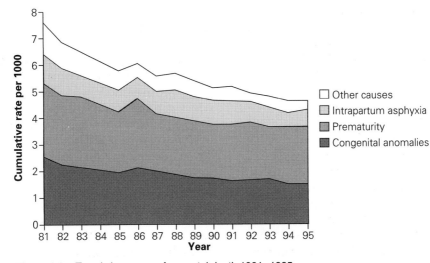

Figure 1.2 Trends in causes of neonatal death 1981–1995.

instance, male infants are at higher risk than females for both stillbirth and neonatal death. Babies of mothers over 40 or under 18 years of age and those born outside marriage are at greater risk, and in Britain the incidence of each of these is rising. In some inner city areas unsupported mothers are in the majority and it is now not uncommon to find a quarter of mothers in an area unmarried and a high proportion of them unsupported by a regular partner.

Although there has been a reduction in perinatal mortality in all social groups over the years, the differences between the rates in the different groups categories remain. The more advantaged sections of the population have low rates, and the more disadvantaged people have the highest rates of perinatal deaths and congenital malformations. Lone parenthood, teenage pregnancy, poor housing, unemployment, poor educational attainment at school and poverty are all associated with higher rates of perinatal mortality and morbidity. In addition, the risks to the offspring of those mothers who fail to make use of the available antenatal care and health education programmes are increased.

Figure 1.3 shows that there are also variations in mortality rates related to the country of birth of the mother, although in second generation ethnic minority mothers born in the UK the risks seem to be diminishing. A total of 8% of British births are from mothers born in the Indian subcontinent, the Caribbean or east Africa. In these infants there is a higher perinatal mortality rate which is greatest in the offspring of mothers originating from Pakistan. Much of this higher perinatal mortality appears to be due to increased rates of congenital malformations. In parts of the UK where a significant proportion of the population is of one of these ethnic groups, the overall perinatal statistics will appear less favourable and such differences must be interpreted with care.

THE QUALITY OF SURVIVAL AND PREVENTION OF HANDICAP

Although perinatal statistics give valuable information about how many babies live or die, it is equally important to establish the incidence of handicapping conditions and in how many of them a potentially preventable perinatal cause can be found. Studies showing the prevalence of handicap relating to such causes are harder to find, but some studies in which all babies born over a period of time have been carefully followed and assessed have provided useful information.

Most severe learning disability without physical handicap is of genetic origin (e.g. Down's syndrome) or due to some fetal insult at a very early stage of pregnancy (e.g. intrauterine viral infections, drugs, genetic disorders), but about 15% result from perinatal difficulties, particularly hypoxic-ischaemic damage associated with placental dysfunction. Milder forms of learning disability have less connection with events at this time and hereditary and socioeconomic factors are predominant. Such conditions as fragile X chromosomes (p. 221) and other recognizable syndromes are increasingly being identified in this group.

On the other hand, cerebral palsy has many different causes, of which around 50% are attributable to problems occurring before the onset of labour and a significant proportion result from complications occurring during the treatment for

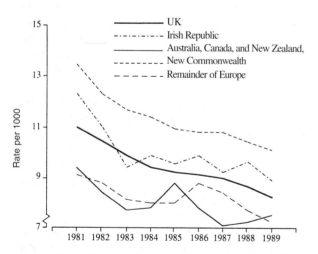

Figure 1.3 Infant mortality in the UK by country of birth of the mother (using a 3 year average centred on the year shown). (By kind permission of the Office of National Statistics.)

extreme prematurity. Others are caused by infection or other diseases occurring after birth, but studies now suggest that only a minority of cases are related to factors operating during labour itself. A significant proportion of children who develop cerebral palsy are born after an uncomplicated pregnancy, straightforward birth and a normal neonatal period.

Published figures showing the trends in the incidence of cerebral palsy may be misleading, since in recent years the diagnosis has been attached to an increasing number of mildly affected children who formerly would not have been included. Some types of the disorder – notably cerebral diplegia – affecting babies born very prematurely (Fig. 1.4), have diminished in numbers whilst others have increased. Concern has been expressed that keeping increasingly immature babies alive is simply adding to the numbers of damaged babies and children. In fact, the incidence of significant cerebral palsy, even in very pre-term infants, remains around

10%, suggesting that babies who would in the past have been affected are now surviving intact. Published reports from Australia show that despite overall improvements in perinatal survival there has not been a reduction in such conditions. Estimates of the proportion by which the number of children with this type of handicap could be reduced if every possible modern development in obstetrics and neonatal care were universally available vary from 20 to 50%, the lower figure probably being the more realistic. Other problems which may be related to perinatal events to a much smaller extent include epilepsy, severe deafness and severe visual impairment.

The introduction of antenatal diagnosis for spina bifida with myelomeningocele, Down's syndrome, cystic fibrosis and an increasing number of other genetic disorders has opened up greatly the possibility of termination of the pregnancy if it is acceptable to the parents (p. 19). In families where there is a history of other inherited diseases, genetic counselling is often able to reduce further the incidence of such handicapping conditions (p. 194).

THE PREVENTION OF ILL HEALTH IN INFANCY

A careful routine examination of all newborn babies in the first few days leads to early diagnosis of many congenital defects, the timely treatment of which can greatly reduce their ill effects. Examples of this are congenital dislocation of the hip, talipes and some forms of congenital heart disease.

The health of normal infants is also affected by maternal factors during the pregnancy and the care of the infant in the first few weeks of life. For example, the infant of a mother who smokes in pregnancy is not only more likely to be growth-retarded at birth but also at greater risk of sudden infant death syndrome (SIDS) or of suffering recurrent wheezing in infancy. Positively promoting breast feeding is of great importance in all circumstances, but particularly where hygienic preparation of artificial feeds is difficult to achieve, since not only does it provide the best nutrition available for the baby, but it

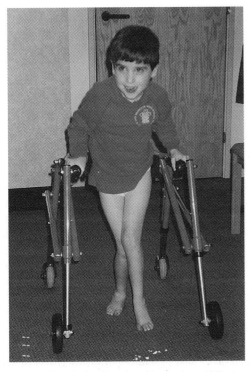

Figure 1.4   Cerebral palsy related to pre-term birth.

reduces the infant's susceptibility to respiratory and gastrointestinal infections. In addition, it improves the attachment between the mother and baby and may, as a result, reduce the risk of child abuse.

There are many other preventable causes of neonatal or infant ill health which, with the appropriate professional advice, can reduce the risk to the growing child. Recent epidemiological research has even linked low birth weight and fetal growth retardation with an increased risk of hypertension, diabetes mellitus and coronary heart disease during middle age. Thus there are great responsibilities on those caring for the developing fetus and newborn infant which reach far beyond the first few weeks of life and may result in better physical, emotional and social health for many years to come.

It is therefore no longer sufficient for those caring for mothers and babies to measure their success on the grounds of mortality figures alone. Such factors as increasing the breast feeding rate (p. 82), reducing the numbers of mothers smoking or drinking alcohol in pregnancy, and successfully teaching parents about diet, clothing and safe sleeping positions for the baby (p. 72) are at least as important.

THE PSYCHOLOGICAL DIMENSION OF PERINATAL CARE

Technological solutions to perinatal problems may also fail if they are not accompanied by an understanding of wider human needs. The wishes of some women for a return to the practice of home delivery, for example, present a challenge to hospital care which needs to be faced. The selection of mothers for home confinement, for intrapartum care in hospital with immediate transfer to home afterwards or for full hospital care must be balanced with the paramount requirement to keep the mother and infant safe and to provide appropriate services for unforeseen emergencies should they arise (p. 41). Making hospital maternity departments more home-like and friendly whilst still maintaining the safety of readily available skills and techniques goes some way to meeting these legitimate requests of mothers but cannot replace the home atmosphere.

The formation of a sound and lasting attachment between mother and child is influenced by what happens in a maternity department or special care baby unit. Observational studies have confirmed that when circumstances interfere with the natural mother–child attachment process during the critical first few hours and days, inadequate 'mothering' is more likely to follow. When adverse social factors are added, the seeds of child abuse may be sown. Bonding and attachment can be greatly assisted by staff in maternity and neonatal units if they understand its importance and adopt sympathetic attitudes towards the mothers.

THE NEED FOR SPECIAL CARE

Although the great majority of newborn infants will be healthy, about 8–10% will need the attention of the paediatric staff for a medical disorder. Traditionally the response to this has been to admit such infants to a special care baby unit for observation, investigation and treatment. Increasingly, however, babies are being nursed at their mothers' bedsides or in 'transitional care units' where mother and baby can be kept together under the supervision of trained neonatal nurses until the baby's problem has been resolved. Clearly there is a small number of infants who do need the special skills of highly trained nurses and paediatricians and it is these infants who now make up a large part of the work of neonatal units. In some areas of the UK, such units are only available in regional centres a long way from the parents' home, which only adds to their concern. In others, intensive care is provided in the majority of district general hospitals in small units. The requirements for intensive care are described elsewhere in this book (p. 123). Whatever additional care the baby requires, it is important for the medical and nursing staff not only to possess skills in the necessary techniques but also to be aware of the broader issues involved. The increasing use of procedures and protocols to guide the care of the mother or baby will not help unless they are interpreted carefully in the light of sound knowledge and experience, with clinical judgement and with a sensitivity to the needs and wants of the parents. Awareness of these factors will contribute considerably to the baby's future well-being, especially as many parents in this situation have considerable anxiety about their infant which adds to the normal emotions of childbirth.

ETHICAL ASPECTS OF PERINATAL CARE

The major developments in perinatal care over the last decade have made it possible to treat increasingly immature infants, and the genetic tests now available enable a greater number of conditions to be identified earlier in pregnancy. Although these advances have resulted in improved outcomes for many babies, they have also raised complex legal and ethical questions which those caring for the mother and baby will face from time to time. It is necessary in some circumstances to consider not only what can be done but also whether it is acceptable or right to do it. These dilemmas may relate to life and death issues such as whether babies of 23 or 24 weeks gestation should or should not be treated because of the high risk of handicap in the small number of survivors. Others may concern if and when to discontinue life support or whether an infant may be suitable as an organ donor. It is necessary in these situations to consider how decisions of this type are to be reached, in particular to what extent the parents should be involved in solving the dilemma. New treatments for newborn infants frequently need evaluation through clinical research which involves subjects who cannot consent to the investigation themselves. Parents may have to decide on behalf of the baby what to do about unexpected abnormalities found on prenatal genetic testing, a situation which may have significant implications for the child's future and often for other family members as well. Those who care for neonates are frequently confronted with these and other ethical dilemmas and it is essential for them to listen to the views of others who are involved, including those with cultural and religious perspectives, and to integrate these opinions into the clinical decision-making process.

The care of the newborn baby is for the most part a rewarding and successful process, and parents will take home the precious new life they had hoped for. However, despite the best efforts of dedicated health care givers, some babies will not have a smooth entry into life and will have an illness requiring immediate treatment, a malformation, be permanently handicapped or even die. The rest of this book seeks to inform the reader about how best to care for the newborn infant, whether well or ill, and the penultimate chapter is a reminder of the family into which the child is born and the way in which the caring team can continue to provide help and support to them when the baby does not progress in the normal way.

FURTHER READING

Alberman E, Botting B, Blatchley N, Twidell A 1994 A new heirarchical classification of causes of infant deaths in England and Wales. Archives of Disease in Childhood 70: 403–409

Boue A (ed) 1995 Fetal medicine – prenatal diagnosis and management. Oxford University Press, Oxford

Nicholson A, Alberman E 1992 Cerebral palsy – an increasing contributor to severe mental retardation. Archives of Disease in Childhood 67: 1051–1055

Office of National Statistics 1990 Birth statistics series FM1 No 19. HMSO, London

Office of National Statistics 1996 Population trends No 85. HMSO, London

Ponsonby A-L, Dwyer T, Kasl S V, Couper D, Cochrane J A 1995 Correlates of prone infant sleeping position by period of birth. Archives of Disease in Childhood 72: 204–208

Roberton N R C (ed) 1992 Textbook of neonatology. Churchill Livingstone, Edinburgh

Schott J, Henley A 1996 Culture, religion and childbearing in a multicultural society. A handbook for professionals. Butterworth Heinemann, Oxford

Stanley F, Watson L 1992 Trends in perinatal mortality and cerebral palsy in Western Australia. British Medical Journal 304: 1658–1663

2

Maternal and fetal health

As methods of assessing the health of the baby
before birth are becoming more sophisticated, it
is increasingly important that all those involved
with the care of a mother and her unborn baby
during pregnancy and after the birth are aware
of their implications and can advise the mother
appropriately. Although the mother may be
aware of her pregnancy long before she feels
fetal movements, professional responsibilities
towards the unborn child may start even before
conception in some cases. Fertilization of the
ovum occurs about 2 weeks before the mother's
first missed period, and by the second, much of
the differentiation of the internal organs of the
fetus is well underway and is virtually complete
by 12 weeks from conception. Subsequently, the
development of function of those organs continues and the baby grows in size until it is able to
live outside the uterus.

The fetus begins to move spontaneously at
about 7 weeks of postconceptional age, but the
mother only becomes aware of movements after
the 16th–21st weeks. Rhythmical kicking is
almost constant from the fifth month onwards
and is distinguishable from the less regular brisk
jumps which increase until the seventh month
and then gradually decline. Kicking increases in
response to maternal emotional stress and
sounds of high frequency. More organized
movement develops at about midterm, including
turning the head towards one hand in response
to contact with it and even fingersucking. The
response to various sounds also becomes well
developed, and this has led to the use of recordings of intrauterine sounds played to pre-term

infants in incubators in an attempt to reproduce some of the features of the fetal environment.

Some light is known to penetrate the uterine wall and, when very bright, it stimulates activity – presumably by reception through the eyes.

PRENATAL FACTORS AFFECTING FETAL WELL-BEING

From the time the fertilized ovum implants in the endometrium to the time of birth, the developing fetus depends on the placenta to maintain growth and development. The placenta is a complex organ which provides a large surface area where the fetal and maternal blood come into close proximity, separated only by a thin membrane across which the mother provides the fetus with appropriate nutrition and adequate oxygenation of the fetal blood, and ensures the excretion of carbon dioxide, urea, hydrogen ion and other waste products of metabolism. In addition, the unborn child is protected from infection by both the physical barrier of the fetal membranes and the immune mechanisms of the mother.

There are many factors which adversely influence the growth and development of the baby before birth or increase the risk during labour, delivery or in the neonatal period. Preventive measures or treatment during the pregnancy can, in some cases, reduce the harm to the infant. However, the effect of poor socioeconomic circumstances (p. 14) cannot be influenced by medical means alone.

Maternal age

The safest maternal age for the baby is between 18 and 30 years. Complications of pregnancy and labour are rather more likely above and below these ages (Fig. 2.1), whilst certain congenital abnormalities also have an increased incidence in older mothers. Down's syndrome, for instance, has a continuously increasing incidence as the maternal age rises (p. 19). Younger teenage mothers have significantly more low birth weight babies because of an increased risk of both premature labour and fetal growth retardation, which is only partly explained by their poorer socioeconomic circumstances and less use of antenatal care.

Parity

Some problems occur more frequently in the first pregnancy than in later ones, e.g. pre-eclampsia, breech presentation and low birth weight. Neural tube defects are also more common. In multiparity, the risks appear to increase independently of maternal age after the second pregnancy, until in the fifth they are as high as in the first, but other social factors associated with larger families account for much of this increase.

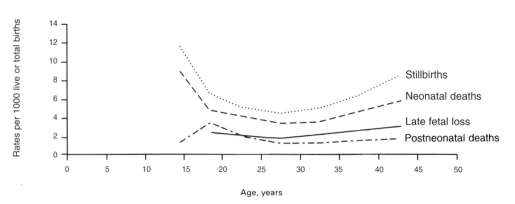

Figure 2.1 Incidence of perinatal deaths by the age of the mother. (By kind permission of the Office of National Statistics.)

Maternal nutrition

Well-nourished mothers of appropriate weight for height who eat a broad diet sufficient to put on around 10–12 kg of weight during the pregnancy should provide the fetus with adequate nutrition for normal growth and health. Studies from developing countries confirm that periods of serious undernutrition during pregnancy can reduce the birth weight of the baby by 300 g and that giving dietary energy supplements to chronically malnourished mothers can increase birth weight significantly. A diet which is relatively high in protein and low in carbohydrate, consisting of meat, vegetables, milk, cereals and fruit, should provide the fetus with all his nutritional needs. A vegetarian diet carries no disadvantage as long as an adequate protein intake is achieved from eggs, cheese, beans and pulses.

Short maternal stature, although frequently genetic, may result from chronic dietary insufficiency in childhood and can reduce fetal size more than a poor diet in pregnancy. Inadequate maternal diet is commonly related to socioeconomic status but also to poor supervision in pregnancy and a failure to make use of antenatal education classes. A contracted pelvis due to rickets secondary to vitamin D deficiency in childhood is occasionally seen in some ethnic minority groups in Britain and may cause obstructed labour from disproportion.

In the absence of clinical or pathological evidence of deficiency of specific dietary components, few mothers require prescribed dietary supplements other than folic acid for the prevention of neural tube defects (p. 21). A physiological anaemia develops during normal pregnancy due to haemodilution, but only when the haemoglobin falls below 10.5 g/dl is the fetus likely to be affected by a lack of oxygen availability, at which point iron supplements are needed to raise it. Studies have shown that British women of Asian extraction are particularly likely to need prescribed iron.

Vitamin D deficiency is also relatively common in pregnancy in women of Asian origin, although it is rare in other ethnic groups. Hypocalcaemia may occur in the newborn infant

if the deficiency is not corrected, so it is wise to investigate such women and prescribe vitamin D if needed.

Some foods such as soft cheeses and patés contain the bacterium *Listeria monocytogenes* which can infect the fetus (p. 162) and should be avoided.

Smoking

Smoking in pregnancy is the major avoidable cause of perinatal and infant morbidity and should be strongly discouraged. In general, the more cigarettes the mother smokes, the higher the risk to the infant. Maternal smoking impairs placental function by reducing its blood flow. This diminishes fetal growth, causing a reduction, on average, of about 300 g in birth weight. There is an increase in the incidence of babies who are small for gestational age and thus more susceptible to perinatal asphyxia and neonatal hypoglycaemia. Increased rates of placental abruption and antepartum haemorrhage also add to the risk of intrapartum asphyxia in the fetus. Although there is also an increase in preterm delivery, the incidence of respiratory distress syndrome is lower than expected, which is likely to be the result of stress to the infant from prolonged placental insufficiency (p. 92). There is no increase in congenital malformations in the offspring of smoking mothers. In infancy, however, the risk of sudden unexpected death is increased; the incidence of recurrent wheezing is much greater even if the baby is not exposed to cigarette smoke after birth; and there is an overall reduction in their educational attainment as they grow older.

Alcohol

Maternal alcohol ingestion in excessive amounts occasionally causes fetal growth retardation and a recognizable facies, the child remaining small throughout childhood and having at least moderate learning difficulties. There is also a small increase in the incidence of congenital heart disease and renal anomalies. There is no clear information about how much alcohol is safe in pregnancy and it is best avoided. Withdrawal symptoms after birth, such as hyperactivity and fits, may occasionally occur in the infant if maternal consumption has been heavy and prolonged.

Radiation

Down's syndrome, and possibly other malformations, seems to occur more frequently during periods of increased environmental ionizing radiation. This effect seems to affect all ages of mothers, although it may be greater in older women and it only accounts for a small proportion of cases of the condition. Irradiation of the ovaries for medical purposes may also have a similar effect.

Social concern during the pregnancy

It is important to realize that psychosocial factors may affect the baby adversely before and after birth. During some pregnancies the family circumstances may suggest that social work support is needed to ensure that the baby will receive proper care after birth. Such situations may include:

- serious or terminal illness in a parent
- a family member with a serious disability
- where the baby is to be placed for adoption
- a concealed or late-presenting pregnancy
- where one or both parents abuse drugs or alcohol
- a parent with a psychiatric disorder
- a history of family violence
- child abuse or neglect in another child
- when one parent has a conviction for offences against children.

In many such cases the social worker can provide sufficient support to ensure the child will receive suitable care. However, where there is a history of child abuse or neglect, a case conference may be held under the local child protection procedures before the baby is born to agree a plan, including court action if necessary, to protect the child from abuse.

Drugs of addiction

There are numerous substances to which a person can become addicted which may have a serious effect on the child before and after birth. The types of drugs involved and their effects are listed in Tables 2.1 and 2.2; it is important to remember that around 25% of women addicted to substances take more than one drug, and many more smoke cigarettes and drink alcohol. Socioeconomic disadvantages which affect the pregnancy and prevent them from making use of the available antenatal care are also common. Some intravenous drug users become infected by hepatitis B virus or human immunodeficiency virus (HIV) (p. 171) from either shared needles or unsafe sexual activity. Unsterile injections may cause septicaemia and there is a higher risk of

Table 2.1 types of drugs of abuse

Group	Examples
Opiates	Morphine, diamorphine(heroin), methadone
Stimulants	Amphetamines, cocaine
Tranquillisers	Benzodiazepines, e.g. diazepam, temazepam
Sedatives	Barbiturates, dichloralphenazone
Solvents	Acetone, butane, trichloroethylene
Cannabis	
Nicotine	
Alcohol	

Table 2.2 Risks to the fetus from drugs of abuse

Risk	Drugs principally involved
Teratogenesis	Cocaine, benzodiazepines, alcohol
Fetal anoxia	Overdose of cocaine,'crack', opiates, solvents
Growth retardation	Opiates, amphetamines, cocaine, nicotine, alcohol, benzodiazepines
Addiction	Opiates, cocaine, barbiturates
Placental abruption	
Pre-term delivery	Too rapid a withdrawal of drugs
Fetal death	

other sexually transmitted diseases in this group of mothers, which may put the fetus at risk or affect the mode of delivery (p. 171). Sudden withdrawal of drugs during the pregnancy can result in intrauterine death. However, if the drugs can be withdrawn progressively from early pregnancy and the mother abstains completely for 4–6 weeks before the birth, withdrawal symptoms in the baby are unlikely. In some centres, regularly decreasing doses of methadone are prescribed as an alternative to the stronger opiates where abstinence cannot be achieved; the lower the dose the mother is taking by the time of delivery, the less severe are the baby's withdrawal symptoms.

Social management of drug abuse in pregnancy

In view of the risk from the abused substances to which the baby is exposed before and after birth, the insecure lifestyle and the social disadvantage of many drug-abusing families, a full multidisciplinary case conference should be held during the pregnancy under the local child protection procedures to ensure the safety of the child through the pregnancy and after birth and to decide what professional support for the mother and baby will be needed to achieve it. This can include court action to obtain one of the care or specific issues orders available under the Children Act (1989), when it is considered that the safety of the child cannot be adequately secured by professional care alone.

Problems for the infant after birth

Opiate addiction. The infant of an opiate-addicted mother also becomes dependent on the drugs, which are powerful respiratory depressants. The baby should not be given naloxone at birth even if his respiratory efforts are diminished, since it causes the rapid onset of withdrawal symptoms. Respiratory support including ventilation may be necessary if breathing is inadequate. In many maternity departments the baby is automatically admitted at birth to the neonatal unit for observation and treatment. Withdrawal symptoms consist of respiratory depression, diarrhoea and vomiting, and autonomic system disturbances such as fever, tachycardia, profuse sweating and nasal blockage. In addition, an encephalopathy develops which is characterized by irritability, tremors, hypertonia, hyperreflexia, wakefulness, a high-pitched cry and, occasionally, fits. These can come on at any time within the first week of life and are managed by giving the infant small and decreasing doses of opiates, or a sedative such as chlorpromazine until the symptoms resolve. Anticonvulsants may be needed for fits. Both hepatitis B immunoglobulin and vaccination should be given to the infant to prevent infection if the mother is known to carry the virus antigen (p. 173). Once the withdrawal programme is complete, the baby usually remains healthy, although there is an increased incidence of sudden infant death syndrome in these children.

Cocaine addiction. Cocaine addiction is becoming more common and has serious consequences for the unborn baby. Spontaneous abortion is common in abusing mothers, as are placental abruption and pre-term delivery which carry their own risks for the newborn baby (pp. 35 and 105). It is a powerful vasoconstrictor and this results in a threefold increase in congenital malformations and a higher risk of intrauterine growth retardation (p. 92). Affected infants have diminished respiratory reflexes in the neonatal period and may require assisted ventilation. Some have cardiac arrhythmias. The drug is also excreted freely in the mother's milk. Later follow-up shows an increased incidence of delay in langauge development and brain growth is often diminished. However, since addicted mothers usually smoke cigarettes and drink alcohol, these too may contribute to the adverse neurological outcome for these children.

Marijuana. Smoking cannabis may slightly increase the risk of pre-term delivery but does not appear to add significantly to the effects of cigarette and alcohol use, young maternal age and the socioeconomic disadvantage which affect many marijuana users. The resin appears in breast milk in sufficient concentration to cause significant effects including constipation in the infant.

Since most of these drugs pass to some extent into breast milk, it is necessary to balance the risk to the infant from formula feeding (p. 77) against the risk from the drugs. In many instances it may be best to allow breast feeding and monitor the progress of the baby closely, although it is not always successful.

Pregnancy-induced hypertension

This common condition, usually defined as the onset of hypertension during pregnancy with a sustained diastolic pressure over 90 mmHg, carries little risk for the mother or fetus. However, if accompanied by proteinuria there is a significant risk of placental insufficiency, which may result in fetal growth retardation, asphyxia, placental abruption or even fetal death. This condition, known as pre-eclampsia, is more likely in primigravidae, multiple pregnancy, diabetes and rhesus isoimmunization. The severity of placental dysfunction does not always correspond to the degree of hypertension, and hypotensive therapy seems to have little beneficial effect on the fetus. β-adrenoreceptor antagonists such as atenolol and labetalol which are used to lower blood pressure may sometimes add to fetal growth impairment and should only be used cautiously in the third trimester. Outpatient hospital observation is the mainstay of treatment, with a careful watch on fetal growth and the mother's health in order to pick the optimal time to deliver the baby. Factors which help in deciding this are a progression to severe hypertension, the occurrence of maternal renal, hepatic and haematological impairment, which carry a risk for the mother, and the results of fetal assessment. These include evaluation of fetal heart rate patterns by cardiotocography, ultrasound scanning for growth, Doppler blood flow studies of the fetal circulation and a biophysical profile (p. 18).

Acute and chronic illness

Any acute severe illness or accident causing significant trauma may affect the pregnancy by precipitating a miscarriage or causing pre-term labour and delivery, or may affect the infant by compromising the placental function. In addition, an infective agent may also cross the placenta and cause fetal infection (p. 158).

Chronic illnesses of many sorts can affect placental function and cause a degree of intrauterine growth retardation. These include urinary tract infection, renal failure, cystic fibrosis, malnutrition, ulcerative colitis and Crohn's disease. Other disorders which have more specific effects on the infant are discussed later in this chapter. It should also be remembered that the course of such conditions as cystic fibrosis, chronic renal failure, congenital heart disease or cancer is sometimes adversely affected by the pregnancy and this may occasionally justify a therapeutic termination.

THE ASSESSMENT OF FETAL HEALTH

The maternity team needs as much information about the health of the fetus as is available in order to assess the need for intervention or to time the delivery of the infant most appropriately. Although the earliest possible antenatal assessment is desirable, it should be remembered that attitudes to antenatal screening and intervention vary greatly. In certain ethnic groups, parents may wish to set limits on the extent to which investigations may be performed and such requests should be respected. Language and socioeconomic difficulties may also affect the uptake of antenatal care. Since many of the available methods of assessment used do not clearly distinguish between the growth, maturity and well-being of the fetus, it is reasonable to consider them together. A complete maternal medical and obstetric history and full clinical evaluation form the basis of the assessment of fetal health which should include the date of the last period, measurement of uterine size using a tape measure, maternal weight gain and assessment of general health. Maternal observations of fetal movements and 'kick counts' may alert the midwife or obstetrician to the need to evaluate the fetus further, but they are too non-specific to be regarded as tests of fetal health and should be supplemented with one or more of the following

Table 2.3   Methods of assessment of the fetus during pregnancy

Method	What it can assess
Ultrasound	Fetal maturity Fetal growth (serial measurements) Malformations of the fetus Placental position Liquor volume
Maternal plasma oestriol or human placental lactogen	Indirect measure of placental function
Maternal plasma α-fetoprotein	Screening for neural tube defects
Amniotic fluid analysis — cytogenetic	Chromosome pattern in fetus Fetal sexing
— lecithin–sphyngomyelin ratio — cells	Fetal lung surfactant production Rare enzyme defects
Chorionic villus sampling	Chromosome pattern in fetus DNA analysis
Doppler blood flow studies	Fetal arterial blood flow Fetal asphxia
External cardiotocography	Fetal cardiac arrhythmias Fetal asphyxia
Fetal umbilical blood sampling	Rhesus isoimmunization Exclusion of haemoglobinopathies Rare enzyme defects

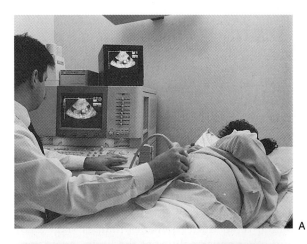

A

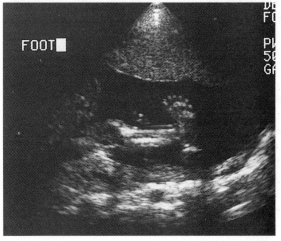

B

Figure 2.2   A: Prenatal ultrasound screening. B: Talipes of the foot shown on prenatal sonography. (By kind permission of Dr Jo Fairhurst.)

methods of evaluating the health of the fetus (Table 2.3).

Assessment of fetal growth and maturity

Ultrasound

Ultrasound (Fig. 2.2A) has become the most accurate method of assessing the gestational age and growth of the fetus and it can also detect some fetal abnormalities. The presence of a fetus can be confirmed and multiple pregnancy diagnosed at about 8 weeks. Gestational age is best established in early pregnancy by measurement of the crown–rump length which predicts the date of delivery more accurately than measuring the biparietal diameter of the head. At 12 weeks of pregnancy, the gestational age can be estimated to within a week either way, and at 18 weeks to within 14 days.

Ultrasound can also identify some fetuses which are failing to grow at the appropriate rate. Usually the biparietal diameter of the baby's head and the abdominal circumference increase at a similar rate, but in about half the 'small for dates' infants the head grows at a normal rate while the abdomen lags behind because of relative malnutrition. Serial measurements of the abdomen can identify growth-retarded infants who require more careful observation, often including umbilical vessel blood flow studies, but it is not always possible to pick out those infants who will be affected. Since these babies are at much greater risk of asphyxia during labour and of developmental problems afterwards, many types of intervention are being tried, such as supplementary oxygen, bed rest and certain drugs, using ultrasound measurements of growth to assess their effectiveness. At present their effectiveness is uncertain.

Structural abnormalities

Ultrasound can also identify polyhydramnios or oligohydramnios, the site of the placenta and an increasing number of congenital abnormalities such as hydrocephalus, anencephaly, spina bifida, renal tract anomalies, talipes (Fig. 2.2B) and other abnormalities of the limbs, some congenital heart disease, prenatal cardiac arrhythmias and many others. Intrauterine treatment of obstructive uropathy and other fetal anomalies is occasionally carried out in specialist centres. Choroid plexus cysts may be seen in the developing cerebral ventricles, the renal pelves may be slightly dilated, and cystic hygromas may be identified in early screening ultrasound examinations. They often resolve spontaneously and only occasionally persist after birth. Increased thickness of the tissues at the nape of the neck occurs in Down's syndrome but is not yet a reliable sign to use to screen for the condition.

X-rays

Assessment by X-rays is used much less now because of the slightly increased risk of leukaemia in childhood in those babies exposed in utero. However, it may be justifiable in identifying some skeletal abnormalities in the fetus which cannot be accurately defined by ultrasound scanning.

Fetal products

Certain substances such as oestriol and human placental lactogen which are synthesized only by the fetus pass through the placenta to the maternal circulation and have been used as indicators of fetal well-being. However, oestriols may be low in anencephaly, Down's syndrome and some congenital heart disease and may be diminished by certain antibiotics and corticosteroids; these tests have been superseded by more direct methods of assessing the fetus (Table 2.3).

The lecithin–sphingomyelin ratio evaluates the quantity of certain phospholipid substances in the amniotic fluid and reflects the maturity of the fetal lungs. The ratio is usually less than 1 until the 26th week of pregnancy, after which it gradually increases. If it is still below 1.5 at a pre-term birth, there is a high risk of respiratory distress syndrome associated with the immaturity (p. 128).

Biophysical profile

The imaging of the infant by ultrasound allows direct evaluation of his reactivity to stimulation, the muscle tone, his breathing pattern, the volume of the liquor and the fetal heart rate. Using these features, a scoring system has been developed where the infant is given a value from 0 to 2 for each feature, 0 being a poor response and 2 a good one. Thus the infant's health is scored out of 10 – the higher the score, the better the infant's state. This biophysical profile, which aims to assess the response of the fetus to the placental function at the time of measurement, is sometimes used to help determine whether the fetus is at greater risk from continuing in utero or whether it would be better to deliver, although its effectiveness in improving the outcome for the baby is as yet undecided.

Doppler blood flow studies

Prolonged fetal asphyxia secondary to placental insufficiency causes changes in blood flow velocity waveforms in the umbilical cord, the baby's aorta and major neck vessels. In experienced hands the fetal circulation can be visualized and blood flow rates measured using Doppler ultrasound. In this way fetal asphyxia may be identified before it becomes clinically apparent. The technique is particularly important when there is evidence of fetal growth retardation or reduced placental function, and its use can improve the outcome of babies in these circumstances. The methods used to detect fetal distress clinically are discussed in chapter 3.

PREVENTION AND ANTENATAL DIAGNOSIS OF FETAL DISORDERS

Since the cause of most abnormalities of fetal development is still uncertain and a clear hereditary pattern is exceptional, intervention to prevent fetal malformations is currently possible in only a minority of cases. The best known examples are the rubella immunization programme for all infants (p. 169) and the dietary supplementation with folate to prevent neural tube defects (p. 21). A careful history taken in early pregnancy may reveal a family pattern of disease, and where an inherited disorder is suspected, genetic counselling plays an important role in reducing the incidence of such diseases. This applies particularly when a mother has already had a baby with a specific disorder known to follow a clear pattern of inheritance or familial incidence, e.g. cystic fibrosis, mucopolysaccharidosis, phenylketonuria, Duchenne muscular dystrophy and others.

Diagnosis for a limited but rapidly increasing number of such disorders is now possible in early pregnancy by biochemical investigation of amniotic fluid or analysis of fetal cells obtained at amniocentesis, or chorionic villus sampling by cytogenetic techniques or DNA analysis at a time when termination of the pregnancy is possible. Ultrasonography can identify some structural abnormalities in the fetus and localizes the placenta accurately. This reduces the risks of amniocentesis and enables a biopsy of the chorion to be taken from about 10 weeks of gestation, yielding fetal cells for examination at a much earlier stage. However, in all invasive investigations of the fetus in early pregnancy, there is a small risk of producing a placental bleed or abortion which, in a Rhesus-negative mother, may stimulate the formation of Rh antibodies (p. 184). These should be neutralized by routinely giving the Rh-negative mother an injection of anti-D globulin after the procedure.

AMNIOCENTESIS AND CHORIONIC VILLUS BIOPSY

Certain types of abnormality can be identified using one or other of these methods.

Chromosomal abnormalities

Cytogenetic analysis of fetal cells in the amniotic fluid or chorionic villi can reveal any deviation from the normal pattern of 46 chromosomes with two sex chromosomes. Using varying techniques, additional or missing chromosomes, structural abnormalities and tiny deletions or duplications of small fragments can be identified. The commonest abnormality found is an extra chromosome 21, indicating Down's syndrome (p. 220). This abnormality usually follows non-disjunction of the parental chromosomes during one of the stages of cell division, and in this situation the risk of recurrence is closely related to advancing maternal age, although there is also an increased risk in teenage pregnancy. The total incidence for Down's syndrome is about 1 in 600 births. At 20 years of age the chance of bearing an affected child is 1:1923; at 25 it is 1:1205; at 30, 1:835; at 40, 1:109; and at 45, 1:32. In spite of this, 70% of babies with Down's syndrome are born to mothers under 35 years of age because childbirth is so much more frequent in the younger age group.

In the minority of cases the abnormality is due to translocation of chromosome material and in about half of these cases the balanced translocation can be identified in one or other parent, the risk of recurrence in this case being as high as 1 in 4. In the rest it arises as a new mutation. It is advisable for all parents of Down's syndrome children to have chromosome studies to identify the small number with a translocational abnormality so that appropriate genetic counselling can be given. Amniocentesis or chorionic biopsy for chromosome analysis can then be offered in subsequent pregnancies, with the option of termination of pregnancy should the baby be found to be affected.

It is calculated that offering amniocentesis and chromosome analysis on the amniotic fluid to all mothers over the age of 35 would detect only 25% of the total number of babies with Down's syndrome, mainly because pregnancies in that age group are greatly in the minority. An improved test on the maternal blood can now be used to assess the likelihood of a baby having

Down's syndrome. This triple test measures the level of α-fetoprotein (which is low in Down's syndrome), β-human chorionic gonadotrophin (which is high) and oestriol (which is low). It must be remembered that this is only a screening test and not diagnostic, but if those mothers identified as being at high risk by the test were all to have cytogenetic studies on amniotic fluid, it is estimated that 66% of Down's babies would be identified. Neither system provides complete identification of affected infants, but provided that a full explanation is given and personal views are respected the introduction of such a policy is justifiable.

Molecular genetic analysis of DNA

This technique reveals abnormalities of the genes on the chromosomes in the cell nucleus and it can identify an increasing number of inherited conditions in early fetal life. It is now widely available and the number of conditions amenable to diagnosis in this way is growing ever larger and it is superseding other methods of diagnosis in many genetic disorders. Some examples of conditions amenable to this method are shown in Table 2.4. It can also frequently identify carriers of the abnormal genes for these conditions in other family members, so that they can be advised with greater certainty of the risk of having an affected infant (Fig. 2.3).

Table 2.4 Some conditions identifiable by cytogenetic and DNA analysis of fetal cells

Cytogenetic analysis	
Down's syndrome	47 XY (or XX)* + 21
Klinefelter's syndrome	47 XXY
Turner's syndrome	45 XO**
Trisomy 18	47 XY (or XX)* + 18
Trisomy 13	47 XY (or XX)* + 13
DNA analysis	
Cystic fibrosis	
Duchenne muscular dystrophy	
Huntingdon's disease	
Myotonic dystrophy	
Fragile X syndrome	
Rhesus D genotyping in rhesus-incompatible pregnancies	
Spinal muscular atrophy	
X-linked retinitis pigmentosa	

* XY in boys, XX in girls.
** XO indicates the absence of a second X chromosome.

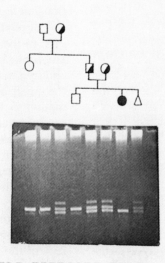

CYSTIC FIBROSIS DELTA F508

Figure 2.3 Family tree and DNA analysis for *ΔF508* gene in a family with cystic fibrosis. (By kind permission of Prof. P Jacobs.)

Recessively inherited metabolic disorders with cell enzyme abnormalities

These are relatively rare diseases in which the enzyme abnormality may be detected by complex histochemical techniques available only in certain specialized centres. The best known examples in this group are the gangliosidoses (e.g. Tay–Sachs' disease), glycogen storage disease (Pompe's disease), the mucopolysaccharidoses, metachromatic leucodystrophy and galactosaemia. These disorders will be increasingly identified by DNA analysis in the future.

X-linked diseases

In these conditions, half of all male fetuses will be affected and sexing of the fetus can be obtained by amnioscopy or chromosomal studies. Some X-linked conditions can be identified from biochemical analysis of fetal blood samples, including Duchenne muscular dystrophy and haemophilia. In these and many other such conditions the abnormal gene has been identified and gene probes can identify affected fetuses from chorionic villus samples even when the underlying biochemical defect is not known.

Neural tube defects

Neural tube defects include anencephaly and spina bifida with myelomeningocele (p. 213) The frequency with which these conditions occur in the UK varies according to geographical location and has reduced considerably as a result of both a natural reduction in incidence and prenatal diagnosis followed by termination of pregnancy. The risk of recurrence is increased if there is a family history of the condition, and the mother who has already had one affected child has a 1 in 20 chance of recurrence. Although the aetiology is not clear, supplementation of the mother's diet with folic acid 0.4 mg daily before conception and during the first trimester reduces both the recurrence rate (from 3.5 to 1.0%) and the occurrence rate in primagravidae, and in order to achieve this intake, the fortification of grain-based foods with folic acid is now required in the USA. In some countries, a dose of 4–5mg is recommended for women at high risk. Such doses of folic acid have no known harmful effects in healthy pregnant women, although they may counteract the anticonvulsant activity of some drugs used in epilepsy. Apart from this, antenatal diagnosis with the offer of termination is the main means of lowering the incidence in liveborn infants.

Raised levels of α-fetoprotein in maternal blood at 16–18 weeks of gestation identify those mothers at risk, 1 in 20 of whom are actually bearing an affected child. An ultrasound examination of those with a positive blood test successfully confirms or excludes an open myelomeningocele in the great majority of cases (Fig. 2.4), although in a minority it may be necessary to confirm the diagnosis by testing a sample of amniotic fluid. The presence of an acetylcholinesterase specific for neural tissue as well as a raised a-fetoprotein level indicates an affected fetus, although the latter on its own may also be found in conditions such as gastroschisis and exomphalos.

Fetal blood sampling

Haematological disorders such as thalassaemia

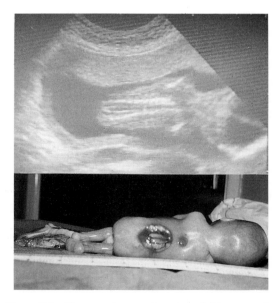

Figure 2.4 Open meningomyelocoele on fetal sonography and after termination of pregnancy.

may be identified by analysis of fetal blood samples obtained by cordocentesis under ultrasound guidance or at amnioscopy, and these techniques open the way to the early identification of many more conditions affecting the blood.

Fetal cardiac monitoring

Fetal cardiac monitoring by means of an external cardiotocograph can sometimes identify cardiac arrhythmias and has also been used to confirm the tachycardia of fetal thyrotoxicosis. In some cases these may respond to appropriate treatment given to the mother. Fetal heart rate patterns and responses to various forms of stimulation have so far proved unhelpful in identifying the infant at risk or improving the outcome for the baby.

DRUGS IN PREGNANCY

Since the thalidomide tragedy in the early 1960s, when children were born with deficient or malformed limbs after their mothers had taken thalidomide in early pregnancy, the medical profession and the general public have been careful about using prescribed drugs in the first 3 months of pregnancy. Some drugs may cause congenital malformations by influencing the development of the fetus in the first 3 months of the pregnancy, whilst others are known to have an effect on the newborn infant when taken in later pregnancy. In general, it is better for the mother to avoid taking drugs for these reasons, although the risk to the fetus must be balanced against the need to provide proper treatment for maternal conditions.

Early pregnancy

Certain outstanding drugs have been associated with developmental malformations in early pregnancy.

Cytotoxic drugs

Cytotoxic drugs for treatment of neoplastic disease, e.g. chlorambucil and methotrexate, are known to be teratogenic.

Anticonvulsants

The babies of epileptic mothers have a two- to threefold increased incidence of congenital malformations. Those treated with phenytoin are at increased risk of having a cleft lip and palate. An excess of neural tube defects, congenital heart disease and several other abnormalities is seen if sodium valproate or carbamazepine is taken, but the drugs are responsible for only a small proportion of these malformations.

Antipsychotic drugs

Lithium, which may be used to treat manic depressive psychosis, can cause malformation of the tricuspid valve in the heart, and also may depress fetal thyroid and renal function when used in later pregnancy. Phenothiazines such as chlorpromazine do not cause malformations, but a syndrome of tremor, hypertonia and hyper-reflexia lasting for some months may affect the baby if the drug is taken near term.

Antibiotics and the like

Streptomycin and neomycin have been known to cause eighth nerve deafness. Tetracycline chelates with teeth and bone, causing yellow-staining and possibly enamel hypoplasia, and the use of chloroquine phosphate may result in retinal damage or deafness.

Steroids

Some progestogens given in the past to prevent premature labour may cause masculinization of the female fetus. Danazol, a drug which raises the level of fetal plasma testosterone, also has a similar effect. Certain preparations containing oestrogen and progestogens were used in the early detection of pregnancy, but an association with congenital malformations led to their withdrawal. Synthetic glucocorticoids, e.g. prednisolone, can occasionally suppress fetal growth when given throughout pregnancy and may increase susceptibility to infection after birth. When given to the mother for 48 hours to accelerate surfactant production in the unborn pre-term infant's lungs, in order to reduce the risk of respiratory distress syndrome, they have no harmful effects.

Hypotensive agents

Methyl dopa has been used for many years and has not been shown to have any adverse effect on the unborn baby. Propranolol and labetolol are able to cause not only fetal growth suppression but also respiratory depression and bradycardia in a small proportion of cases, which can reduce the ability of the infant to respond to resuscitation at birth. There is also an increased risk of neonatal hypoglycaemia in the infant. ACE inhibitors should be avoided as they may cause intrauterine growth retardation, fetal renal failure and oligohydramnios. Nifedipine, a calcium channel blocker appears to be a safe alternative. Although all antihypertensive drugs appear in human milk, breast feeding is normally permissable.

Habit-forming drugs

The effects of the most commonly used drugs, alcohol and tobacco, have been described on page 13. Heroin and other 'hard drugs' are a potent cause of stillbirths in some areas. Lysergic acid diethylamide (LSD) has been known to cause chromosome aberrations.

Anticoagulants

Warfarin is a potent teratogen in the first 3 months of pregnancy and may give rise to stunting of growth, with abnormalities of the eyes and skeleton in up to a quarter of cases. If it is given to the mother in the last month of pregnancy, the baby may be born with a serious lack of vitamin K-dependent clotting factors. In these circumstances, the newborn infant should be given vitamin K intravenously and the clotting status checked to confirm that the defect has been corrected. Heparin may be used in the last month since it does not cross the placenta and has no direct effect on the infant. It is, however,

associated with a higher rate of pre-term labour which may leave the infant at risk of the complications of prematurity.

Late pregnancy

Drugs given to the mother in late pregnancy may often cause problems to the baby immediately after birth. A few known examples are given in Table 2.5.

Psychotropic drugs

Antidepressants. Tricyclic drugs such as imipramine and amitryptilline are generally safe in pregnancy, although occasionally neonates may have a mild withdrawal syndrome.

Sedatives and tranquillisers. The increasing use of these drugs is a cause for concern because of their possible effects on the baby after delivery. Most of them are capable of causing sufficient central nervous system depression to affect the onset of breathing at birth and cause general lethargy in the first 24 hours or more. The benzodiazepines, e.g. diazepam, can enhance the effect of other depressant drugs and, besides lethargy and muscular hypotonia, can cause defective control of body temperature and thus hypothermia in the infant. The solvent used in the diazepam preparations for injection contains a substance which may potentiate neonatal jaundice. If the drugs have been used regularly or frequently by the mother, withdrawal symptoms may occur (p. 15).

Tocolytic agents

Ritodrine and other beta-2 stimulants are commonly given to the mother to suppress uterine contractions in pre-term labour in order to prolong the pregnancy until the fetus is more mature. If used for long periods these drugs can cause neonatal tachycardia and hypokalaemia, and may sometimes accentuate neonatal hypoglycaemia.

Anaesthetics and analgesics used in obstetrics

When a drug is given to the mother in labour, the

Table 2.5 Some problems caused by drugs in late
pregnancy

Drugs	Possible effects on the infant
Antimicrobial drugs	
— tetracycline	Staining of deciduous teeth
— chloramphenicol	Inhibits protein synthesis
— streptomycin	Damage to eighth cranial nerve
— sulphonamides (including co-trimoxazole)	Severe neonatal jaundice (by competing for albumin-binding sites)
— isoniazid	Fits from pyridoxine deficiency
— quinine	Bleeding from thrombocytopenia
— chloroquine phosphate	Retinal damage
— nitrofurantoin	Haemolysis
Anticonvulsant drugs	Blood coagulation defects (relieved by vitamin K)
— phenobarbitone	
— phenytoin	
Anticoagulants	Bleeding at delivery
— phenindione	
— warfarin	
Analgesics	
— salicylates (aspirin) in large doses	Jaundice, by competing with albumin-binding sites and bleeding from decreased platelet function; premature closure of the ductus arteriosus
Indomethacin	Premature closure of the ductus arteriosus
Oral antidiabetic drugs, e.g. tolbutamide	Hypoglycaemia, thrombocytopenia
Antithyroid drugs, e.g. carbimazole	Goitre and hypothyroidism
Antihypertensive drugs	
— reserpine	Hypotonia, lethargy, excessive nasal mucus
— propranolol	Respiratory depression, bradycardia, hypoglycaemia
Psychotropic drugs	
— chlorpromazine	Tremor, hypertonia, hyperreflexia
— lithium	Thyroid and renal dysfunction
— imipramine	
— amitryptilline	Mild withdrawal symptoms
— diazepam	Hypotonia
Diuretics	Electrolyte disturbances
— thiazides	Bleeding from thrombocytopenia
— caffeine	Jaundice
Vitamins	
— K (water-soluble forms)	Jaundice and kernicterus
— D (in excess)	Hypercalcaemia
Oxytocin	Jaundice, hyponatraemia
Ritodrine	Tachycardia and hyperglycaemia

extent of its effect on the baby depends on several variable factors. The blood level of the drug may remain higher for a longer time if the maternal liver or renal function is impaired, the drug thus passing more readily to the fetus. If the maternal serum protein level is low, any drug which normally binds to protein reaches the fetus in greater amounts. The reduction of blood flow to the placenta during contractions may partially protect the fetus from large doses of a drug such as an anaesthetic agent, but the depression of maternal respiration caused by any such drug may contribute significantly to fetal hypoxia.

Anaesthetics by inhalation. Used for analgesia or light anaesthesia, nitrous oxide has no measurable effect on the baby at birth. Deeper anaesthesia for caesarean section or forceps delivery requires other agents, the most commonly used being halothane and enfluorane. All anaesthetic agents cross the placenta and depress the baby's respiratory mechanisms to some extent and can delay the onset of respiration at birth. The effect is minimized by using the lowest effective concentration of the drug for the shortest possible time.

Morphine and pethidine. Morphine and pethidine given to the mother as intrapartum analgesics both cause central nervous system depression and are contributory causes of neonatal asphyxia (p. 35). The duration of the effect is longer with pethidine than with morphine and is maximal when given about 3 hours before delivery.

Local anaesthesia. The use of epidural anaesthesia in labour has increased considerably in Britain. A local anaesthetic agent which is injected into the mother's lumbar and sacral epidural space abolishes the pain of labour and can even enable a caesarean section to be performed without a general anaesthetic. Consequently, the risk of respiratory depression often seen in the baby at birth after the use of either opiates or general anaesthesia is reduced. The drug most commonly used for this purpose is bupivacaine, which appears to have relatively little effect on the infant, although respiratory depression and reduced activity may be seen for up to 24 hours after birth. Lignocaine, which passes rapidly across the placenta and may cause fetal central nervous system depression and bradycardia, is mainly used for pudendal blocks.

MATERNAL DISEASE AND THE FETUS

Almost any disease in the mother is capable of affecting the progress of the fetus to some degree, if only indirectly through impaired nutrition. In certain maternal diseases, specific effects may be anticipated which are potentially serious for the infant and merit a separate description.

Diabetes mellitus

The outlook for the baby of a diabetic mother is now good, some 95% surviving compared with 70% some 30 years ago, but if the mother has diabetes of long standing or already has complications of the disease herself, the infant is at greater risk. Much of the improvement in outlook is due to ensuring better control of the diabetes during the pregnancy. In those pregnancies where control is less good, the placenta is usually large and has evidence of vasculitis and multiple infarcts. The infant grows more than expected in weight and length, some internal organs also become enlarged and excess adipose tissue is laid down. This large size can cause difficulties during delivery of the shoulders, when excessive traction on the neck may stretch or tear the cervical nerve roots causing an Erb's palsy (p. 153). Unexpected and often unexplained fetal death may occasionally occur towards the end of pregnancy, but surviving infants are also at increased risk during the first week of life. The chance of a serious congenital abnormality is doubled, these most commonly appearing in the heart. However, if strict control of the diabetes is achieved before conception and maintained throughout pregnancy, the risk is lower.

In the few days after birth the main problems for the baby are:

- hypoglycaemia, which may or may not provoke symptoms in the baby (p. 97)

- respiratory distress syndrome with all the clinical features seen in the pre-term baby (p 129).

Obstetric management

If maternal blood glucose is maintained within the physiological range throughout the pregnancy, by meticulous attention to the mother's diet and frequent adjustment of her insulin requirements, delivery of the baby can usually be allowed to proceed normally at term but this depends on the estimated size of the fetus. When control is poor, early delivery may be considered and the estimation of the lecithin–sphingomyelin ratio or the level of phosphatidyl glycerol or other components of surfactant (p. 128) in the amniotic fluid will indicate whether respiratory distress syndrome is likely (p. 128). A 48 hour course of corticosteroids to reduce this risk may be needed before 34 weeks of gestation. Delivery by caesarean section may be advised to avoid a prolonged and difficult labour with an oversized baby.

The management of the infant of the diabetic mother is described on page 94.

Epilepsy

Around one pregnancy in 200 occurs in women taking anticonvulsants for recurrent fits. An episode of status epilepticus during pregnancy is associated with a significant fetal mortality, but in controlled epilepsy the pregnancy is usually uneventful and the baby healthy. Occasionally fetal growth is diminished, although this appears not to affect the infant's later development. Congenital malformations occur two to three times more frequently than in the general population. Neural tube defects (p. 213) occur in 1–2% of infants exposed to sodium valproate or carbamazepine; cleft lip and palate occur with increased frequency with phenytoin or phenobarbitone. A combination of unusual facial features and abnormalities of the fingers may also occur in over 5% of infants. The drugs may affect blood-clotting in the newborn infant and all should receive vitamin K intramuscularly after birth. An occasional infant may be irritable or have a fit from 'withdrawal' of the drugs.

Thyrotoxicosis

Maternal thyrotoxicosis can very occasionally cause fetal hyperthyroidism through the over-stimulation of the baby's thyroid gland by a maternal IgG immunoglobulin known as long-acting thyroid stimulator, which crosses the placenta into the fetal circulation. Persistent fetal tachycardia is the cardinal sign of this condition which may be treated by giving the mother antithyroid drugs such as carbimazole to suppress the fetal thyroid gland. More frequently, though, the baby will develop thyrotoxicosis in the few days after birth when he may become alarmingly ill with the rapid onset of hyperactivity, tachycardia and exophthalmos and may even go into cardiac failure. The condition usually responds to treatment with carbimazole, with or without propranolol, which should continue for about 6 weeks.

If the mother's thyrotoxicosis is treated in pregnancy with antithyroid drugs and her thyroid function is monitored carefully, the baby is usually unaffected, but he may be born with a goitre if the treatment is too vigorous. Iodides given to the mother can also have the same effect. The goitre results from the effect of thyroid-stimulating hormone which is secreted in excess by the pituitary gland as a reaction to inhibition of the baby's own thyroid hormone synthesis.

Parathyroid dysfunction

Maternal hypoparathyroidism can affect the fetus by producing secondary increased fetal parathyroid hormone secretion, which may cause demineralization of the baby's bones at birth. Conversely, maternal hyperparathyroidism may cause neonatal hypocalcaemia and tetany by suppression of fetal parathormone production.

Myasthenia gravis

About one-third of the babies born to mothers with myasthenia gravis show a temporary form of the disease, presenting a few hours after birth with severe muscular hypotonia and weakness. This may extend to the muscles of respiration and swallowing and may thus threaten life. Confirmation of the diagnosis can be obtained by the response to an injection of edrophonium chloride 100–200µg/kg intramuscularly. The condition is self-limiting and is usually over in 2 days, although it can occasionally last up to 1 month.

Idiopathic thrombocytopenic purpura

In this condition the maternal IgG antiplatelet antibodies responsible for destroying her own platelets cross the placenta and cause neonatal thrombocytopenia. It is most frequently transient but the platelet count may remain low for several weeks until the baby loses the maternal antibodies. Corticosteroids are often ineffective in increasing the platelet count when given either to the mother in pregnancy or to the baby after birth, and their prolonged use may result in neonatal adrenal insufficiency when they are withdrawn. Treatment of the mother with immunoglobulin injections prior to delivery will frequently raise her platelet count and that of the fetus to a level at which the risk of bleeding is minimal and which will allow a normal delivery to proceed safely. When the infant's platelet count remains below $50 \times 10^9/L$, there is a risk of serious bleeding and the baby should be treated with intravenous immunoglobulin.

Phenylketonuria

There is an increasing number of girls now reaching adult life with normal development, having been treated for this disorder in childhood. Experience has shown that unless they return to a diet which keeps the serum phenylalanine level within or near the normal range before conception, and continue it through the pregnancy, there is a greatly increased risk of damage to the fetus, causing malformation and resulting in developmental delay.

MATERNAL INFECTIONS AND THE FETUS

Antenatal infection

Transmission of the common bacterial infections across the placenta to the fetus is a remarkably rare event, but any infection which produces severe illness in the mother may affect fetal growth by interference with nutrition. Stimulation of the fetal immune defences does take place, as shown, for instance, by the rise in immunoglobulins in cord blood when the mother has had pyelonephritis. Certain microorganisms do pass the placental barrier, infect the fetus and interfere with its growth, differentiation or development, resulting in a seriously handicapped baby. Rubella, cytomegalovirus, toxoplasmosis and syphilis are the best known examples. They are described in detail on page 169. Exceptionally, transplacental infection occurs from Coxsackie, measles, varicella, poliomyelitis, vaccinia, influenza, herpes simplex and hepatitis viruses, whilst the bacteria causing tuberculosis, typhoid fever and listeriosis (p. 158) have been known to spread to the fetus in the same way.

Intrapartum infection

Infection of the amnion surrounding the fetus may occur as a result of prolonged pre-labour rupture of the membranes, and the organisms may spread to the baby through the infected amniotic fluid before delivery. Contamination of the infant by pathogenic organisms colonizing the birth canal may also occur during labour. These conditions are discussed in detail in Chapter 11.

Pneumonia due to inhalation of infected liquor into the infant's lungs may be apparent at birth, presenting as respiratory distress with grunting respirations, tachypnoea and costal recession. Septicaemia and meningitis can also be acquired from infected liquor. The microorganisms most commonly involved are *group B β-haemolytic streptococci* and *Escherichia coli* (p. 162). It is very difficult to distinguish these on clinical grounds but infection with either organism can be catastrophic. If the membranes rupture before the onset of labour and a *group B β-haemolytic streptococcus* has been isolated from the mother's genital tract, it is possible to reduce significantly the risk of infection in the baby by treating the mother with ampicillin during labour. However, without routine culture of vaginal swabs it is difficult to tell which mothers carry the organism, and it is not yet clear whether antibiotic treatment of a carrier during a normal pregnancy affects the risk of infection in the infant after birth.

The acquired immune deficiency syndrome (AIDS) is a fatal infectious disease caused by the human immunodeficiency virus (HIV). Pregnancy appears to reactivate the virus, and in up to 25% of HIV-positive mothers the baby will be infected. Although this does not cause apparent fetal or neonatal disease, a high proportion of infected babies will develop the full syndrome and die in infancy. Of those not infected many will lose one or both of their parents from the disease and in some parts of Africa many children have been orphaned as a result. The subject is discussed in detail on page 171.

Other organisms which can be acquired from the birth canal during labour include *Candida albicans*, gonococci and *Chlamydia trachomatis*, echoviruses, hepatitis B and herpes simplex virus. Table 2.6 shows the effect of various maternal infections on the infant.

Postpartum spread of infection from mother to infant

The newborn baby starts life with immunity to some infections due to the transmission of maternal antibody in the form of immunoglobulin G (p. 157). He has, for example, a good resistance to the common viral infections of childhood, providing the mother possesses that immunity. However, should she be suffering from one of these at the time of birth, no antibody will have been passed to the baby who will then be highly susceptible. A normally mild infection, such as chickenpox, if developed at the age of 3 weeks, may be fatal. The common respiratory virus infections are rarely transmitted from mother to baby after birth but there are exceptions.

Table 2.6   Maternal infection and the fetus

Organism	Effect on the infant
Rubella	Congenital malformations
	Growth retardation
	Mental retardation
Toxoplasmosis	Hydrocephalus
	Choroidoretinitis
	Jaundice
	Mental retardation
Cytomegalovirus	Microcephaly
	Hepatitis
	Mental retardation
Herpes simplex	Encephalitis
HIV	AIDS
Hepatitis B	Hepatitis
	Chronic carrier of virus
Coxsackie B virus	Myocarditis
Chickenpox virus	Chickenpox fetopathy
	Severe chickenpox
Chlamydia	Conjunctivitis
Candida albicans	Oral and perineal thrush
Gonococcus	Severe conjunctivitis
Syphilis	Snuffles
	Skin lesions
	Congenital malformations
Malaria	Congenital malaria
Tuberculosis (TB)	Miliary tuberculosis
	TB meningitis
Group B β-haemolytic streptococcus	Pneumonia
	Septicaemia
	Meningitis
Escherichia coli	Meningitis
	Septicaemia
Listeria monocytogenes	Meningitis
	Septicaemia

Respiratory syncytial virus, for example, may cause a relatively mild rhinitis with a snuffly nose which is quite unlike the more familiar bronchiolitis due to the same virus later in infancy. Occasionally bacterial infections such as *E. coli* gastroenteritis and staphylococcal skin infection are passed to the baby from the mother but are more often derived from other sources. Considerable protection against many of these infections is afforded by the cells, antibody and lactoferrin in the mother's milk in the exclusively breast fed baby (p. 158).

Maternal tuberculosis in the active state is now rare in Britain, although in some ethnic minority groups such as those from the Indian subcontinent and the Far East, there is still a significant number of cases. If intrauterine infection occurs the infant has no transmitted immunity and is exceptionally vulnerable. It usually presents some 6 weeks after birth as described on page 171. Protection of the infant by treatment with isoniazid may be necessary until the immunization with BCG vaccine has had time to take effect. Almost always, however, the maternal disease is quiescent or cured and BCG alone is sufficient. In communities where the prevalence of tuberculosis is increased, neonatal immunization using 0.05 ml of BCG vaccine intradermally should be given to those considered at risk, but it should not be used if the baby has HIV infection or is taking steroids.

FURTHER READING

Autti-Ramo I, Gaily E, Granstrom M-L 1992 Dysmorphic features in the offspring of alcoholic mothers. Archives of Disease in Childhood 67: 712–716

Boue A 1995 Fetal medicine – prenatal diagnosis and management. Oxford University Press, Oxford

Briggs G 1994 Drugs in pregnancy and lactation: a reference guide to fetal and neonatal risk. Williams and Williams, Baltimore

Carrera J M, Torrents M, Mortera C, Cusi V, Munoz A 1995 Routine prenatal ultrasound screening for fetal abnormalities: 22 years experience. Ultrasound in Obstetrics and Gynaecology 5: 174–179

Chalmers I, Enkin M, Keirse M 1992 Effective care in pregnancy and childbirth. Oxford University Press, Oxford

Chamberlain G, Wright A, Steer P (eds) 1993 Pain relief in childbirth. Churchill Livingstone, Edinburgh

Clarke A, Rudd P 1992 Neonatal BCG immunisation. Archives of Disease in Childhood 67: 473–474

Cleland P G 1996 Management of pre-existing disorders in pregnancy – epilepsy. Prescribers Journal 36(2): 102–109

Dallaire L, Lortie G, Des-Rochers M, Clermont R, Vachon C 1995 Parental reaction and adaptability to the prenatal diagnosis of fetal defect or genetic disease leading to pregnancy interruption. Prenatal Diagnosis 15: 249–259

Das G 1994 Cocaine abuse and reproduction. International Journal of Clinical Pharmacology and Therapeutics 32(1): 7–11

David T J (ed) 1991 Infants of drug dependent mothers. Recent advances in paediatrics 9. Churchill Livingstone, Edinburgh

Finnegan L P 1994 Perinatal morbidity and mortality in substance using families: effects and intervention strategies. Bulletin of Narcotics 46: 19–43

Franks S (ed) 1990 Clinical endocrinology and metabolism: endocrinology of pregnancy 4. Baillière Tindall, London, ch 2

Gregory R, Scott A, Mohajer M, Tattersall R B 1992 Diabetic pregnancy 1977–1990: Have we reached a plateau? Journal of the Royal College of Physicians of London 26: 162–166

Levene M, Liford R (eds) 1995 Fetal and neonatal neurology and neurosurgery. Churchill Livingstone, Edinburgh

National Health and Medical Research Council of Australia 1994 Revised statement on the relationship between dietary folate and neural tube defects such as spina bifida. Journal of Paediatrics and Child Health 30: 476–477

Ornoy A, Cohen E 1996 Outcome of children born to epileptic mothers treated with carbamazepine during pregnancy. Archives of Disease in Childhood 75: 517–520

Rubin P C 1996 Management of pre-existing disorders in pregnancy: principles of prescribing. Prescribers Journal 36: 21–27

Russell J 1982 Early teenage pregnancy. Churchill Livingstone, Edinburgh

Toeh T G, Redman C W 1996 Management of pre-existing disorders in pregnancy: hypertension. Prescribers Journal 36: 28–36

Wald N J, Bower C 1995 Folic acid and the prevention of neural tube defects 310: 1019–1020

Whiteman V E, Reece E A 1994 Prenatal diagnosis of major congenital malformations. Current Opinion in Obstetrics and Gynaecology 6: 459–467

3

Care of the infant at birth

BIRTH AND ADAPTATION TO INDEPENDENT LIFE

The care of the baby at birth should ensure a safe transition from the intrauterine environment to the point where her parents can safely take care of her without professional help. Even with careful preparation, the parents will often feel a mixture of anxiety and anticipatory wonder during the birth, and unnecessary actions by the midwife, obstetrician or paediatrician can adversely affect the development of the relationship between the parents and their infant and should be avoided. Planning for the birth is a vital part of antenatal care, and increasingly the parents' wishes about the place, mode of delivery and the care of the infant after birth are incorporated into a plan agreed with the midwife for the birth. Yet, although about two-thirds of deliveries progress in a natural manner and the baby is born without medical intervention, it is not always possible to identify in advance the baby who may suffer harm, and all care givers must watch for potential hazards and act when necessary.

Two major hazards for the baby are the development of asphyxia during birth, which can prevent the onset of breathing, and excessive heat loss resulting in hypothermia after it.

PROCEDURE AT A NORMAL BIRTH

In the normal course of events, the baby is delivered after only a minor degree of oxygen deprivation caused by interruption of blood flow through the placenta at each uterine contraction, and breathing starts spontaneously within a few seconds. The only immediate actions required are to ensure that the airway is clear, so that debris and fluid from the mouth and nose are not inhaled into the lungs with the baby's first breaths, and to dry the baby with a warm towel to prevent her from losing heat.

As soon as the head is delivered, therefore, the nose and mouth are gently wiped clear of mucus and debris. Vigorous nasal suction with a catheter can damage the mucosa and cause the heart rate to fall from vagal stimulation and is not often necessary. Vernix and blood should be wiped away from the eyes. As long as the vessels are pulsating, some blood continues to flow into the baby through the umbilical cord supplementing her blood volume. This provides her with additional red cells which maintain a higher haemoglobin level and extra iron stores. Even if the baby is delivered up onto the mother's abdomen (Fig. 3.1), the cord may be left unclamped until cord pulsation stops, unless asphyxia or the risk of hypothermia necessitate immediate resuscitative measures. Two cord clamps should then be applied 5 and 6 cm from the umbilicus and the cord divided between them.

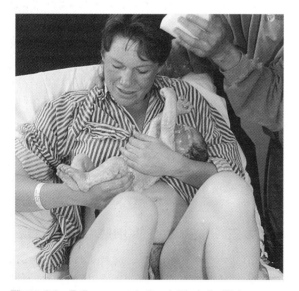

Figure 3.1 Delivery up onto the abdomen facilitates attachment to the baby.

Fluid material from the fetal lungs will often accumulate in the baby's mouth and pharynx and this should be removed by a soft suction catheter attached to a mechanical sucker regulated to a pressure of no more than 100 cmH$_2$O. Higher pressures may damage the mucous membranes. Mouth-operated mucus extractors should not be used unless there is no alternative and should have a filter fitted to protect the operator from aspirated material. When there is a risk that blood or mucus is infected, they should not be used.

Maintaining body temperature

Although the newborn infant has a temperature-regulating mechanism, it is less efficient than that of an older child and there is a much greater risk of excessive cooling or overheating. Because babies are small and have a large surface area in relation to volume, they are likely to lose heat rapidly and this applies even more when birth weight is low (p. 92).

Heat loss occurs through evaporation from exposed wet skin, direct radiation to surrounding objects, conduction through coverings and convection in the surrounding air. A surprisingly large amount is lost from the head, which justifies the use of an insulating bonnet if the baby is exposed to any extra risk of cooling. Heat production is governed by the rate of metabolism, the amount of muscular activity and by a chemical process of heat liberation in the specially large store of brown fat around the back and neck peculiar to the newborn. The capacity of newborns to produce heat by muscular shivering is poorly developed. A drop in body temperature leads to stimulation of the metabolic rate and a steep increase in consumption of oxygen which has to be provided by augmenting respiratory function, which constitutes an additional strain on any infant already having trouble breathing. This increase in metabolic activity may also use up all the available glucose and render the baby hypoglycaemic (p. 97).

Prevention of hypothermia immediately after birth is therefore essential. Any necessary attention given at delivery must be in a warm, draught-free environment with a radiant heat source above the resuscitation site. Drying the baby immediately and wrapping her in a warm dry blanket will substantially reduce the risk of hypothermia. Heat loss during transport from the labour ward to the neonatal unit can be reduced by wrapping the baby in a metal foil sheet, although this should not be used as a substitute for a warmed incubator and warmed blankets for longer journeys.

As soon as the baby is dry and breathing normally, she should be given to her mother to hold and caress. Provided that the surrounding temperature is warm enough, the mother may be encouraged to hold the baby naked and allow her to suck at the breast, since the skin-to-skin contact diminishes the drop in the baby's temperature. Otherwise, she should be wrapped in a warm towel to prevent heat loss. Bonding should not, however, take precedence over other immediate needs of the infant, such as any resuscitative measures.

Fostering the bonding and attachment process

The development of love between parents and their baby originates long before birth. For some mothers it starts at the moment pregnancy is confirmed, for others at the time of quickening, at about 16–20 weeks. In other cases it is not until the baby is seen that the real feeling develops. Attachment to the infant gradually develops over the early months of life and the ease with which it grows can be greatly influenced by the events during pregnancy, delivery and the first few hours and days of the infant's life. Although safety of the infant must be paramount at all times, it is important to recognize and respond to the emotional needs of the parents and infant throughout this time. Observational studies suggest that physical contact between mother and baby encourages the attachment between them, and research shows that putting the baby to the breast immediately after birth improves the chances of successful breast feeding.

This time offers the parents their first opportunity to look at, feel, hear and wonder at their new infant. A brief initial examination by the midwife can reassure the parents that there is no visible abnormality. It should not be necessary to hurry this phase of care and after the infant is wrapped up warmly again it should be possible for her to stay close to her mother for as long as she wishes.

If the baby has a visible abnormality, is sick or of low birth weight, this procedure may have to be modified or curtailed. The general principles, however, apply even more strongly and meeting emotional needs of the parents and family without physical risk to the baby is a matter for careful judgement in each individual case.

The midwife or doctor may usefully carry out the preliminary brief examination of the baby in the view of the mother, before wrapping her again in warm blankets and placing her in her cot. In maternity units, identification bracelets or security devices should be put on and the infant given 1 mg of vitamin K intramuscularly or orally to prevent haemorrhagic disease of the newborn (p. 179) before the baby leaves the delivery room.

SIGNS WHICH MAY INDICATE A SICK INFANT

Following the birth there may be an indication that the baby is not completely healthy. Such signs as a delay in the onset of breathing, grunting respiration, tachypnoea, cyanosis, hypotonia, hypothermia and pallor may indicate a serious underlying condition. They should all be taken seriously and their cause diagnosed if necessary by investigation in the neonatal unit (Table 3.1).

Selection of babies for admission to the neonatal unit

In general, newborn babies should be allowed to stay with their mothers unless some action needs to be taken for which facilities are only available in the neonatal unit. Babies at high risk of developing serious illness or needing highly trained nursing should be cared for in a special unit, but ideally services should provide as much care as possible on the postnatal wards. For example, most babies requiring phototherapy for jaundice,

Table 3.1 Common warning signs at birth

Syptom	Some causes
Delayed onsert of breathing	Maternal sedation
	Anaesthesia
	Cerebral asphyxia
Respiratory distress	Choanal atresia
	Pneumothorax
	Diaphragmatic hernia
	Respiratory distress syndrome
Cyanosis	Congenital heart disease
	Respiratory disorders
	Persistent pulmonary hypertension
Hypotonia	Cerebral asphyxia
	Other CNS disorders
	Benign hypotonia
	Down's syndrome
Pallor	Asphyxia
	Haemorrhage
	Haemolytic disease
Hypothermia	Inadequate temperature management
Small size	Prematurity
	Growth retardation
	Congenital malformation

observation for hypoglycaemia and some needing tube feeding can be nursed at their mother's side and those with uncomplicated congenital malformations should not be removed.

There is no justification for admission for observation alone since even temporary separation can interfere with the growth of the normal parent–child relationship and the development of good parenting. It may also reduce the chance of successful breast feeding and give the parents the incorrect impression that their baby will continue to be frail or vulnerable after discharge from the unit. Although the exact criteria for admission will vary from one unit to another, babies with the following conditions are at sufficient risk to justify separation from their mothers:

- under 1800 g birth weight
- less than 34 weeks of gestation
- respiratory symptoms such as grunting, tachypnoea or costal recession
- severe rhesus haemolytic disease
- symptoms from a congenital abnormality
- convulsions
- persistent vomiting or abdominal distension
- hypoglycaemia which does not respond to oral or nasogastric feeding
- any ill baby (pp. 33 and 161).

For some infants, such as those that are dying, an individual decision about where and how to care for the baby will need to be made, remembering to take account of and respect the parents' wishes (p. 229).

PERINATAL ASPHYXIA AND RESUSCITATION OF THE NEWBORN BABY

The onset of respiration

The change from the intrauterine environment to the more independent life outside involves large changes in physiological function, the most vital of which is the use of the lungs for oxygenation of the blood. Precisely how breathing is started so efficiently is imperfectly understood, but breathing movements occur before birth and the lungs contain a liquid which differs from amniotic fluid. These movements gradually lessen towards term and only become deep enough to draw in amniotic fluid when the fetus is significantly hypoxic from placental insufficiency. During a normal vaginal delivery the thorax is compressed and some of the lung fluid is expelled, the rest being absorbed and removed by lymphatic channels (all of it in the case of caesarean section).

The first breath the baby takes after birth is initiated by nerve impulses arising in the brain stem and triggered by several kinds of stimulus. Normally, when oxygenation of the brain has not been impaired during labour, contact of the skin with the cold air and harder surfaces outside the uterus, stimulation by light and sound together with the lowered pH and raised CO_2 content of the blood acting through chemoreceptors in the aorta and carotid arteries are enough to initiate an inspiratory gasp and a subsequent cry followed by strong breathing movements.

The negative pressure in the thorax required to take the first few breaths to expand and fill the alveoli is greater than that needed later, due to surface tension produced by the film of intra-alveolar fluid. Sometimes this pressure can be as high as 60 cmH$_2$O, but it is usually between 20 and 30 cmH$_2$O. Phospholipid substances lining the alveoli reduce this tension and prevent them from collapsing completely between each expansion. The negative pressure required for breathing after the first few minutes is smaller – in the region of 5 cmH$_2$O.

Factors predisposing to birth asphyxia

When there has been a period of oxygen deprivation during the birth, the resultant asphyxia renders the infant's brain less responsive to the stimuli which normally initiate breathing. After minor degrees of asphyxia during labour, the baby may be born apnoeic but recover rapidly with relatively little resuscitation ('primary apnoea'). Greater degrees of asphyxia are followed by irregular slow gasping breaths or a state of 'terminal apnoea' in which none of the ordinary stimuli are effective, and a progressive acidosis develops from which only vigorous resuscitation can rescue the infant.

Although an occasional baby fails to breathe without an apparent cause, the great majority of infants requiring resuscitation are born after a complicated labour or delivery. Known predisposing causes before labour are:

- placental dysfunction from pre-eclampsia or smoking
- growth retardation of the fetus
- prolongation of pregnancy
- retroplacental haemorrhage
- congenital abnormalities
- congenital infections.

During labour they are:

- prolongation of the second stage
- prolapse of the umbilical cord
- excessive maternal analgesia
- malpresentation (especially breech)
- cerebral injury.

These risks are greatly increased if the fetus is pre-term, has suffered from prolonged partial asphyxia or is growth-retarded from chronic intrauterine malnutrition, especially if unfavourable patterns of fetal blood flow have been found on Doppler ultrasound studies.

RECOGNITION OF THE ASPHYXIATED FETUS – FETAL DISTRESS

Several clinical and biochemical features may indicate that the fetus is asphyxiated during labour. Meconium staining of the liquor often, but not always, results from fetal hypoxia, but not all asphyxiated babies pass meconium before birth. A more consistent finding is a fetal brady-cardia of less than 120 beats/min or a tachycardia of more than 160 beats/min. This has led to the practice of fetal heart monitoring which can be done by a direct electrocardiographic recording from a fetal scalp electrode or more commonly from external cardiotocography in which a sensitive microphone, placed over the mother's abdomen, picks up the fetal heart sounds whilst a pressure transducer records uterine contractions. The apparatus identifies patterns of change in heart rate with contractions and records them on moving paper. A recording in which the heart rate varies with activity within a range of 110–160 beats/min and in which there is good beat-to-beat variation usually excludes asphyxia (Fig. 3.2A). During uterine contractions there is often a fall of the fetal heart rate which returns to the resting level immediately the contraction is over (type 1 deceleration). This is usually of no significance, but a delay in the recovery of the heart rate to the resting level (type 2 deceleration; Fig. 3.2B) is considered particularly indicative of asphyxia. Other patterns which may signify fetal distress are a drop in the heart rate which continues after the height of the uterine contraction, profound deceleration to a rate of less than 80 beats/min and a loss of the normal beat-to-beat variation in the heart rate. A persistent fetal bradycardia of less than 100 beats/min is almost always associated with a poor fetal cerebral circulation and demands urgent delivery of the baby.

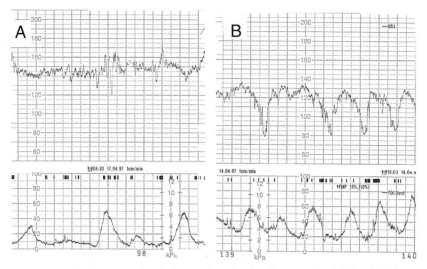

Figure 3.2 Cardiotocography. A: A recording showing the normal variability of fetal heart rate (above) with uterine contractions (lower trace). B: Episodes of fetal heart rate deceleration continuing beyond the uterine contraction with slow return to the baseline level (Type II dips) indicating fetal asphyxia. (By kind permission of Mr Michael Dooley.)

During episodes of hypoxia the fetus derives her energy from the breakdown of glycogen stores by anaerobic metabolism which is relatively inefficient. The consequent accumulation of lactic acid and other acidic products of this metabolism lowers the fetal blood pH. Repeated sampling of capillary blood from the fetal scalp through the dilating cervix and measurement of its pH provide a direct measure of the degree of fetal acidosis and give the clearest indication of the state of the baby's health. A pH of 7.20 or less indicates severe asphyxia. However, this method should not be used in mothers infected with HIV or hepatitis B virus, to prevent infection of the baby (p. 172). If asphyxia is clearly demonstrated on clinical or instrumental evidence, steps must be taken to deliver the baby as rapidly and safely as possible and this may mean an emergency caesarean section, forceps or Ventouse assisted delivery.

Predicting the need for resuscitation

A large study in Sweden has demonstrated that only 1% of babies of greater than 2500 g birth weight and 0.2% of babies born at more than 32 weeks of gestation after an apparently normal delivery needed any resuscitation. Of those who did require assistance, between 80 and 90% responded to bag and mask resuscitation alone. For term babies born after an uncomplicated pregnancy and delivery, therefore, advanced resuscitation is required in only about 1% of cases.

The majority of babies who require resuscitation at birth are born after a complicated pregnancy or delivery. The following circumstances require the presence of a professional who is competent at assessment and resuscitation of the newborn even though many babies in these categories will establish normal breathing spontaneously:

- pre-term babies under 36 weeks of gestation
- fetal distress or meconium staining of the liquor
- prenatal diagnosis of fetal growth retardation
- prenatal diagnosis of a congenital abnormality
- multiple pregnancy
- breech presentation
- caesarean section
- instrumental delivery other than lift-out forceps
- Rhesus haemolytic disease

- prolapsed cord
- where a perinatal complication has occurred in a previous delivery.

Assessment at birth

At birth the state of the baby depends on the duration and degree of asphyxia before and during delivery. The healthy baby who has not suffered any asphyxia will emerge as an active, pink baby who cries immediately after birth. A mild degree of asphyxia will cause the baby to be cyanosed and apnoeic, although she remains responsive to skin stimulation, has good muscle tone and a heart rate above 100 beats/min. More prolonged asphyxia results in the onset of circulatory failure in which the baby becomes a pale grey-blue colour, is limp, unresponsive to skin stimulation and has a heart rate below 100 beats/min.

A quantitative and objective clinical evaluation of the state of the baby directly after delivery is desirable because it serves as an immediate indicator of whether resuscitation is required and, if so, what form it should take. The most widely used scoring system is that devised by Apgar (Table 3.2) in which each of five features is given a score of 0, 1 or 2. The higher the total, the less likely it is that resuscitation will be required. The evaluation is made 1 and 5 minutes after birth but can be repeated every 5 minutes if the baby has not responded adequately. Although some infants with an Apgar score of 5 or more

have inadequate breathing, a score of 4 or less at 1 minute suggests a degree of asphyxia for which immediate active resuscitation should be implemented, and low values persisting after 5 or 10 minutes suggest that asphyxia has been prolonged and that resuscitation should continue. Unfortunately the scoring system predicts less than half of the babies with a significant degree of acidosis from intrapartum asphyxia, and there is little correlation between Apgar scores and long-term neurological outcome.

Apparatus required for neonatal resuscitation

Since only about 80% of babies needing resuscitation will be identified before birth it is essential for a resuscitation service to be available for all deliveries. A trained midwife or doctor should be present or immediately available solely to resuscitate the infant. The room itself should be well illuminated, draught-free and warmed to at least 25°C; warm towels are required to dry the infant and maintain her temperature; a suitable padded surface at table height is needed and there should be a telephone or emergency call system to summon more assistance. Ideally the equipment required includes (Fig. 3.3):

- overhead radiant heater
- a clock with a sweep second hand
- mechanical suction apparatus adjustable up to 100 cmH$_2$O
- infant oral airways of several sizes
- oxygen supply with facilities to regulate the pressure and flow rate
- face masks
- self-inflating bag
- laryngoscope with infant blades
- endotracheal tubes sizes 2.5, 3.0 and 3.5 mm
- syringes and needles
- umbilical venous catheterization set
- drugs for intravenous administration:
  — naloxone
  — sodium bicarbonate 4.2%
  — 10% dextrose
  — calcium gluconate
  — adrenaline 1:10 000 for tracheal instillation.

Table 3.2 Apgar's method of scoring in the evaluation of asphyxia in newborn infants

Sign	Score		
	0	1	2
Heart rate	Absent	Under 100 beats/min	Over 100 beat/min
Respiratory effort	Absent	Weak, irregular	Strong, regular
Reflex response to stimulation of the feet	None	Weak movement	Cry
Colour	Blue or pale	Body pink, extremities blue	Completely pink
Muscle tone	Limp	Partial flexion	Active movement

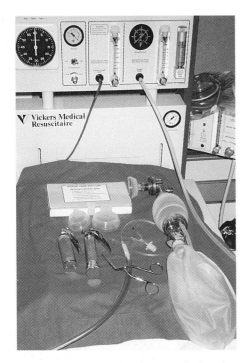

Figure 3.3 Equipment required for resuscitation of newborn babies.

RESUSCITATION OF THE ASPHYXIATED INFANT

When respiration does not immediately start, or when after a preliminary gasp it fails to become established, the action taken must depends on the condition of the baby, evaluated as described above. The following scheme gives an idea of how to proceed and is summarized in Table 3.3.

Initial step

In all cases the first step is to note the time and then apply gentle skin stimulation to the back or the soles of the baby's feet. This alone may encourage her to breathe or cry. The nose and pharynx should then be cleared of mucus, liquor and blood by gentle suction to prevent aspiration into the lungs when breathing starts. This procedure also often stimulates the sensory areas known to provoke the onset of breathing. Since mouth breathing is not possible at this age

the clearing of the nasal passages is vital if respiratory efforts are being made but are obviously failing to inflate the lungs.

Meconium in the liquor

Meconium can cause considerable inflammation in the bronchi if aspirated into the lungs during or after labour. Light meconium staining of liquor usually causes few problems. If thick meconium is present, it may indicate that the baby has been asphyxiated or that meconium has been inhaled into the lungs. At birth, meconium should be aspirated from the mouth and nose as soon as the head is delivered using a mechanical sucker with a large suction tube. If the baby is vigorous and cries, no further action is normally needed after birth, but if it is not, the larynx and trachea should be sucked out under direct vision with a laryngoscope using a large suction tube. The next step will be determined by the severity of the asphyxia.

Mild asphyxia

If the baby has good muscle tone, makes some movement in response to stimulation, has a heart rate of over 100 beats/min and yet breathing is inadequate (Apgar score 5 or more), stimulation of the skin may be adequate, but if breathing fails to start after 60–90 s, gentle inflation of the baby's lungs with air or oxygen by means of a close-fitting mask and self-inflating bag (Fig. 3.4) at a rate of one breath every 2 s should be carried out while checking that the chest wall moves with each breath. This should continue until the baby starts to breathe spontaneously. Subsequently, if pethidine has been administered to the mother within the 4 hours prior to delivery, naloxone hydrochloride 10–30 mcg/kg body weight should be given intravenously, or 70 mcg/kg intramuscularly, to reverse the respiratory depressant effect of the drug, but this is not an alternative to adequate ventilation of the lungs.

If effective bag and mask ventilation has been

Table 3.3 Resuscitation of the newborn. *Using the chart:* assess the baby's condition using the features at the top left of the chart, then follow the actions indicated by the flow arrows (after Handbook on the resuscitation of babies at birth 1997)

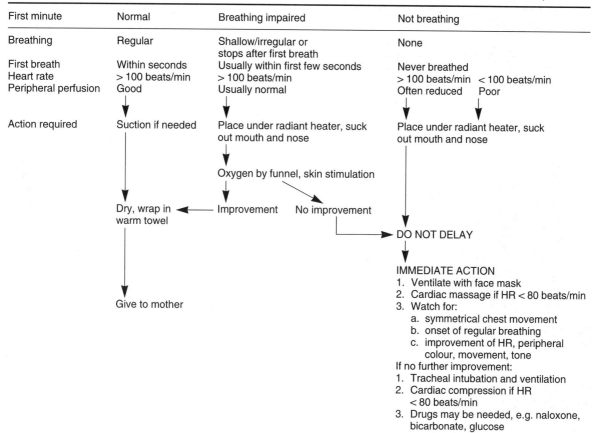

First minute	Normal	Breathing impaired	Not breathing	
Breathing	Regular	Shallow/irregular or stops after first breath	None	
First breath	Within seconds	Usually within first few seconds	Never breathed	
Heart rate	> 100 beats/min	> 100 beats/min	> 100 beats/min	< 100 beats/min
Peripheral perfusion	Good	Usually normal	Often reduced	Poor
Action required	Suction if needed	Place under radiant heater, suck out mouth and nose	Place under radiant heater, suck out mouth and nose	
		Oxygen by funnel, skin stimulation		
	Dry, wrap in warm towel ← Improvement	No improvement		
			DO NOT DELAY	

IMMEDIATE ACTION
1. Ventilate with face mask
2. Cardiac massage if HR < 80 beats/min
3. Watch for:
   a. symmetrical chest movement
   b. onset of regular breathing
   c. improvement of HR, peripheral colour, movement, tone
If no further improvement:
1. Tracheal intubation and ventilation
2. Cardiac compression if HR < 80 beats/min
3. Drugs may be needed, e.g. naloxone, bicarbonate, glucose

Give to mother

used for a period of 1–2 minutes but the baby has not started breathing he may have been more asphyxiated than the initial assessment suggested and endotracheal intubation and positive pressure ventilation is then essential.

Severe asphyxia

If at birth the baby is limp and pallid with poor muscle tone and a heart rate of less than 100 beats/min (Apgar score 4 or less), bag and mask ventilation should be instituted at once, inflating the lungs at a rate of 60 per minute since she will not respond to anything less. If the heart rate falls below 80 beats/min, this should be combined with external cardiac massage since the circulation to the baby's brain becomes compromised below this rate. The heart should be com-

pressed at a rate of twice a second using a squeezing motion with the two thumbs on the lower sternum and the fingers around the chest. If ventilation is inadequate and the heart rate remains below 100 beats/min after 2 minutes, endotracheal intubation and intermittent positive pressure ventilation should be undertaken. This should continue until the heart rate rises well above 100 beats per minute, the baby becomes pink, vigorous and shows clear signs of spontaneous breathing.

When this procedure is followed closely without delay, there is rarely a need for any further treatment. However, in the absence of a rise in heart rate after 2 minutes of effective positive pressure ventilation, 5 ml of 4.2% sodium bicarbonate solution should be given slowly into the umbilical vein, using an umbilical catheter rather

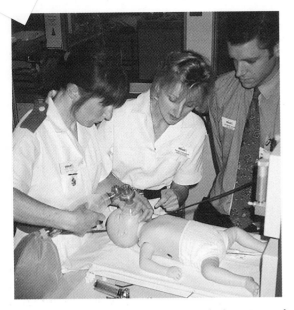

Figure 3.4 Bag and mask resuscitation – the importance of both good technique and adequate training.

For this technique to be effective the mask should be large enough to cover the mouth and nose and flexible enough to obtain a leak-free seal on the face to ensure that the inflation pressure produced is able to reach baby's lungs. With the baby lying on her back and the neck slightly extended, the mask, with the bag already attached, is applied to the face, the operator using the thumb and forefinger to press down on the mask while the other fingers elevate the chin, both to ensure a good contact between the mask and the face and to open the baby's airway. The bag is then fully and sharply squeezed at a rate of 30 per minute to inflate the chest. The chest wall should rise and the trachea bulge in the suprasternal notch with each inflation. If adequate chest movement cannot be achieved, the insertion of an infant oral airway may improve air flow by preventing the tongue from obstructing the laryngeal opening.

Endotracheal intubation and ventilation

With the infant lying on her back and the neck slightly extended, the baby laryngoscope is inserted to the back of the tongue so that the tip of the blade elevates the epiglottis and the vocal cords can be seen through the oval glottis. After clearing the pharynx of accumulated mucus by gentle suction, the endotracheal tube is inserted 1–2 cm through the opening. A fine catheter may then be quickly passed through the tube and suction applied to clear the trachea, after which intermittent positive pressure ventilation with oxygen is started using either a self-inflating bag or a Y connector operated with the thumb. Resuscitation equipment has a gauge to indicate the pressure being applied and a valve which limits the pressure to a maximum of 30 cmH$_2$O, since higher pressures can damage the lungs. After a few slow sustained puffs to expand the lungs, 10–15 cm H$_2$O is usually sufficient pressure to maintain ventilation until spontaneous breathing is fully established. The oxygen flow rate must not exceed 2 L/min since higher flow rates may render the pressure regulation inaccurate. As soon as spontaneous breathing starts, the infant becomes pink and the

than attempting needle puncture, to correct the persisting acidaemia which can cause additional brain damage.

Pre-term infants

Endotracheal intubation and positive pressure ventilation as a first step immediately after delivery are recommended for all pre-term infants under 34 weeks of gestation who do not cry vigorously at birth, in order to reduce the incidence and severity of respiratory distress syndrome (p. 128). It may also be needed when a baby (usually after caesarean birth) breathes immediately but then becomes apnoeic.

Methods of artificial ventilation

Bag and mask (Fig. 3.4)

The technique of bag and mask ventilation is easy to learn, safe and almost free of complications. Everyone involved in the care of a baby at birth should become proficient in the method and be prepared to use it as and when needed.

heart rate rises above 100 beats/min, the tube may be withdrawn.

Resuscitation at home deliveries

Since most home births will be low-risk deliveries, resuscitation will only ocasionally be needed. A second midwife or a doctor trained in bag and mask resuscitation should be present at the birth and must have available a portable resuscitation kit including an oxygen supply with a flow regulator, suction equipment and a suitable neonatal bag and mask. Immediate access to a telephone is essential to summon more expert help if required. Only rarely will intervention be needed beyond the bag and mask technique, except in such emergencies as those which precipitate pre-term delivery. Even in these circumstances, adequate ventilation can usually be maintained with a bag and mask until a paediatrician with advanced resuscitation skills arrives.

The baby who fails to improve with resuscitation

A poor response to resuscitation should prompt an immediate check that the chest is moving with each breath given with the bag, or that the endotracheal tube is correctly placed in the trachea and not the oesophagus, that it is large enough to be effective and that the pressure is sufficiently high to inflate the lungs. The occasional baby may fail to breathe or remain cyanosed despite apparently adequate resuscitation. In these infants, an additional cause, such as cyanotic congenital heart disease, diaphragmatic hernia, pneumothorax, severe anaemia or a neurological disorder, should be suspected.

Care of the baby after resuscitation

The majority of infants requiring resuscitation respond rapidly, becoming active and starting to cry. Once it is clear that the baby's condition is stable, she should be wrapped in a warm towel and given to the parents. Since very few of these infants develop hypoxic-ischaemic encephalopathy (p. 144) as a complication of their transient asphyxia, the infant should normally stay with the mother, only being admitted to the neonatal unit if there is another reason to do so (p. 33).

FURTHER READING

David T J (ed) 1994 Birth asphyxia. In: Recent advances in paediatrics 13. Churchill Livingstone, Edinburgh, ch 2
Handbook on resuscitation of babies at birth 1997 College of Paediatrics and Child Health, London
Kinmond S, Aitchison T C Holland B M, Jones J G, Turner T L, Wardrop C A 1993 Umbilical cord clamping and preterm infants: a randomised trial. British Medical Journal 306: 172–175
Marlow N 1992 Do we need an Apgar score? Archives of Disease in Childhood 67:765–767
Levene M 1993 Management of the asphyxiated term infant. Archives of Disease in Childhood 68: 612–616
Palme-Kilander C 1993 Methods of resuscitation in low-Apgar-score newborn infants – a national survey. Acta Paediatrica 81: 739–744

Perlman J, Risser R 1993 Severe fetal acidaemia: neonatal neurological features and short term oucome. Paediatric Neurology 9: 277–282
Roberton N 1992 Textbook of neonatology, 2nd edn. Churchill Livingstone, Edinburgh
Roberton N 1995 Clinical paediatrics. Baillière Tindall, London, vol 3, no 1
Sinclair J, Bracken M 1992 Effective care of the newborn infant. Oxford University Press, Oxford
Whitelaw A 1989 Intervention after birth asphyxia. Archives of Disease in Childhood 64: 66–68 (review)
Yu V Y H (ed) 1995 Clinical paediatrics: pulmonary problems in the perinatal period and their sequelae. Baillière Tindall, London

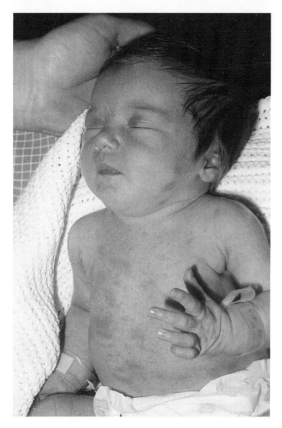

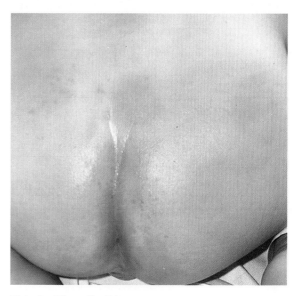

Plate 2   'Mongolian' blue spot.

Plate 1   Urticaria neonatorum.

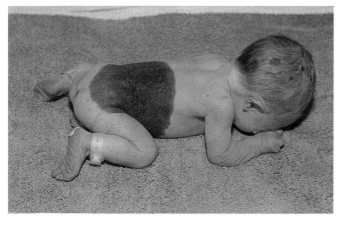

Plate 3   Giant pigmented naevus with satellite smaller lesions.

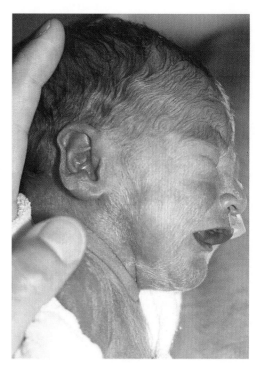

Plate 4   Lanugo.

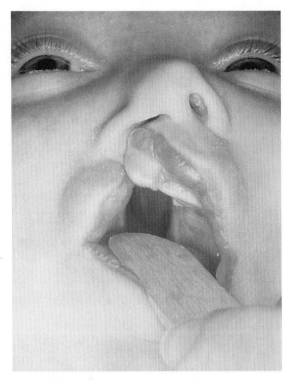

Plate 5 Cleft lip and palate.

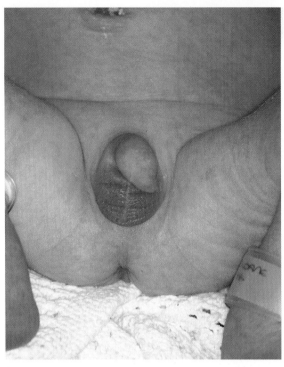

A

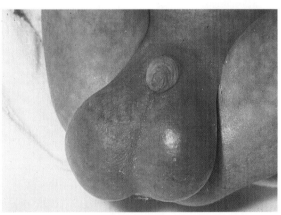

Plate 6 A: Bilateral undescended testes. B: Bilateral hydroceles.

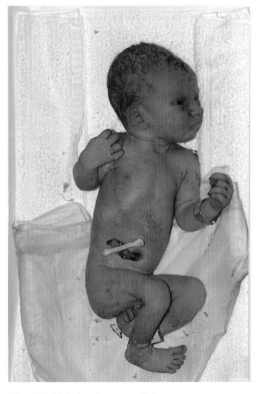

Plate 7 Light for dates term infant.

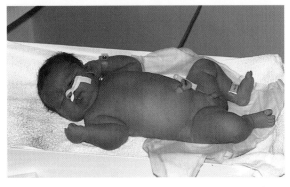

Plate 8 Infant of a diabetic mother showing macrosomia and polycythaemia.

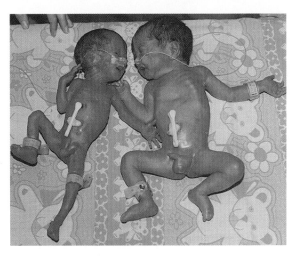

Plate 9 Growth retardation in one of a pair of twins.

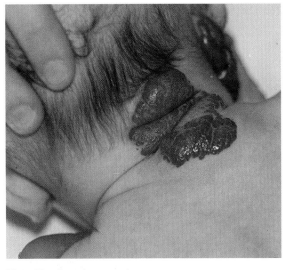

Plate 10 Strawberry marks.

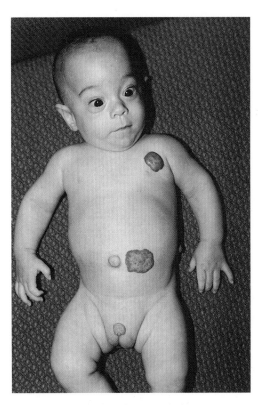

Plate 11 Multiple strawberry marks in a pre-term infant.

4

Physiology of the neonate

SIZE AND GROWTH OF NORMAL INFANTS

Those who work with the newborn soon come to realize that no two infants are alike and that there is a wide range of size, proportion, nutritional state and patterns of growth among healthy 'normal' infants. It is by becoming aware of this variability that it is possible to assess which infants require closer observation and investigation and which are more likely to be normal. It is not always easy to define the limits of normality in the neonate, but as far as growth is concerned, those falling outside the range of the 5th to 95th percentiles are more likely to have problems than those nearer to the average.

Weight

The average term infant in Britain weighs 3500 g at birth; 95% of babies are between 2500 and 4250 g. Those of 2500 g or less are classified as 'low birth weight' and about half of these are small because they are pre-term (born before the end of the 37th week of pregnancy). The remainder are unusually small for their gestational age and, if their weight falls below the 10th percentile on the growth chart, they are referred to as light (or small) for dates (LFD or SFD) babies (p. 92). The weight at birth is influenced by many factors in addition to the length of gestation. Maternal disease such as pre-eclampsia which affects placental function reduces the size of the baby, whereas inadequately controlled diabetes mellitus results in excessive fetal growth. Mothers of shorter stature usually have small babies, although taller women do not necessarily have big infants. Extreme maternal malnutrition may restrict fetal growth. Ethnic differences also occur. The British born babies of mothers of West Indian origin tend to be larger than ethnic white babies. A higher percentage of Asian-origin British births are below the 10th percentile, but in the second generation their birth weights seem to be rising. The average boy at term weighs nearly 250 g more than the average girl. Birth weight bears some relation to size in later childhood, mainly through the common factor of parental height, but the connection is less clear in those infants towards the extremes of the centile ranges.

Growth

During the first 3–5 days of life, the infant usually loses up to 10% of his birth weight as the kidneys excrete a small physiological excess of body fluid but regains it by the 7–10th day as real weight is gained through adequate feeding. In the following month, weight gain is usually between 180 and 210 g each week but it is seldom an even rise; days of slow progress are followed by days of compensatory gain. Babies who are light at birth due to growth retardation caused by intrauterine malnutrition may catch up to their expected weight by accelerated gain in the first few weeks, and conversely those who are heavy at birth due to excessive intrauterine growth may at first grow more slowly and thus fall towards their intended (genetic) size (p. 95). Plotting the weight of the baby about once or twice a week on a chart such as the one shown in Figure 4.1 is a valuable guide to growth and progress, and the majority of infants grow along their birth centile. Provided the baby's health is not judged on this alone, consistent growth usually indicates a healthy infant, but one whose weight centile continues to fall, a condition referred to as 'failure to thrive', may either be receiving inadequate nutrition or have some medical condition preventing him from growing.

Length

The average length of a term baby is 51 cm and 95% measure between 46 and 56 cm. Increase in length gives an indication of skeletal growth, but it is much more difficult to measure accurately than weight even if special apparatus is used. Little useful information is gained from measurement of length at intervals of less than 3 months.

Length should be measured at birth to serve as a baseline against which to judge future growth. This should be done with the infant in the supine position, with the head held straight by one person and the legs held fully extended by another. The distance is measured between the topmost point of the head and the heels, with the feet held at a right angle to the table. A simple apparatus consists of a flat measuring mat with two end-plates at right angles to the base, one of which is fixed at the end while the other slides along its length (Fig. 4.2). Table 4.1 shows average dimensions of babies at different gestational periods and the growth chart in Figure 4.1 gives a guide to the changes in length, weight and head circumference usually seen in healthy infants from birth to 2 years of age, indicating the 3rd, 10th, 50th, 90th and 97th percentiles.

THE HEAD
Size

The head circumference is the greatest measurement around the forehead and the occiput (the occipitofrontal circumference) and should be recorded 2–4 days after birth when the effects of moulding during delivery have resolved. The circumference normally lies between 33 and 37 cm, with an average of 35 cm, the head size reflecting weight and length. However, if the baby's weight is low for his gestational age because of the effects of late intrauterine malnutrition, the head growth is often preserved and appears to be relatively large. During the first month of life the head circumference normally grows by about 2 cm, although growth-retarded infants may show catch-up growth. Abnormally rapid head growth may be seen from weekly charting of the head circumference and, if accompanied by widened cranial sutures and increased tension of

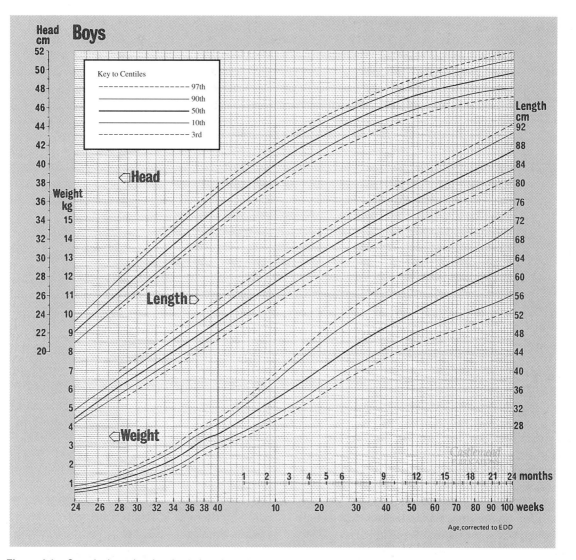

Figure 4.1   Growth chart showing the 3rd, 10th, 50th, 90th and 97th percentiles for weight, length and head circumference from 24 weeks of gestation to 2 years of age. (By kind permission of Castlemead Publications.)

the anterior fontanelle, it may indicate raised intracranial pressure (p. 215).

The eyes

Vision

The term infant can see from the first day of life and it is possible to demonstrate that the eyes follow a moving object or turn towards the light. Fixation of the gaze is at first slow and patience is required to show that it is present at all. Gradually it improves and the baby obviously fixes and follows with the eyes at about 6 weeks of age. It is worth noting that a human face is often followed some time before a brightly coloured object or a light.

Eye movements

Eye movements are at first poorly coordinated

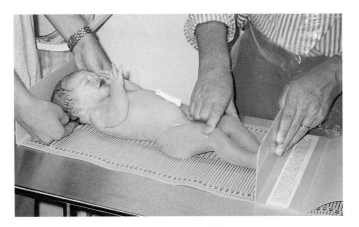

Figure 4.2 Portable mat for measuring the length of babies.

Table 4.1 Average dimensions at different periods of gestation

Weeks of gestation	Weight g (±2 SD)	Length cm (±2 SD)	Head circumference cm (±2 SD)
24	700 (±200)	32 (±4)	22 (±2)
28	1200 (±350)	37 (±4)	26 (±2)
32	1800 (±500)	43 (±5)	30 (±2)
36	2700 (±800)	49 (±5)	33 (±2)
40	3600 (±750)	53 (±6)	35 (±2)

and the eyes may sometimes move independently, producing a squint. However, it is only a persistent squint which requires urgent referral for surgical correction, to prevent permanent loss of binocular vision, since the majority resolve spontaneously. The pupils react to light from birth. Tears are rarely seen during crying in the newborn baby.

The nose and mouth

The importance to the baby of his nasal airway is not always appreciated. The control of breathing and swallowing is so arranged that he can breathe through his mouth only with difficulty. This can result in severe respiratory distress in the rare infant born with congenital obstruction of the nose (p. 99). Care must therefore be taken not to damage the delicate nasal mucosa by vigorous insertion of nasal catheters. The alae nasi muscles are normally used in the first few days, and flaring of the alae with breathing does not always signify respiratory distress.

THE SKIN

The skin is one of the largest organs in the body and has several functions which are vital for protection and maintenance of homeostasis. It is the most important structure in the maintenance of body temperature. By varying the state of the arteriolar circulation, the skin can enable the baby to lose or retain heat as needed. Sweating, which increases heat loss by evaporation of water from the skin surface, is also well developed in the newborn infant, although it is only in rare situations (e.g. acute heart failure) that it is visible. Smaller babies are more likely to become cold than larger ones because of the relatively larger surface area of skin, and the ambient temperature should be adjusted to take account of this during resuscitation, nappy changing, bathing and radiological examination in order to prevent a drop in temperature.

Larger babies in incubators and normal babies in hot climates can overheat equally easily, because their smaller skin surface in relation to weight limits their ability to lose heat. The subject of maintenance of body temperature is discussed more fully on page 32.

The skin also acts as a physical barrier which prevents both the loss of body fluid through surface evaporation and the absorption of toxic substances into the body. This function is not fully developed until the stratum corneum, the superficial layer of the epidermis, thickens and dries to form a barrier on the surface of the skin. This process, known as cornification, takes several days in the term infant but up to 2 weeks in the very pre-term baby. Prevention of invasion of pathogenic bacteria is achieved both by this physical barrier and by the maintainance of an acidic pH by the skin secretions.

The protective greasy vernix caseosa which covers the skin and which decreases in amount after term should be left alone as it protects the underlying skin until is is cornified and will come off within a few days.

Skin colour varies widely and depends on the state of the capillary circulation at the time. It may change from a pale pink during sleep to a deep red while crying. The hands and feet are often slightly blue in the first 48 hours, especially after being changed or washed, which may indicate that the baby has become cold.

Rashes are common and are often of no great significance. They are discussed on p. 57.

THE CHEST
Shape and appearance

The ribs slope downwards to a lesser extent in the newborn than in later childhood and thus the chest is relatively deeper from back to front and narrower from side to side.

Breathing

The physiology of the onset of respiration at birth and those factors which delay it are discussed on p. 35. Once respiration is established, much useful information can be gained by critical observation of the baby's breathing from the moment of birth onwards. Although regular rhythmic breathing at about 30–50 breaths/min is often established within a few minutes, irregular breathing at rates from 15 to 100 breaths/min are not uncommon. The greater the rate varies from the average, the more likely it is to be abnormal, and a consistent rate above 60 breaths/min

may be caused by lung disease, metabolic acidosis or congenital heart disease. Decreased rates may be caused by suppression of the respiratory centre by drugs or cerebral asphyxia.

More important than the rate is the manner of breathing. The normal infant breathes more with the diaphragm than the thorax so that indrawing of the soft lower ribs is often seen. This costal recession (Fig. 9.2, p. 129) is accentuated in any form of lung disease, particularly in the pre-term infant, the baby with upper airway obstruction and also in some forms of congenital heart disease (p. 208). Backward movement of the head on inspiration is often seen when respiratory difficulty arises and may be accompanied by a short 'grunt' which results from closure of the glottis during expiration.

The volume of air taken with each breath (the tidal volume) is 6 ml/kg body weight and this ensures that the baby receives the 6ml/kg per minute of oxygen required to keep the blood gases within the normal range (p. 53). Control of the depth and rate of breathing is achieved by the respiratory centre in the medulla of the brain, which is fully mature in most term infants and responds to changes of the carbon dioxide and oxygen levels in the blood and its pH. Occasionally during sleep a healthy baby will have brief self-limiting apnoeic spells caused by immaturity of the respiratory centre which last up to 12 seconds and resolve spontaneously as the carbon dioxide in the blood rises and stimulates breathing again. As long as they are not accompanied by a slowing heart rate or cyanosis, they do no harm and usually cease within a few weeks.

THE HEART AND CIRCULATION
The change from fetal life to independence

Figure 4.3 is a diagram of the fetal circulation. This is arranged such that the deoxygenated blood returning to both sides of the heart is directed down the aorta to the umbilical vessels and thence to the placenta to oxygenate the haemoglobin and discharge the carbon dioxide

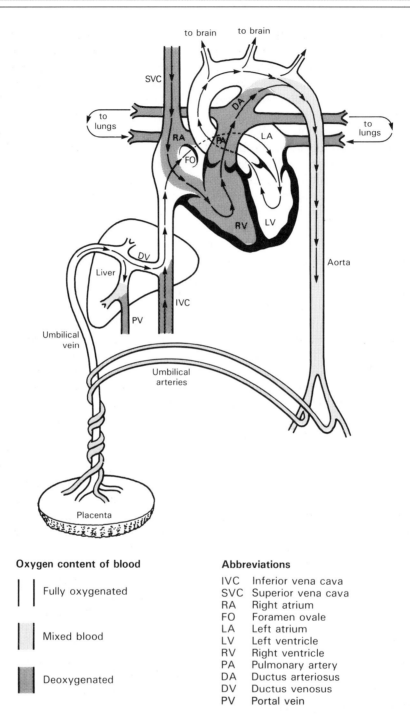

Oxygen content of blood

Fully oxygenated

Mixed blood

Deoxygenated

Abbreviations

IVC   Inferior vena cava
SVC   Superior vena cava
RA   Right atrium
FO   Foramen ovale
LA   Left atrium
LV   Left ventricle
RV   Right ventricle
PA   Pulmonary artery
DA   Ductus arteriosus
DV   Ductus venosus
PV   Portal vein

Figure 4.3   Fetal circulation showing the patterns of blood flow and distribution of oxygenated and deoxygenated blood.

to the maternal circulation, whilst the most oxygenated blood is available to the developing brain. To achieve this, the oxygenated blood returning via the umbilical vein and ductus venosus to the right atrium is directed through the foramen ovale to the left atrium and thence to the left ventricle and aorta. The developing brain thus receives the most oxygenated blood through the carotid arteries. Deoxygenated blood returns to the heart via the superior vena cava into the right atrium. The right ventricle is hypertrophied in the fetus and the systolic pressure it achieves is equal to that in the left ventricle. Hence it can pump the deoxygenated blood across the ductus arteriosus to reach the aorta through which it returns to the placenta.

The amount of blood flowing through different parts of the circuit varies inversely with the resistance encountered, which depends on the degree of constriction of the blood vessels. This is regulated by changes in pH and oxygen saturation in the blood. High resistance in the pulmonary vessels maintains minimal blood flow through the functionless fetal lungs until the first breath is taken and the vessels dilate.

The placenta usually receives about half of the cardiac output, but if its blood supply is reduced by infarction or failure to grow, a significant reduction in oxygen supply and nutrition to the fetus ensues. Whilst oxygen tension in the fetus is only about 3–4 kPa (20–30 mmHg) compared with the healthy newborn value of 12–13 kPa (90–100 mmHg), this is offset by the higher oxygen-carrying capacity of fetal haemoglobin and an increased number of red cells produced by the fetal bone marrow.

At birth the expansion of the lungs with the baby's first breaths leads to a reduction of the pulmonary vascular resistance and allows most of the right ventricular output to flow through the lungs. The flow from the placenta having ceased, pressure in the inferior vena cava and right atrium falls, and rising pressure in the left atrium caused by the increased blood flow from the lungs closes the flap valve of the foramen ovale, thus separating the pulmonary and systemic circulations. A very small shunt of blood across the foramen ovale may continue for 4–5 days normally but is greatly increased where the dynamics are altered by such disorders as the respiratory distress syndrome or certain cardiac malformations. The ductus arteriosus constricts and closes in response to the rising oxygen tension in the aortic blood, thus preventing the blood from the aorta and the pulmonary artery from mixing. However, it is anatomically patent for 2 or 3 days and may open up again in situations of arterial desaturation from any cause. A systolic murmur can often be heard from a patent ductus at this stage. The change from the fetal to the neonatal circulation is so effective that arterial blood oxygen saturation normally reaches 90% within an hour of delivery.

The electrocardiogram (ECG)

At birth, the ECG pattern reflects the hypertrophy of the right side of the heart which has ensured the effectiveness of the fetal circulation. As the baby rapidly adapts to independent existence, alterations occur in the ECG within the first 24 hours (Fig. 4.4). Thereafter, the pattern becomes fairly stable, although certain characteristics differ from those in later infancy. The electrical axis of the normal neonatal heart is between +110° and +180° (as shown by a dominant S wave in lead I, and R wave in lead III) caused by the dominant right ventricle which is represented as prominent R waves in the V_4R and V_1 chest leads and by S waves in V_5 and V_6. Notching of the R wave in V_1 is a common variation of normal. The T waves in the right chest leads are usually upright for the first 24 hours but become inverted by the fourth day.

Disorders of conduction and rhythm, particularly atrial premature beats, are present in about 1% of newborn infants, although rarely do they cause clinical disturbance and usually they disappear by 3 months of age. They may also be seen on fetal heart recordings in labour.

Blood pressure

It is very difficult to measure the blood pressure by auscultation or even by palpation. The most accurate measurements are made by placing a

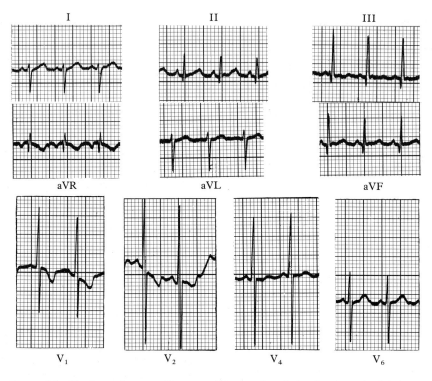

Figure 4.4 Electrocardiogram of the normal term newborn baby showing a dominant right ventricular force and right axis deviation (see text for details).

Doppler ultrasound probe over the brachial or tibial artery below the cuff. Automated electronic apparatus using a pressure-sensitive transducer can make repeated measurements in even the smallest infant and is now a standard part of intensive neonatal care, particularly of the sick baby with respiratory distress syndrome. A blood pressure recording may also help in the diagnosis of aortic coarctation where the pressure in the legs is significantly lower than in the arms.

The normal range of blood pressure is wide and varies with gestational age. In a term baby, the systolic pressure in the arm rises from about 70 mmHg on the first day to around 85 mmHg by the second week and 95 mmHg at 6 weeks. Variation in the size of the cuff causes big differences in the readings, too small a cuff giving too high a value. The inflatable section should cover over half the length of the upper arm and more than two-thirds of its circumference. For the term newborn infant, a width of 5 cm and a length of

7–10 cm is ideal, with relatively narrower cuffs for smaller babies.

ALIMENTARY TRACT FUNCTION

Feeding

Whether the baby is breast or bottle fed, the milk is obtained by a wave-like movement of the tongue compressing the nipple from front to back while the areola is held in a firm grip by the lips. When the milk hits the palate it induces swallowing, which is completed before the next suck occurs. The coordination to 'latch on' and obtain the feed in this way develops near term, and most infants over 35 weeks of gestation are able to suck adequately to obtain enough milk to grow. The normal infant swallows a variable quantity of air during feeds, most of which is expelled afterwards, sometimes with a little milk. Vomiting of a more persistent nature should be regarded as abnormal and a cause sought (p. 88).

Digestion and absorption

There is relatively good development of secretory and absorbing surfaces in the infant gut from well before term. This results in efficient absorption of food, but the gut may become distended with wind because of a lack of supportive tissues in the bowel wall. Digestive enzymes are fully active at term except for pancreatic amylase, so that digestion of starch is theoretically not possible.

Faeces

Meconium is a viscid semifluid substance consisting mainly of mucus with an accumulation of swallowed amniotic fluid, desquamated epithelial cells and bilirubin, which gives it the characteristic blackish-green colour. The first stool is normally passed within the first 24 hours, but exceptionally it may be delayed for up to 3 days in normal infants. A firm plug of meconium may obstruct the anus and cause abdominal distension which is relieved after gentle stretching of the anal sphincter by rectal examination.

If feeding is taking place normally, 'changing stools' of a light greenish brown colour replace the meconium on about the third or fourth day. Thereafter, there is a gradual change to the mustard-coloured stools of the breast-fed, or the paler yellow stools of the formula-fed, infant. There is great individual variation in the number and consistency of the stools which bears little relation to the rate of the infant's weight gain. A vigorous gastrocolic reflex may cause the breast-fed baby to pass one or two stools at each feed, but occasionally infants pass only one large soft stool as infrequently as once every 2 or 3 days. Much more regularity is found in formula-fed babies, and variations in the number and consistency of stools are more likely to reflect an alimentary disorder.

RENAL FUNCTION

Urine secretion takes place in the latter half of pregnancy and much of the amniotic fluid is fetal urine. The baby may also micturate during delivery, when it may go unnoticed. Normally, a baby first passes urine at any time up to 48 hours, or even exceptionally as late as the third day, although most infants will do so within 12 hours. Serious causes for delay are rare in the absence of other clinical signs such as enlargement of the bladder. The nature of the urinary stream should be observed, since dribbling micturition is the most useful sign of urethral valves in a boy or ectopic ureters in a girl.

The amount and frequency of urine passed gradually increases with the quantity of feed taken during the first week and the bladder may empty up to 20 times a day during the second week. The volume is immensely variable and depends on the fluid intake. In a study of breast-fed infants it averaged 20 ml on the first day, rising to 200 ml on the 10th day.

Urate crystals may colour the urine at this age, leaving a brick-red stain on the nappy which can be mistaken for blood. Albumin is not normally present in more than slight traces, but false-positive tests due to urates can sometimes be misleading.

The normal term infant has a glomerular filtration rate of about 40 ml/min per 1.73 m^2, or about one-third of adult values, and it only slowly increases over the first year of life. The kidneys can neither rapidly excrete a water load nor concentrate the urine to conserve fluid well in the first month, although the tubules are capable of responding normally to antidiuretic hormone. The term infant can conserve sodium but the premature baby's kidney often leaks sodium even when the serum level is low. Because of these facts it is important that the term baby is not given feeds with too high a sodium concentration, as these could render him hypernatraemic and damage the developing brain. The pre-term baby, by contrast, may need sodium supplements to prevent hyponatraemia. Hydrogen ion excretion by the renal tubules is also limited and an excessive protein load can cause a metabolic acidosis which may show itself as lethargy or poor feeding.

This immaturity of renal function may affect the duration of action of some drugs which are mainly excreted by the kidney, and the dose or frequency of administration may be different from that given to an older child (pp. 168 and 233).

BEHAVIOUR AND RESPONSE TO ENVIRONMENT

No two healthy newborn babies behave in exactly the same way, even when they are identical twins, but there is a broad pattern which can be regarded as normal, from which only minor deviations occur. At first it is a relatively simple pattern of sleep, wakefulness and semi-purposeful movements with some reflexes, such as sucking and swallowing, which enable the baby to survive. From the moment of birth, however, the infant is able to respond to his carers and the environment in his own individual way and begin the process of learning which will enable him to progress in his development (p. 69).

At times during the day the baby lies awake and quiet, at others he is active and crying. For between 16 and 20 hours each day he will be asleep, although the depth and duration of sleep vary considerably from one baby to another. Some arouse easily and are wakeful even though well fed, whilst others wake only to be fed and changed. In most cases the early sleep pattern has no predictive value in assessing later characteristics.

Sucking

The normal term infant can suck and swallow almost immediately after birth. The touch of the nipple on the baby's face initiates rooting, latching onto the nipple and the coordinated movements of lip, tongue, palate and pharynx required to feed successfully (Fig. 4.5). Failure to suck when the stomach is empty always means something is amiss and is an important sign of brain stem damage.

Crying

Crying is the baby's main means of communicating his needs in the first weeks of life. He cries vigorously and spasmodically without tears and

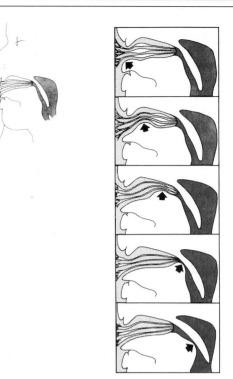

Figure 4.5 Diagram showing the rolling action of the tongue during breast feeding. The nipple is compressed between the tongue and the anterior part of the palate from which a wave of compression (arrowed) progresses backwards towards the pharynx, thus expelling the milk and initiating swallowing. (From *Successful breastfeeding*, with permission from the Royal College of Midwives.)

often without any obvious reason. At birth, crying is a response to the dramatic sensations of light, sound, cold and gravity experienced for the first time. Thereafter, it generally means hunger, thirst or pain, but may also indicate a need for protection or comfort. Most mothers will rapidly learn to recognize their own baby's need from the types of cry he makes, although such factors as negative experiences around the time of birth or maternal depression afterwards may diminish her sensitivity to the infant's needs and perpetuate the crying.

Various other discomforts can initiate crying, for instance contact with a cold hand, sudden movement or a bright light. Infants appear to be more sensitive to visceral pain (e.g. distension with wind) than to somatic pain, although there is clear evidence to suggest that they feel significant pain from invasive procedures such as heel pricks and venepuncture (p. 140).

It is unusual for an adequately fed baby who is given sufficient attention to cry for more than a total of 2 hours a day in the first 2 weeks. Occasionally a baby may be unusually sensitive to disturbances of any sort, may cry for long periods and may be difficult to pacify. Parents may be spared much unnecessary worry if it is made clear to them that to pick up and comfort a crying newborn infant will not spoil him, but rather is to satisfy a natural instinctive need in both mother and child.

THE BLOOD AND BODY COMPOSITION

A term baby weighing 3500 g consists of 70% water (of which half is in the cells), 16% fat, 11 % protein and 1% carbohydrate. A 1000 g pre-term infant may be 85% water, only 1% fat, 8% protein and 0.5% carbohydrate. These figures emphasize the fact that the pre-term baby has very limited stores of fat and glycogen, and thus of available calorie sources, and stress the importance of adequate early feeding in such infants to avoid hypoglycaemia and its serious consequences. The same applies to the mature 'light for dates' infant who has suffered from poor nutrition before birth.

Haematological values

Large changes take place in the constituents of the blood during the first few hours and days of life, and the range of variation from one baby to another is also relatively wide compared with the adult. The values given here refer to those commonly seen in healthy term infants.

The blood volume is about 85 ml/kg body weight (40 ml/lb), giving the average baby a total blood volume of 240–300 ml. Thus the loss of 40–50 ml of blood from a newborn infant is roughly equivalent to a loss of 500 ml from an adult.

The haemoglobin content of cord blood in 95% of infants ranges from 15 to 20 g/dl, with a mean value of 17 g/dl. The figure is slightly lower in pre-term infants, and higher values are found in post-term infants or those who have suffered fetal growth retardation or hypoxia. The value is influenced greatly by the volume of the placental transfusion received before the cord is cut. During the first 6 weeks of life, few red cells are produced and the haemoglobin level falls by around 1g/week (p. 177). About 80% of the haemoglobin at term is of the fetal type, which permits a better uptake of oxygen at a relatively low partial pressure, and it is gradually lost at the rate of 3–4% per week and replaced by adult haemoglobin.

The packed cell volume rises to an average maximum of 70% at about 3 hours of age and then falls to 50% in 2 days (range 36–60%).

The red cell count at birth is somewhat above adult levels (average $6 \times 10^{12}/L$) but relatively less so than the haemoglobin because the cells are large. The numbers fall at a slower rate than the haemoglobin, reaching about $4.5 \times 10^{12}/L$ by 4 weeks. These changes are due to reduced red cell production in the bone marrow which fails to keep pace with the natural loss of red cells.

The white cell count is extremely variable,

Table 4.2 Blood chemistry values at 1–2 weeks of age in healthy term infants

Constituent	Range
Sodium	130–145 mmol/L
Potassium	3.6–5.8 mmol/L
Calcium	1.90–2.85 mmol/L
Magnesium	0.59–1.05 mmol/L
Chloride	92–109 mmol/L
Phosphate	1.8–3.2 mmol/L
Urea	1.0–5.0 mmol/L
Creatinine	62–106 μmol/L
Glucose (fasting)	3.2–4.9 mmol/L
Other units	
Blood gases:	
— pH	7.33–7.47
— P_aCO_2	4.4–6.0 kPa
— P_aO_2	6.0–9.0 kPa
— base deficit	−5 mmol/L
Total protein	43–76 g/dl
Albumin	28–49 g/dl
Immunoglobulins:	
— IgG	4.8–13 g/L
— IgA	15.6–124 mg/L
— IgM	140–603 mg/L

ranging from 6 to 22 $\times$ 10^9/L. Neutrophils predominate at first, but after the second day, as the total count falls, lymphocytes become predominant and by 14 days amount to about 60% of the white cells. Although an infection will cause a rise in the neutrophil count, the variability of the count in healthy babies is so great that a single measurement is of little value in identifying the infected infant.

Biochemistry

The blood biochemistry for those constituents commonly estimated in the newborn period is summarized in Table 4.2. The concentration of many of these alters with almost every hour after birth and varies widely from one baby to another, but the quoted figures may be regarded as the normal range of values for term infants at 1–2 weeks of age (Clayton & Round 1984).

FURTHER READING

Clayton B, Round J 1984 Chemical pathology and the sick child. Blackwell, London
Gluckman P, Heyman M 1996. Paediatrics and perinatology: the scientific basis. Arnold, London
Heine R, Jaquiery A Lubitz L, Cameron D J, Catto-Smith A G 1995 Role of gastro-oesophageal reflux in infant irritability Archives of Disease in Childhood 73: 121–125

Levene M, Liford R (eds) 1995 Fetal and neonatal neurology and neurosurgery. Churchill Livingstone, Edinburgh
Roberton N 1992 Textbook of neonatology, 2nd edn. Churchill Livingstone, Edinburgh

5

Examination of the newborn and detection of abnormality

Since most babies are healthy, have no congenital malformations and behave normally, it may be thought that routine medical examination is an unimportant chore. However, if its purpose is understood and it is carried out and recorded carefully, it forms an accurate record of the state of the baby at birth which becomes the initial record for continuing child health and development surveillance programmes. It also identifies most babies who need further observation, although some significant malformations in the heart and renal tracts are not identifiable at this stage. It can also give important clues about the relationship between the mother and her infant.

The health of the baby may be adversely affected during intrauterine life and a search of the mother's notes should reveal relevant information about factors which could affect the fetus (p. 12). The family history may reveal a genetic disorder, and prenatal diagnosis may have been undertaken (p. 19). The mother herself may have a complication of the pregnancy or a medical condition which could, either through the disorder itself or through its treatment, cause a malformation, alter fetal growth or affect the health of the baby in the first few days of life (p. 25).

The mother's age, family structure and the support available from others will be noted from the social history. This information should be supplemented by a discussion with the parents which may reveal previously undisclosed facts which could affect the care or health of the baby.

INSPECTION AT BIRTH

A brief examination of the baby should be carried out following its safe delivery, to confirm the sex and identify any visible abnormalities such as spina bifida, hare lip or talipes. It is important to provide a sympathetic explanation to the parents of any major defect noted at this time. If the baby is vigorous, alert and well she should be given to the mother and a fuller examination should be left until 24–48 hours of age. If it is clear that the baby is unwell or needs more urgent attention, this should be explained to the parents, but as long as she is well enough, it is more important for the parents to see, touch and hear her at this moment than to carry out nursing or medical tasks.

ROUTINE EXAMINATION

The first examination of the baby should always be carried out in the presence of the mother and she should be invited to participate by undressing and dressing the baby. While observing how she performs these tasks, an assessment can be made of the mother's confidence in handling her baby and how well she relates to her. It also gives an opportunity to discuss with her any concerns she may have about the baby. Reassurance can be offered about features related to the birth, such as a caput succedaneum or moulding of the head, which will resolve completely leaving no lasting effect on the baby. This is also a good time to discuss the programme of immunizations which the baby should receive and recommend exclusion of pertussis vaccine if there is a perinatal contraindication to its use (p. 151).

Although in most cases the intended method of feeding the baby will have been determined before she is born, some additional guidance may be needed. Breast feeding may not be appropriate if the mother has to take certain drugs (p. 79). For the baby with a cleft palate, for instance, the method of feeding may be found only by trial and error, some managing to breast feed surprisingly well while others need specialized teats and must be bottle fed. This information can also be very important to those who will be giving continued support to the family after discharge from the maternity unit.

The purposes of the physical examination are:

1. To confirm that the infant is well grown, healthy and behaving normally, and to reassure the parents.
2. To assess the baby's adaptation to extrauterine life and her response to any resuscitation which may have been necessary.
3. To identify any effects of the process of birth on the baby.
4. To confirm the maturity of the infant by an assessment of her gestational age.
5. To detect any congenital anomalies which may be identifiable at this time, to discuss their management with the parents and initiate the appropriate treatment. It may be helpful to explain to some parents that not all abnormalities show themselves at this time and that further routine clinical assessments will be carried out after discharge from the maternity unit.
6. To recognize the baby who is ill and arrange the necessary investigation and treatment, admitting the baby to the neonatal unit if this is appropriate.

Observation of the baby as a whole

The growth and state of nutrition of the baby can be assessed both by observation and by plotting the weight, length and head circumference on standard growth charts suitable for the ethnic group from which the baby comes. Most well-grown babies will have a moderate covering of fat, but in poorly controlled maternal diabetes mellitus the baby will have a gross excess of fat. By contrast, the baby who has suffered from late intrauterine malnutrition will be noticeably thin, although head growth is often spared and the head circumference centile may be greater than the weight centile. More prolonged fetal growth retardation can result in a small but apparently healthy baby with reduction of all parameters of growth, the degree of which may only be seen when the figures are plotted on the growth chart.

The baby's maturity should be assessed (p. 106) and compared with the mother's dates.

The size and shape of the limbs may be out of proportion to the body size in achondroplasia and other rarer bone dysplasias, although asymmetry and some postural deformities resulting from the effect of the cramped intrauterine environment are common and usually resolve rapidly.

Combinations of odd features, particularly on the face, hands and feet, may constitute a syndrome and should always be investigated further (p. 222). Racial and familial features will also be visible and should be taken into account when assessing the facies.

SYSTEMATIC EXAMINATION

The skin

The colour and texture of the skin give much useful information. In most mature infants from white ethnic groups the skin is pale over the body, but within the first 24–48 hours the hands and feet may be slightly blue. Central cyanosis, jaundice or unusual pallor should always be regarded as abnormal and explored further. In darker-skinned infants such features must be sought on inspection of the mucous membranes, particularly in the mouth. Racial colouring, particularly in babies of mixed race, may not be obvious at birth but the scrotum is often more pigmented. Birth marks should be noted.

Rashes

Urticaria neonatorum (Plate 1). Urticaria neonatorum or erythema toxicum is a very common and rapidly varying blotchy red rash occurring mainly on the trunk which sometimes has yellowish pinhead spots resembling pustules, but which are actually sterile and contain eosinophil cells. It usually occurs between the second and eighth days and, although alarming in appearance, it is harmless. Its cause is uncertain and it disappears usually within a few days.

Superficial skin peeling. Superficial peeling of the skin, particularly over the extremities, is common at some stage in the first week and is seen at its maximum in post-term babies or in babies who have suffered intrauterine malnutrition (p. 93). It requires no treatment and gives no indication of the future condition of the baby's skin.

Milia. Milia, the whitish pinhead-sized spots which are really tiny sebaceous retention cysts and can be felt with the finger, are concentrated mainly on and around the nose. They last for only a few weeks.

Subcutaneous fat necrosis. Also known as pseudosclerema, this is a localized area of induration, usually on the back but sometimes over the face or thighs. The skin has a blotchy reddened appearance and is hardened so that it is impossible to pick up a fold of it between the fingers. Sometimes it may be shown to be the result of pressure, as on the face after forceps delivery, but often there is no known cause. It has no serious significance and gradually resolves spontaneously within the first year, but it must be clearly distinguished from sclerema neonatorum which is an entirely different condition with a much more serious outcome (p. 120).

Traumatic cyanosis. This is a term used to describe the appearance of cyanosis of the face and head which is produced by masses of very small petechial haemorrhages in the skin. It can occur after there has been congestion of the head, perhaps due to the nature of the delivery or the presence of a tight umbilical cord around the neck at one stage. The local nature of the condition distinguishes it from true cyanosis, and examination with a lens easily reveals the petechiae.

Occasionally transient skin flushing of one-half of the infant is noticed, with a clear demarcation down the midline separating it from the normal half. Known as the harlequin change, this odd phenomenon has no serious significance.

Birthmarks

'Oriental' or 'Mongolian' blue patch (Plate 2). A bluish-black coloration of the skin over a circumscribed area in the sacral region or over the buttocks is common in dark-skinned races and occasionally it may be seen on fair-skinned babies. It is sometimes mistaken for a bruise although the lack of colour change over a few days is distinctive.

'Stork marks' or 'pressure marks'. These are names traditionally given to the reddish-purple areas of skin which are superficial capillary hae-mangiomata. They are visible in about one-third of normal babies over the midline of the lower forehead just above the nose, on the nape of the neck and sometimes on the upper eyelids. They always fade and usually become practically invisible after the first year.

Naevus flammeus. Naevus flammeus or the 'port wine' naevus is flat and dark reddish pur-ple in colour. The overlying skin is coarse and thickened. Laser therapy can reduce the colour to a moderate degree but this is not usually advised in infancy, and careful cosmetic covering later in life is often the best solution. The occasional asso-ciation of such a lesion over the trigeminal nerve area of the face with an intracranial haeman-gioma on the same side, constituting the Sturge–Weber syndrome, is worth bearing in mind.

Strawberry marks are described on page 102.

Pigmented naevi. Pigmented naevi may involve a wide area, as illustrated in Plate 3, and may have a covering of hair. Excision and skin grafting later in childhood is a possibility if they are not too large. Pigmented moles do not occur at birth, nor are such marks as café-au-lait or depigment-ed patches present until later in infancy. Thus the diagnoses of neurofibromatosis and tuberose sclerosis, both of which are inherited conditions, cannot be reliably excluded by neonatal exami-nation.

Head and neck

The skull and head

The bones of the cranial vault, being relatively soft and connected only by fibrous tissue, alter in shape readily in response to external pressure. The mode of presentation can often be deduced by observation of the moulding that has taken place, the vertex being prominent in cephalic delivery but rather flattened after a breech birth. These changes are more marked in infants of primipara than multipara and are sometimes accompanied by overriding of the cranial bones. The *caput succedaneum* is the oedematous thick-ening of the scalp in the presenting area (usually one parietal region), which is more obvious after prolonged labour and disappears within 2 days.

The *anterior fontanelle* is a diamond-shaped depression at the point where the frontal and parietal bones converge and is variable in size – from just admitting the tip of the forefinger, to an area 5 cm across. The size of the fontanelle is less informative than its tension. Normally it is slightly concave and may visibly pulsate, where-as if there is increased intracranial pressure it becomes first tense, then convex. It is continuous with the sagittal suture which passes from the posterior angle towards the occiput, and the coronal sutures which proceed laterally towards the ears. Their position is identifiable but there is not usually a palpable gap between the bones. A persistent metopic suture (felt as a gap running forward from the anterior fontanelle and divid-ing the frontal bone) is common. If the sutures are palpably separated, hydrocephalus should be excluded by regular plotting of the head circum-ference or ultrasound examination of the ventri-cles (p. 215).

A softening of the skull bone known as cran-iotabes is demonstrable by easy indentation on light pressure with the fingers over localized areas near the suture lines. It is a common nor-mal finding, but when it is more generalized it may be a sign of one of the rare disorders of bone calcification such as osteogenesis imperfecta or early rickets. In the rare condition of cleidocra-nial dysostosis the fontanelle may be enormous and the sutures very wide from a dysplasia of the membrane bone of which the skull is formed and which is the underlying abnormality in the con-dition. The clavicles, which are also formed from membrane bone, are impalpable and their absence can be confirmed by an X-ray of the chest.

The face

Facial features strongly reflect the characteristics of both the family and racial groups from which the baby comes. Some infants, however, have features which are obviously unusual, the best-known example being the child with Down's syndrome. There are many such dysmorphic syndromes and each baby should be investigated (p. 222) since some are genetically determined and associated with developmental delay.

Hair

The fine facial and body hair known as *lanugo* (Plate 4), which is a feature of pre-term infants and may be seen in dark-haired infants at term, is gradually lost during the first month along with some scalp hair. In ethnic white babies, the hair colour at this stage is not much of a guide to its future shade.

Ears

The upper margin of the ears should be at the same level as the eyes and complex in form. Occasionally accessory auricles, in the form of small pedunculated skin tags, will be seen in front of the ears. These can be dealt with by tying them off at the base (Fig. 5.1).

Nose

The nose varies in width and depth of the nasal bridge and it frequently forms epicanthes over the inner borders of the eyes, giving the false impression that the baby has a squint. Many babies have snuffles due simply to retained nasal mucus and not to a cold, although if there is respiratory distress, obstruction of the nasal passages from choanal atresia should be excluded by passing a fine polythene tube through the nose into the pharynx.

Eyes

Examination of the eyes can be difficult and little useful information can be obtained if the eyes are forced open. Holding the baby upright often results in spontaneous opening of the eyes. Their size and position and the angle of the palpebral fissures should be noted (Fig. 5.2). A fixed squint or nystagmus is always abnormal. Most normal newborn babies can fix their gaze on the examiner's face briefly. Crescentic subconjunctival haemorrhages are often seen on the sclerae around the margins of the iris, particularly after a difficult vaginal delivery, but they are benign and resolve within 2–3 weeks. Sticky and crusted

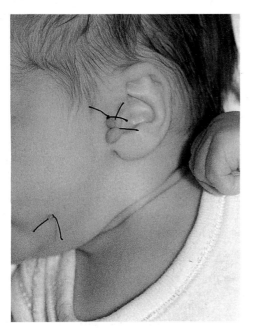

Figure 5.1   Preauricular skin tags showing ties.

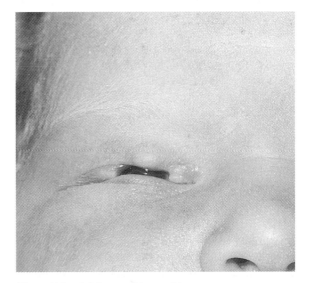

Figure 5.2   Coloboma of the eyelid.

eyes commonly occur in normal infants but pus indicates an infection which needs urgent attention. The iris should form a complete ring around a black pupil. A grey or white pupil, or loss of a red reflex on shining a light into the eye, may indicate that cataracts are present, and unusually large eyes may be caused by congenital glaucoma (p. 216). Tears rarely appear with crying in the neonatal period.

Examination of the optic fundi should be carried out when other congenital abnormalities are found to identify associated eye defects. Congenital infections (p. 169) often cause a retinopathy. Examination is much easier if each pupil is dilated with cyclopentolate hydrochloride. Compared with the older child, the neonatal fundus has a pale greyish tinge and is relatively streaky, especially at the periphery.

The mouth

The mouth is normally held closed and should open symmetrically. If it is drawn to one side during crying, this may indicate a facial palsy. A small receding jaw may cause feeding difficulties. To exclude a cleft, the palate is best inspected while the infant is crying (Plate 5) since it is often difficult to depress the tongue sufficiently with a spatula. Small white retention cysts on the palate, known as Ebstein's pearls, are common normal findings which require no treatment. Rarely a submucosal mucus retention cyst under the tongue, called a ranula, may be seen. An epulis is a firm fibrous swelling protruding from the gum margin which may interfere with feeding and require surgical attention.

Tongue tie is often suspected through lack of knowledge of the wide variation of the normal frenulum. True limitation of movement sufficient to interfere with sucking or later speech development is uncommon. Where a thickened frenulum grooves the tongue tip and obviously limits protrusion or upward movement, it is best dealt with by surgical division later in the first year.

Rounded thickened areas are often present on the lips (particularly the midline of the upper lip) and are known as sucking blisters. They are easi-ly distinguished from true blisters since they contain no fluid.

Teeth. The eruption of one or more lower incisor teeth before or soon after birth occurs about once in 2000 births. They are usually loose and do not interfere with feeding, and so, unless they are obviously about to become detached, they may safely be left alone.

Macroglossia. A large protruding tongue can be a feature of congenital hypothyroidism (p. 222), but is more likely to be an isolated feature. It may form part of Beckwith's syndrome in which there is also either an exomphalos or a large umbilical hernia, together with hypoglycaemia which, if untreated, may lead to mental retardation in a minority of cases.

The neck

The neck is commonly rather short at this time but it should be fully mobile. Where the baby prefers to hold the head to one side, the sternomastoid muscle should be palpated for a swelling known as a sternomastoid tumour (p. 103), although in most cases it simply results from an unusual intrauterine posture. Webbing of the neck posteriorly and an excess of skin at the nape of the neck commonly accompany some chromosome disorders and should prompt a search for other dysmorphic features which may suggest Turner's syndrome (p. 222). In other cases an X-ray may identify anomalies of the cervical vertebrae. The clavicles should be palpated to identify fractures which may occur during difficult deliveries. *Dermoid cysts* and *thyroglossal cysts* are uncommon and show as midline swellings, whereas *branchial cysts* or sinuses appear just in front of the upper third of the sternomastoid muscle.

Chest and heart

Watching the baby's breathing pattern identifies most abnormalities and conditions affecting the lungs, since most will present with grunting respirations, tachypnoea, or indrawing of the sternum, intercostal spaces or ribs on inspiration. If any of these features are present, a chest X-ray is needed to identify the underlying cause (p. 98). Little additional information is gained from auscultation of the lungs, but a knowledge of normal breath sounds is useful in intensive care of the newborn. They are usually bronchovesicular, inspiration and expiration being similar in pitch and duration. Fine râles (crackles) may be present if a part of the lung is consolidated. Percussion is of value in diagnosis when there are gross lung changes such as complete collapse of one lobe or a major pneumothorax, but even then it can be misleading. Detection of mediastinal shift by an alteration in the site of the maximal heart sounds is more useful diagnostically.

The heart lies relatively transversely and if the apex can be detected (which is difficult by palpation) it is in the midclavicular line in the left fourth intercostal space. There is often an easily palpable parasternal cardiac pulsation at this stage, due to the dominance of the right ventricle during intrauterine life.

The *pulse* is best felt either at the elbow from the brachial artery or in the groin from the femoral artery, but it is easier to count the rate using a stethoscope over the heart. The heart rhythm should be regular, but the rate is extremely variable, especially over the first 2 days. At birth it usually rises to about 180 beats/min and thereafter a rate from 80–120 is normal at rest, rising with stress and activity up to 200 beats/min. If it is consistently outside these limits when the infant is quiet, a cause should be sought.

Abnormalities of the heart rate conducting system are not uncommon and may even be detected before birth from observing irregularity of the fetal heart rhythm. Continuous bradycardia below 80 beats/min should prompt the investigation of congenital heart block. Supraventricular tachycardia, where the heart beats continuously at a rate of over 200 beats/min can lead to heart failure and requires immediate referral for treatment (p. 209).

Auscultation also requires a quiet baby and is best carried out while she is sucking on a teat. The heart sounds are of about equal intensity at both the apex and the base of the heart. Heart murmurs are common and can be heard in about 50% of all infants at some time during the first week,

although most are variable and transient. They are usually not loud and are thought to arise from variations in the dynamics of the circulation, or sometimes from a functionally persistent ductus arteriosus. A cardiac murmur is a common indication of a congenital cardiac malformation, although in many cases the murmur cannot be heard until the second week or later (p. 209).

The brachial and femoral pulses should be palpated. Impalpable femoral pulses suggest the diagnosis of coarctation of the aorta; they are always difficult to feel in the first few days of life, but with practice can usually be detected if the baby is lying quietly on a firm base with the hips gently flexed and abducted.

Breasts

At term in both sexes, a firm nodule of breast tissue 6–8 mm in diameter can be felt under the nipple which may enlarge and even produce a little colostrum after the third day of life, due to changes in hormonal balance after birth. It usually resolves within a few weeks but may occasionally last a few months. No treatment is needed and handling should be avoided to prevent an infective mastitis from developing.

Abdomen

Initially the abdomen should be inspected for distension and the umbilicus checked for unusual features. Three vessels – one vein and two arteries – should be identified on the cut end of the umbilical cord. The groins should be checked for herniae. On abdominal palpation it is usual to find the liver edge 1 cm below the costal margin, and both kidneys can frequently be felt between fingers of the two hands palpating simultaneously deep in the upper abdomen and in the loin. The spleen is also commonly felt superficially at the left costal margin. The rectus muscles are often separated in the midline of the upper abdomen at this time, allowing some bulging of the abdominal structures between them. The full bladder is often palpable in the neonate, which facilitates suprapubic aspiration of urine (p. 165). The identification of other abdominal masses or a palpable bladder which persists after micturition always indicates a serious abnormality which requires immediate investigation.

Genitalia

The scrotum in the male and the labia minora in the female are relatively large in the newborn, an appearance which is exaggerated in the pre-term infant or temporarily by transient oedema in a breech baby.

Male infants

The penis varies in size and shape, but the fore-skin should form a complete covering to the glans. No attempt should be made to retract it, as it adheres to the glans in infancy, gradually separating until 90% are retractable by the age of 3 years. There are no medical indications for circumcision in the neonatal period. The shaft of the penis should be straight and this can be seen most clearly if the baby has an erection. In hypospadias, the urethral meatus opens on the underside of the penis at some point below the tip (p. 211). If the baby micturates it is useful to confirm that he has a good urinary stream to exclude urinary obstruction but often the mother will be able to give a good description of it.

The scrotum varies in size and should contain both testes in the full-term infant. If they are not in the scrotum, it is important to note whether the testes are ectopic, in the inguinal canal or absent (Plate 6A). The testes normally descend from the abdomen at the eighth month of fetal life, and by 36 weeks they lie at the neck of the scrotum. In 98% of boys at term, they lie in the scrotum or can easily be manipulated there on examination. The majority of those which are not down descend within the first month, but those which do not are the true undescended testes. The degree of descent helps to determine the gestational age of pre-term infants (p. 107) and fully intra-abdominal testes will usually emerge at the appropriate gestational age. The testes are often surrounded by soft transillu-minable fluid swellings known as congenital hydroceles (Plate 6B). These need no treatment and resolve within the first few months of life.

Female infants

In the term infant, the labia majora completely cover the labia minora but they can be easily separated revealing a mucoid hymen. Occasionally, some endometrial bleeding occurs from the hormonal changes after birth, reaching its maximum between the third and fifth days and generally ceasing during the second week.

Ambiguous genitalia

Ambiguous genitalia which are neither clearly male nor clearly female are always an indicator of a serious underlying abnormality such as congenital adrenal hyperplasia or testosterone insensitivity and need urgent investigation (p. 212). They are also very worrying for the parents who naturally wish to know the sex of their child, but it is vital to avoid guessing the sex of the baby despite the parents' natural desire to know.

Spine

The spine should be inspected for evidence of a scoliosis or kyphosis, either of which may indicate malformation of the vertebrae. A dimple at the base of the spine is a common finding and is usually of no significance as long as the base is visualized and skin-covered and there is no noticeable discharge from it. A hairy patch or haemangioma over the lower lumbar region may indicate an underlying spina bifida occulta which should be investigated radiologically later in the first year.

Limbs

The arms and hands should be checked for normal shape and posture, for deformities or limitation of movement of the joints, and to confirm normal symmetrical movements. Accessory digits may be found, often at the base of the little fingers. Unless the baby has Down's syndrome,

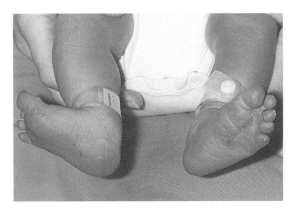

Figure 5.3   Postural right talipes calcaneovalgus.

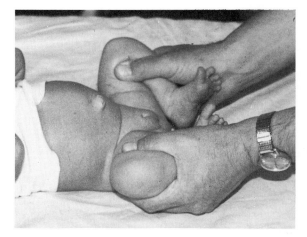

Figure 5.4   Ortolani's test for instability or dislocation of the hips.

there is no significance in the isolated finding of single transverse palmar creases.

The legs often retain the flexed fetal posture for some days after birth and often cannot be extended completely at the knee. The feet should be examined for talipes, although in many cases this is purely postural and will resolve without intervention (Fig. 5.3). If the foot cannot be easily placed in a normal position without force, talipes is confirmed and treatment will usually be needed. Overriding toes and syndactyly are common benign features needing no more treatment than reassurance to the parents.

Hips

The importance of identifying the dislocated or unstable hip cannot be overstated and it is vital for all those involved in assessing babies to become proficient in the examination techniques. This is probably the most difficult part of the neonatal examination and reliable only in experienced hands. For the examination to be successful the baby must be relaxed and this can be facilitated greatly by allowing her to suck on an empty sterile feeding teat and by ensuring that the examiner's hands are warm. Great gentleness is essential if damage to the joint or its capsule is to be avoided. If it is carried out in this way, it should cause the baby minimal discomfort. Shortening of the leg or asymmetrical skin creases on the posterior thighs are sometimes

present when there is established dislocation of one hip.

The infant is examined lying on her back with her hips flexed to a right angle and knees flexed. The examiner should first note any inequality of length of the thighs and then proceed to Ortolani's test (Fig. 5.4). The legs and thighs are grasped between the thumb and first finger while the middle finger is placed over the greater trochanter of the femur at the hip. Both hips are then gently abducted as far as they will comfortably go. If a hip is unstable it may relocate in the acetabulum with a palpable 'clunk' during the manoeuvre under the gentle pressure exerted on the trochanter from behind. Ligamentous 'clicks' are normal findings and can be ignored. In Barlow's test an attempt is made to push the head of the femur backwards out of the joint with a similar 'clunk' as the abducted hip is slowly adducted.

The range of abduction is then tested. If the baby is relaxed it should be possible gently to abduct each hip through 80–90°, i.e. to move the thigh to a position with its outer side almost flat on the table. A definite restriction of this movement usually indicates established congenital dislocation, although if it is bilateral it may be caused by adductor muscle spasm (spasticity). The management of the unstable hip is discussed on page 217.

NEUROLOGICAL EXAMINATION

A great deal of information about the neurological state of the baby can be deduced from simple observation and a discussion with the mother about her behaviour. The ability of the infant to latch on and suck at the breast, how much she cries, how well she sleeps and how readily she wakes all suggest how her brain is functioning. The maturity of the baby affects the response to the environment and handling, and progressive maturation of such activities is used in the assessment of gestational age (p. 107). Considerable experience of the newborn child is needed to evaluate the normality of her movements and reactions to stimuli. They change with development and gestational age, so what is normal at, say, 34 weeks of gestation may be quite abnormal at term – hence their value in assessing maturity.

The formal neurological examination must be interpreted in the light not only of the gestational age of the infant but also her degree of arousal, and wherever possible the assessment of an individual baby should be carried out some time after a feed with the infant in a state of quiet wakefulness. The muscle tone of the infant is best assessed by confirming that she flexes her head on arm traction from the supine position and briefly holds her head up to the horizontal on ventro-suspension (see below). Noticeable floppiness or hypertonia is abnormal and should be investigated further (p. 151). She should respond to handling without distress and be alert and suck well. She should gaze at the examiner's face at least briefly.

Normal posture, movements and general responses

When lying on her back at rest, the legs of the normal infant are semiflexed and the head turns to one side (Fig. 5.5A). If the arms and legs are extended, they should recoil readily and the elbow should not cross the midline when the arm is 'wrapped' around the neck.

When prone, the legs are even more flexed and tend to be drawn up under the abdomen

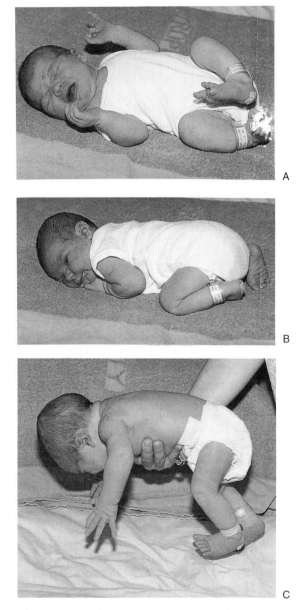

Figure 5.5 Normal posture of a newborn term infant when placed supine (A), prone (B), and in ventrosuspension (C).

(Fig. 5.5B). The arms are held flexed to the chest. If the infant is held up by a hand under the chest (ventrosuspension), the posture is semiflexed and the head is momentarily extended in line with the trunk (Fig. 5.5C).

Spontaneous movements of all four limbs occur when the baby is awake, usually alternating flexion and extension which can appear to be semi-purposeful. The degree of these movements is very variable and sometimes may be so wild as to resemble choreoathetosis, but this usually subsides after a week or two without sequelae.

Jittering movements of the limbs often accompany a general increase in the deep reflexes and should bring to mind the possibility of hypoglycaemia or hypocalcaemia. Slight jittering is very common, and in the absence of other signs of a neurological disorder it is of no serious significance.

The fingers are often fully flexed at rest but open spontaneously when feeding or when the back of the hand is stroked. The thumb is often tucked in under the fingers.

Specific responses

Certain stimuli produce consistent response patterns. Some of those that are well known, like the Moro response, are elicited regularly during routine examination of the newborn in the belief that the neurological integrity of the baby has thereby been tested. Certainly, persistence of these primitive reflexes beyond their normal time may indicate an emerging cerebral palsy, but since they depend only upon spinal reflexes they give little useful information about the future developmental progress of the infant. Some of the responses depend on the state of alertness at the time and the maturity of development.

The feeding responses are present from birth and are most easily elicited when the baby is hungry. The rooting reflex (Fig. 5.6) is the deviation of the opened mouth and turning of the head towards a touch on the cheek, seeking the nipple. Stimulation of the upper lip causes opening of the mouth, pouting of the lips and tongue movements. Latching on, sucking and swallowing are reflex responses and the whole coordinated pattern of feeding movements of the lips, tongue, palate and pharynx is developed by 32 weeks of gestation, although it becomes strong enough for adequate feeding only around 36 weeks. Failure of this complex mechanism in a hungry term infant may indicate severe neurological damage at a midbrain level, for surpris-

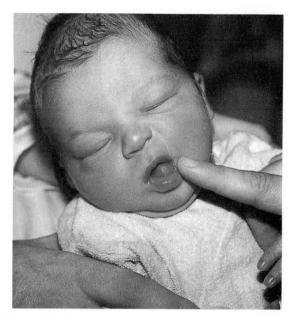

Figure 5.6   Rooting reflex.

ingly it remains intact when most of the forebrain is absent.

Cranial nerves

The cranial nerve responses are not all easy to obtain, but with patience a considerable amount of information can be gained.

Vision (II). The healthy term infant will turn her head towards a bright light, and will often fix her gaze on the observer's eyes and follow through a few degrees. Initially the baby can see clearly only to about 30 cm but this increases rapidly over the next few weeks. The pupils respond to light from 30 weeks of gestation.

Eye movements (III, IV, VI). When the head is turned to one side, the eyes tend not to move with it ('doll's eye phenomenon'). If the baby is held erect facing the observer, who then rotates himself, the eyes move in the direction of the movement, but at times the gaze may be briefly fixed. This is known as *optico-kinetic nystagmus* and shows that the baby has adequate vision, and can be used to demonstrate which ocular movements are abnormal if the baby has a squint.

Glabella tap (V, VII). A tap just above the bridge of the nose causes the baby to blink. This reflex appears at 32–34 weeks.

Bulbar reflexes (IX, X, XII). These include the gag reflex, sucking and swallowing.

Primitive reflexes

Grasp responses. The palmar and plantar grasp responses are spinal reflexes. The 'grasp', with flexion of the fingers and adduction of the thumb when the palm is touched, is developed as early as 12 weeks' gestation and is very strong in the term infant (Fig. 5.7). Similarly, the toes flex in response to stimulation of the sole.

Traction response. The traction response – the flexion of the elbows in response to pulling the baby by the hands towards the sitting position – reflects the development of flexor tone at around 37 weeks.

Asymmetric tonic neck reflex. The asymmetric tonic neck reflex is seen most prominently during the phases of development when the extensor tone is dominant, from 30 to 36 weeks of gestation and again some 4–6 weeks after term. If the head is turned to one side, the arm and leg on that side extend whilst the others remain flexed. Although this is a normal response requiring only an intact medulla and spinal cord, if it is very obvious and obligatory in a baby at term, it is an indication of abnormal extensor hypertonia. This can be due to many different forms of neurological disturbance, including metabolic disorders such as hypocalcaemia, increased intracranial pressure, cerebral birth injury or asphyxial brain damage (p. 144).

The Moro reflex. This reflex, although easy to obtain, has limited value except as a means of demonstrating a unilateral nerve lesion such as an Erb's palsy (p. 153). The body is supported in the supine position whilst the other hand supports the head. The head is suddenly allowed to drop back a little way by lowering the hand while the baby is relaxed. The reflex consists of a rapid outward flinging of the arms, opening of the hands and extension of the legs, followed by a return of both the arms and the legs to the flexed position. During the manoeuvre the baby will look startled and may cry. It may be absent in severe asphyxial brain damage or heavy sedation. The flexion component is absent in many pre-term infants.

Progression responses

Crossed extension reflex. The crossed extension reflex is obtained by stimulation of the sole of one foot which causes withdrawal of that leg and flexion of the other leg followed by strong extension and adduction.

The stepping response. The stepping response has a similar mechanism; when the baby is held in the standing position with the sole of one foot on a firm surface, the leg extends and the opposite leg makes a stepping movement, which can be continued on alternate feet. The trunk and head tend to straighten at the same time. Present by 34 weeks, these reflexes are not always easy to elicit until near term and they indicate only the presence of mature extension and flexion mechanisms.

Interpreting the neurological examination

The changes in neurological function which accompany development of the baby before term and the way in which certain reflexes seem to be appropriate for certain stages of gestation make these observations a valuable means of assessing

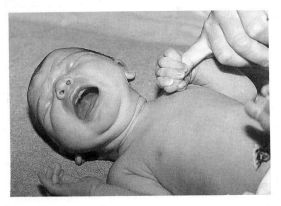

Figure 5.7   Grasp reflex.

maturity when maternal dates are uncertain (p. 106). However, predicting the future development of a child from neurological signs around the time of birth is more difficult. The neonatal reflexes do not depend on higher (cortical) brain function and therefore may be normal in the presence of quite serious cerebral damage. It is more often through a combination of predisposing features and an altered pattern of behaviour that the baby who will have lasting cerebral damage can be identified. The risk factors include low birth weight, abnormal delivery, asphyxia, congenital abnormalities such as hydrocephalus, and those infants with unusual facial features (p. 222).

The following features may be associated with significant cerebral injury and indicate that the baby should be evaluated more fully:

- persistent failure to latch on to the breast or suck
- irritability, staring or fisting (persistently clenched fists)
- a high-pitched cry
- persistent head retraction
- hypotonia or hypertonia
- lack of spontaneous activity or asymmetry of movements
- convulsions.

Any baby showing such signs should be investigated for underlying causes in a neonatal unit.

Neurological assessment at this early stage of life cannot always detect those babies who are at risk of developing a handicap later. Some who appear quite normal in the neonatal period will be brain-damaged, whereas many with clear signs of cerebral dysfunction in the first days of life, such as cerebral irritability (p. 145), will have no permanent sequelae. It is important that, in counselling the parents, unnecessary anxieties should not be generated by attributing too much significance to minor variations in neurological signs or behaviour. Moreover, there is some evidence that early developmental treatment directed by a skilled paediatric physiotherapist and implemented at home can improve the eventual outcome for their child (p. 149). This subject is also discussed in Chapter 10.

SPECIFIC SCREENING TESTS

In addition to the clinical examination of the baby, certain potentially treatable metabolic disorders can be identified in the neonatal period, long before they produce any detectable harm to the baby, by employing specific screening tests on a small sample of blood. It is theoretically possible to detect many disorders, but so far only a few tests have been shown to be sufficiently accurate, economical and beneficial to the infant to justify introduction as a universal routine procedure. The reasons for carrying out such screening procedures are:

- to detect the disorder at an early enough stage to introduce effective treatment to prevent the disease from affecting the baby's development, for instance in phenylketonuria
- to enable genetic counselling to be given to the parents at an early stage with the possibility of prenatal diagnosis in any subsequent pregnancies
- to give the parents advice on the prognosis for the condition
- to reduce the morbidity of the condition by early detection, for instance in cystic fibrosis or sickle cell disease.

Phenylketonuria

The blood test is fully established for this rare inherited biochemical disorder which, if untreated, results in the accumulation of phenylalanine in the blood; this causes progressive brain damage and severe learning difficulties which may be prevented by dietary restriction from a few weeks of age and continuing throughout childhood (p. 223). The incidence is estimated to be about 1 in 10 000 births in Britain and about half this figure in the USA. The test is made on dried blood spots taken from a heel prick onto absorbent paper on the 5th to 10th day (Fig. 5.8). A central laboratory estimates the blood level of phenylalanine, either using the bacterial inhibition method of Guthrie or by amino acid chromatography.

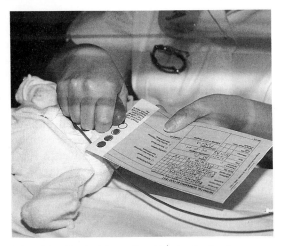

Figure 5.8 Heel prick capillary blood collection for hypothyroidism and phenylketonuria screening.

Primary congenital hypothyroidism

This condition has a fairly universal incidence of about 1 in 4000 births and, although some cases are diagnosable clinically in the first week, about a third are missed until some degree of brain damage is already established which cannot be reversed by treatment (p. 222). There is clear evidence from clinical trials that the incidence of learning difficulty from the condition is substantially reduced by early treatment of those babies identified by the screening programmes. Not all babies so identified will have permanently reduced thyroid function, and a review of thyroid function of all children with positive tests should be carried out after a year to find those who need to continue with treatment. Most authorities favour estimation of thyroid-stimulating hormone (TSH) on dried blood spots (as for phenylketonuria testing) for routine use, although it fails to detect the exceptional case of

secondary hypothyroidism (incidence about 1 in 100 000).

Cystic fibrosis

In some regions, screening is carried out for cystic fibrosis by means of estimation of immunoreactive trypsin from a dried blood spot taken from the baby at 7 days of age. Although cystic fibrosis is more common than some of the other conditions for which screening is routine, there is insufficient evidence to show that the eventual prognosis for the children with this disease is improved by early diagnosis, and although screening is carried out in Australia and some parts of the UK, it has not yet been accepted for general use.

Other conditions amenable to biochemical screening

Congenital galactosaemia, maple syrup urine disease and homocystinuria (incidences from 1 in 60 000 to 1 in 100 000 births) are now included in some screening programmes in the USA, since all these conditions are at least partially treatable by dietary restriction.

Haemoglobinopathies such as sickle cell disease and thalassaemia can be identified by haemoglobin electrophoresis on neonatal blood, and screening has been introduced in parts of the USA where a sizeable part of the population is from ethnic black groups or other predisposed races.

Many other conditions are suitable for neonatal screening programmes and may be taken up in the future as gene therapy becomes more sophisticated and able to treat a greater variety of enzyme deficiency disorders.

FURTHER READING

Clayton B, Round J 1984 Chemical pathology and the sick child. Blackwell, London
De Vries L 1992 Routine neurological examination of the newborn. Current Paediatrics 2: 183–185
Gluckman P, Heyman M 1996 Paediatrics and perinatology: the scientific basis. Arnold, London

Levene M, Liford R (eds) 1995 Fetal and neonatal neurology and neurosurgery. Churchill Livingstone, Edinburgh
Morrisey R 1990 Paediatric orthopaedics, 3rd edn. Lippincott, Philadelphia
Roberton N R C (ed) 1992 Textbook of neonatology. Churchill Livingstone, Edinburgh

6

Care of the normal infant

CARING FOR THE NEWBORN INFANT

After birth, the baby should normally be allowed to stay with the mother at her bedside so that she can get to know him, have the opportunity to enjoy his company and learn to love and care for him. She will also learn the way he behaves, how he expresses his feelings, and the significance of the sounds and cries he makes, since no two babies are the same. It also offers the mother the opportunity to express her feeling for the baby as and when she wishes and to learn how often he wants a feed or other attention. In hospital maternity departments this 'rooming-in' works well provided that the ward units are small (six beds or under), but one really fretful baby can interfere with the much needed sleep of many mothers, and therefore good nursery accommodation is still an asset.

The baby's needs in the first few days of life are to be kept warm and comfortable, to be fed and cleaned, clothed and protected, but above all to be loved, cared for, cherished and enjoyed. Both physical and emotional care are vital for the infant's future health and development, and from the start these should take precedence over any other routine procedures required by professional carers.

Good parenting involves providing the baby with his physical needs, ensuring a consistent caring relationship which avoids confusion, and understanding the baby's wants and responding promptly, appropriately and sensitively to them. It is not always an easy task and both parents may need much encouragement and support before they become confident in caring for their infant. Many parents will have experienced how to provide good care for a baby within their own families, although poor practices may be learned if their own childhood was emotionally deprived. It is therefore wise to allow most parents to develop their own ways of caring for and responding to their baby, based upon their own experience and cultural practices and influenced by the information gained from the midwife or antenatal classes during the pregnancy. By encouraging the good features, the parents' confidence in nurturing their baby can be effectively increased. The risk of 'spoiling' the infant by responding promptly to his needs is small, and both mother and baby will become more content if they are met appropriately. It should only be necessary to recommend to a mother that she changes the way she handles her baby if it is clear that her ways are detrimental to the baby's well-being.

The medical and nursing care of healthy babies consists of teaching the parents the necessary skills to enable them to prevent avoidable illness, to provide proper nutrition, to encourage appropriate developmental stimulation of the infant and to ensure that the parents' love for the child can evolve and grow. As long as this is happening satisfactorily, little intervention is needed, although it is important to respond appropriately to the parents' requests for help or advice and to provide encouragement when new parents lack confidence in caring for their new baby.

Factors which affect parenting ability

The psychological well-being of the mother before and after birth can have a profound effect on the care she can provide for the baby, and where her confidence is diminished by unhelpful or negative remarks from professional care givers or unsupportive family members, inadequate mothering can follow. The baby needs good eye contact with the parents, gentle affectionate handling, to hear the sound of the parents' voices and to be given the opportunity to see and hear what is going on around him while he is awake. If the parents are not able to provide

this stimulation, his developmental progress may be hindered. Social factors may also adversely affect the infant's progress. Poor maternal educational attainment, young maternal age, lone parenthood, the reduction in family income which often accompanies the arrival of a baby, unemployment and social isolation may also take their toll. When several of these factors are present there may be an increased risk of the infant failing to thrive or suffering delayed psychosocial development.

Not all mothers have a straightforward puerperium, some having had a medical complication of the pregnancy or an abnormal delivery, while others may develop the 'blues' or true puerperal depression or psychosis. These can seriously impair the mother's ability to care for her infant and it is vital for him that such conditions are recognized by the midwife or health visitor and the mother referred for treatment or given additional support. It is often at this time that a supportive father can make a most important contribution to the care of the baby and mother. Sometimes it is only through noting that the baby is failing to thrive, that he is less responsive than expected or that he is unsettled or miserable that the maternal condition is identified, or other adverse social factors come to light. Further enquiry into this situation with appropriate counselling and advice from the health visitor could reduce the risk of child abuse or neglect.

MAINTAINING BODY TEMPERATURE

Although the newborn infant has a temperature-regulating mechanism, it is less efficient than that of an older child and there is a much greater risk of excessive cooling or overheating. The mechanisms of heat loss and temperature regulation have been described on page 32.

The maintenance of a normal body temperature is important since prolonged hypothermia can lead to neonatal cold injury, and hyperthermia has been identified in some cases of sudden infant death syndrome (cot death). The healthy term baby has a remarkably stable temperature at 37°C and significant variations from this figure require an explanation. Both high and low temperature may indicate an infection, and appropriate examination and investigations should be carried out (p. 162). If the baby is not infected, the probable explanation is that he has either too much or too little clothing for the surrounding room temperature. Although most parents clothe their babies with an appropriate number and type of garments instinctively, a more formal assessment can be made by calculating their 'tog' values, which give a numerical figure to the insulating quality of the clothes. The higher the value the greater the heat retained. Table 6.1 gives the tog values of commonly used baby wear and bedclothing. For most infants, a value of 6–10 tog will keep them safe from hypothermia and hyperthermia in an ambient temperature of 16–20°C, although it must be remembered that in cold weather the room temperature of an unheated room may fall considerably during the night. In practice this means that, at night, an average well-nourished baby should have a vest, nappy, babygro, cardigan and two blankets (tog value, 8.2–9.2), or if the cardigan is replaced by a sleeping suit only one blanket is needed (tog value, 8.7–9.2). A very slim baby may need more, and a fatter baby fewer, clothes to keep warm. If the temperature falls significantly or the infant feels cold, additional coverings should be used. Blankets are preferred since it is easier to adjust the tog value of this type of bedding than it is when a duvet is used. On the other hand, swaddling the infant with blankets and covering the head increase the risk of overheating by preventing the baby from adjusting his own temperature through increasing heat loss from the head.

If a steady room temperature cannot be maintained it is usually possible to ensure a stable body temperature during the night by clothing the infant for the cooler rather than the warmer expected room temperature. It must be remembered, however, that cold clothes will initially take heat from the baby, so it is preferable to put on warmed garments if the room is cool. Heating the cot itself is not necessary, apart from the initial warming before the baby is placed there. For a well fed thriving infant there is probably more risk of hyperthermia from overwrapping than hypothermia from too little clothing. Midwives and health visitors now check on these features routinely.

During the first week, regular temperature recording, either by a rectal thermometer or from the axilla, ensures that a harmful drop in temperature, which can be one indication of neonatal infection, is not missed. Thermometers which read as low as 30°C are an essential part of the midwife's equipment.

Hypothermia

Neonatal cold injury has become less common in the last few years. There is a recognizable clinical picture associated with hypothermia which may remain undetected for several days unless the condition is kept in mind. Although sepsis, underfeeding or intracranial bleeding may all be associated causes, the principal factor is usually inadequate heating or clothing in the home in winter. The baby makes good initial progress but in the first week or two of life begins to show apathy, refuses some of his feeds and fails to gain weight. The cry becomes feeble and whimpering. At this time, if felt, the skin is cold to touch, although surprisingly enough the baby may not look ill and there is often a misleading redness of the face and extremities. The rectal temperature is found to be below 34°C (94°F), sometimes in the region of 30–32°C (85–90°F). Hard oedema or sometimes true sclerema (p. 120) develops and, if untreated, death ensues. Pulmonary haemorrhage is the usual terminal complication.

Table 6.1 Tog values of baby clothing and bedding

Item	Tog value
Vest	0.2
Babygro	1.0
Jumper	2.0
Cardigan	2.0
Trousers	2.0
Disposable nappy	2.0
Sleeping suit	4.0
Sheet	0.2
Old blanket	1.5
New blanket	2.0
Quilts	Variable, but approximately 9

The treatment involves rewarming the body gradually, maintaining the infant's nutrition by giving tube feeds of milk with additional glucose to counteract the associated hypoglycaemia – using a glucose intravenous infusion with hydrocortisone in severe cases – and treating any identified infection by giving an appropriate antibiotic. The warming process must be slow and is probably best done by simply keeping the infant lightly dressed in a surrounding temperature which is just a few degrees above his body temperature, and allowing the metabolic processes of the body to produce heat by metabolizing the administered glucose.

Ventilation

Fresh air is important, but obviously at home open windows are only appropriate if the room conditions and outside temperature allow it. An excessively dry atmosphere is to be avoided and, when an extra source of heating like a gas fire is used, a bowl of water placed in front helps to increase the humidity.

SLEEPING POSTURE AND PREVENTION OF COT DEATH

Recent research in Britain and several other countries has confirmed a connection between sudden infant death syndrome (cot death) and placing babies face down to sleep. In Britain the overall incidence of the condition halved after it was recommended that all infants should be placed on their backs to sleep, and this reduction has been maintained. Although the exact reasons for this are not clear it is known that hyperthermia from overheating, which has been found in some cot death victims, is more likely in the prone position, particularly if the infant has a virus infection. All infants should be placed on their side or back to sleep unless there is a clear medical reason to do otherwise, such as gastro-oesophageal reflux. There is no evidence of a serious risk of inhalation in the supine position.

Other factors which recent research has shown to be related to cot death include overheating the infant, postnatal exposure of the baby to tobacco smoke, low birth weight and poor socioeconomic circumstances.

Action which can be recommended to parents includes the following measures, although there is no complete guarantee that they will prevent sudden unexpected death:

- The baby should be placed on his back to sleep (Fig. 6.1).
- Clothing should be sufficient to prevent hypothermia but should avoid overheating the infant.
- Duvets, loose bedding and head coverings should be avoided.
- The baby should not be exposed to cigarette smoke nor share a bed with parents who smoke.
- Prompt medical advice should be sought if the baby is feverish or unwell.
- The infant should be placed with his feet near the foot of the cot and the blankets tucked in so that the head is exposed and cannot be covered if he moves during sleep (Fig. 6.1).

MINIMIZING THE RISK OF INFECTION

During the process of a vaginal birth, the infant encounters the bacterial flora of the mother's birth canal and perineum with which he becomes colonized harmlessly during the first few days of life. Unless the mother has an active infection with a pathogenic organism, she is unlikely to be the source of serious infection for the baby, since he has received her antibodies through the placenta (p. 157). The infant's main sources of infection in hospital are other members of the hospital staff, clothing, feeding utensils and, occasionally, other infants. In maternity hospitals where the babies may be cared for in large nurseries, ensuring that there is sufficient space between cots reduces the risk of cross-infection from other infants. The main practical precautions to prevent infection after birth are as follows:

- Where possible the mother should give the baby all the necessary care. Handling of the baby by health professionals should be limited to essential care, e.g. bathing, changing nappies, feeding.

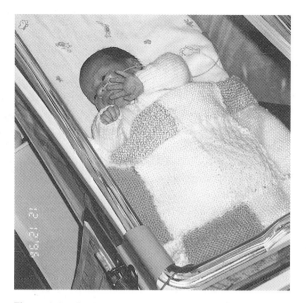

Figure 6.1 'Back to sleep and feet to foot'. Recommended sleeping posture to reduce the risk of cot death.

• Hand washing is the single most effective measure against cross-infection of infants in hospital (Fig. 6.2). Mothers should wash their hands with ordinary soap before handling their infant. All other care givers must wash their hands thoroughly with an antiseptic soap or apply a suitable antiseptic lotion before dealing with each baby.

• Umbilical cord stumps may be treated with an antibiotic application at birth or an antiseptic powder at each nappy change.

• Good facilities are essential for preparation of sterile feeds. Where bottles and teats must be re-used (e.g. special teats for an infant with a cleft palate), they should be used only by the same infant and sterilized carefully (p. 86).

• Nappies and excreta should be carefully disposed of in sealable identifiable bags.

• Cot blankets and infant clothing must be effectively sterilized in laundering. Cotton blankets are found to be greatly preferable to wool ones in this respect.

• Special attention is paid to minor infections in those who come into contact with the babies, e.g. a nurse, midwife or doctor with a bacterial skin infection, throat infection or mild gastroenteritis should be excluded temporarily.

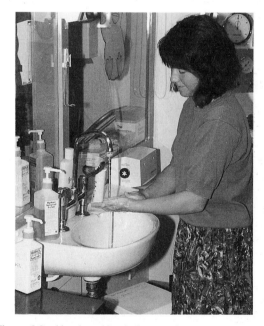

Figure 6.2 Hand washing is the most important means of preventing cross-infection in hospital.

• Wherever possible, any infected infant must be isolated from the others, preferably being cared for by the mother in a single isolation ward. If circumstances make this impossible, extra precautions against cross-infection (barrier nursing techniques with gowns) should be used whenever the baby is handled. Disposal of infected material, particularly faeces, must be carried out with great care.

• Any infant admitted from outside the hospital should be regarded as a potential source of infection and isolated until it is clear that he is not infectious.

• Healthy visitors, including the young siblings of the new baby, are rarely a source of infection, although parents should be encouraged to report minor illnesses in family members to the hospital staff so that advice can be given to deter those with significant infections from visiting (Fig. 6.3).

The use of face-masks and the routine wearing of gowns by hospital staff or the parents does not protect the infants from infection.

Cleansing

Any faecal soiling should be wiped gently from the skin as soon as possible after it occurs, particularly in the nappy area to prevent nappy rash, using cotton wool and sterile water only. Most modern paper-based disposable nappies soak up urine and prevent the skin from remaining in contact with it. However, the nappy must be changed and the skin washed approximately 4-hourly as the urea in the urine can be broken down by faecal organisms to form ammonia which may cause nappy rash.

The first full bath should be given only when feeding is well established, since before this time there is a risk of the baby becoming cold. For the term infant this may be at the end of the first week of life, whereas for the pre-term infant it may be delayed for several weeks. The use of a moisturizing baby soap will prevent the skin from becoming dry and uncomfortable especially in babies who are post-term or growth-retarded. The infant should be gently patted dry and wrapped in a warm towel to prevent heat loss. After the first week or so, bathing becomes largely a social event which should be pleasurable for both mother and baby.

The umbilical cord

Soon after the initial clamping with forceps, a sterile disposable clamp is placed on the cord 1–2 cm from the umbilical skin. The possibility of a single umbilical artery and its associated congenital malformations (p. 196) should be re-checked at

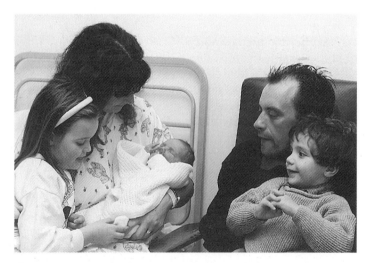

Figure 6.3 Healthy family visitors rarely cause infection in newborn babies.

this time. The cord is then cut about 1 cm beyond a clamp which is left on until the stump is dry, usually around 2 or 3 days. Separation usually occurs between 7 and 10 days of life. The stump is occasionally moist when the cord separates and it can become colonized by potentially pathogenic bacteria. Cord care practices vary, some units allowing the stump to dry naturally with no interference, some wiping with water only, others using isopropyl alcohol swabs and application of 0.3% hexachlorophane powder with each nappy change, while others recommend an antibiotic spray at birth with no other active intervention. Whichever method is chosen, it is important to inspect the cord daily and to note any periumbilical erythema or discharge so that an infection can be treated before it becomes generalized.

WEIGHING

The baby must be weighed accurately (Fig. 6.4) within a few hours of birth and thereafter on alternate days. Weighing should always be carried out immediately before a feed and at the same time of day on each occasion so that weights are comparable. All babies will lose a little weight in the first 4 days, but if this exceeds 10% of birth weight an explanation should be sought. As long as the weight begins to rise from

the fourth day, alternate daily measurements can be reduced to weekly weighing after 10 days of age. Rates of weight gain vary considerably and apparently slow gain must be interpreted carefully (p. 95).

FEEDING THE BABY

It is important at the outset to realize that feeding is not only a process designed to provide nutrition for the baby, but it also contributes to the protection of the infant from infection, fosters and develops the relationship between the baby and its parents and, in the case of breast feeding, assists in the mother's recovery from the pregnant state. Much could be written about infant feeding, but there is no intention to discuss it fully here. Only those features which are thought to be most important in the newborn period will be described, and ways of facilitating more effective feeding patterns and alleviating some of the common difficulties encountered will be discussed.

PRINCIPLES OF NEONATAL NUTRITION

At birth a baby has stores of brown fat and glycogen which are metabolized to produce heat, which in turn maintains body temperature. The

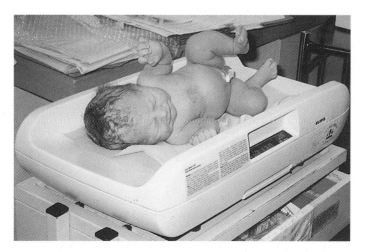

Figure 6.4 Accurate weighing of newborn babies is essential.

principal nutritional importance of the feeds given within the first few hours of life is to maintain a safe blood glucose level, whereas after the first few days the provision of sufficient calories, proteins and minerals for growth and increasing activity becomes more important. From the end of the first week, the rate of growth and weight gain of the infant are faster than at any other time, and the average term baby gains between 180 and 210 g each week. To achieve this gain, at least 1.5 g/kg per day of protein are required with sufficient calories from carbohydrate to utilize it, and approximately one-third of the total calorie intake is expended on growth. An inadequate supply of energy will, therefore, decrease weight gain, although brain growth is usually spared until intake is grossly deficient. Human milk contains appropriate amounts of all the necessary nutrients, minerals and vitamins, including fats which provide about half the baby's energy needs and the essential fatty acids, such as arachidonic and linoleic acids, which are needed for optimal brain development. These are also present in all reputable baby milk formulae as currently recommended by international bodies such as the World Health Organization. Recent research suggests that long chain polyunsaturated fatty acids are also important for optimal brain growth, particularly in the pre-term infant, although their importance in the term infant has not yet been determined.

The amount of feed required varies from one baby to another, depending on the rate of metabolism, how active he is and on the need to produce heat to keep warm. In addition, a baby whose intrauterine growth was reduced may need to make 'catch-up growth' which requires additional nutrients. These differences cannot be accurately calculated, but fortunately, except when the baby is ill or pre-term, he usually obtains the amount he needs by showing when he is hungry or satisfied.

The feed must meet all the metabolic needs of the baby without exceeding the capacity of the body to handle specific components. The kidneys have a limited ability to dispose of the urea produced by protein metabolism and an excessive intake may result in the baby becoming uraemic.

Table 6.2 Selected daily nutritional requirements of a newborn baby at 1 week of age

Nutrient	Quantity
Calories	120–140 kcal/kg
Protein	1.5–4.0 g/kg
Carbohydrate	8–15 g/kg
Sodium	2.5 mmol/kg
Calcium	0.5–1.0 mmol/kg
Phosphate	2–3 mmol/kg
Vitamin A	5000 IU
Vitamin D	400 IU

Too much lactose in the gut can cause diarrhoea. Excess vitamin D produces hypercalcaemia.

Average daily requirements of some important nutrients in the neonatal period are shown in Table 6.2.

BREAST OR BOTTLE?

When asked the question, those concerned with the care of the newborn generally express no doubt that breast feeding is the method of choice. Yet, although it is the cheapest and most convenient way of feeding, and despite having been promoted vigorously by health professionals and others, only around 63% of mothers start breast feeding in Britain, fewer than 50% successfully breast feed beyond 2 weeks and less than 25% are breast feeding at 4 months. The factors affecting the parents' decision about whether to breast or bottle feed have more to do with social and cultural attitudes, whether or not the mother encountered problems breast feeding previous babies, support from the family and whether the mother needs to work after the birth than with professional recommendations. For example, it has been shown that mothers are less likely to choose to breast feed if they already have several children, have no partner, completed their education before the age of 16 or smoked during pregnancy. Nevertheless, doctors, midwives and health visitors should discuss with parents the advantages of breast feeding, and should encourage more mothers to choose it and support those already committed to it to continue, although undue pressure on the parents to make a decision to breast feed may be counter-productive.

There is now good evidence that locally based initiatives can also increase the rates of breast feeding if midwives and medical staff are committed to them (see Box 6.4, p. 82). Mothers who are undecided know that bottle-fed babies thrive and may feel tempted to bottle feed because they can see how much the baby has taken; they also know that someone else will be able to take over if they are unable to give an occasional feed themselves, particularly at night, and these factors may sway the mind of those uncertain about which method of feeding to choose. To assist in the promotion of breast feeding, the United Nations Children's Fund (UNICEF) has suggested a number of factors which may be introduced into a hospital to make it more 'baby friendly' and to encourage more mothers to start and continue to breast feed their babies (Box 6.1).

The benefits of breast feeding are summarized in Box 6.2.

Why should breast feeding be encouraged?

The nutritional advantages of human milk are

> **Box 6.2**   The benefits of breast feeding
>
> - Provides optimum nutrition for growth and development
> - Content of the milk adapts to baby's changing needs
> - Protects the baby against some infections
> - Promotes a good relationship between mother and baby
> - Reduces risk of later childhood eczema and diabetes
> - Assists the mother to lose weight
> - Reduces the risk of some breast and ovarian cancers in the mother

---

numerous. It has a varying composition which alters over the days and weeks to provide for the changing needs of the growing baby. Initially, the energy content of the milk provides around 115 cal/kg per day, falling to 100 cal/kg per day after about 3 months. The proteins, initially consisting predominantly of lactalbumin with little casein, are readily digested and absorbed. The relative amounts change, and as breastfeeding continues the proportion of casein increases. Breast milk contains the correct amounts and ratios of certain lipids, including long chain polyunsaturated fatty acids which are essential for optimal development of the brain and retina. Other individual components of breast milk, including iron, are in a form well suited to the healthy full-term baby's requirements so that deficiency states rarely emerge. The low concentration of sodium prevents the development of hypernatraemia which can cause brain damage. Neonatal convulsions from hypocalcaemia and hypomagnesaemia are prevented by the low phosphate content of breast milk (p. 150).

Colostrum and breast milk contain numerous factors, including secretory IgA immunoglobulin, lysozymes, lactoferrin, and white cells which have a considerable protective effect against gastroenteritis and infections of the middle ear, respiratory tract and urinary tract, which is particularly important in babies in developing countries. The high lactose content, by producing a relatively acid pH in the large intestine, favours the growth of lactobacilli and inhibits that of potentially harmful *Escherichia coli*, and the

---

> **Box 6.1**   UNICEF-designated 'baby friendly' initiative: 10 steps to successful breast feeding
>
> Every facility providing maternity services and care for newborn babies should:
>
> - Have a written breast feeding policy which is routinely communicated to all health staff
> - Train all health staff in skills to implement this policy
> - Inform all pregnant women about the benefits and management of breast feeding
> - Help mothers initiate breast feeding within half an hour of birth
> - Show mothers how to breast feed, and how to maintain lactation even if they are separated from their infant
> - Give newborn infants no food or drink other than breast milk, unless medically indicated
> - Practise rooming-in 24 hours a day
> - Encourage breast feeding on demand
> - Give no artificial teats or pacifiers (dummies) to breast feeding infants
> - Foster the establishment of breast feeding support groups and refer mothers to them on discharge from the hospital

oligosaccharides, which form about 15% of the carbohydrate in mature breast milk, also inhibit bacterial growth. The stools are inoffensive and constipation is rarely a problem. Other factors such as hormones, growth factors and certain enzymes are also present although their precise function is as yet unknown.

Breast feeding, exclusively and from the start, reduces substantially the risk of introducing the allergens of cow's milk protein which, if taken in the first few weeks of life, can be a contributory cause of later atopic disease such as eczema. Thus it is especially important to encourage breast feeding in cases where there is a strong family history of allergic disease. In pre-term infants it is associated with better neurodevelopmental outcome and it reduces the risk of necrotizing enterocolitis (p. 136). The incidence of insulin-dependent diabetes mellitus in later childhood is lower if the infant has been breast fed.

Breast feeding also has psychosocial advantages. Not only is the milk readily available whenever the baby requires it, but the mother is likely to lose any excess weight gain more readily. However, perhaps the main value of breast feeding lies in the act itself, for when it goes well there is often an emotional satisfaction to the mother which is reflected in the reactions of the baby and can strengthen the strong attachment between the two (Fig. 6.5). Although bottle feeding by no means precludes this, the closer contact of breast feeding often provides an easier way of fostering the normal stable relationship.

The disadvantages are few. Haemorrhagic disease of the newborn due to vitamin K deficiency occurs mainly in breast-fed babies, but can be prevented by giving a supplement of the vitamin at birth (p. 179). Extra vitamin D may be required to prevent the possible onset of rickets after 6 months of age and it is probably wise to supplement those infants from dark-skinned ethnic groups and those living in cities in temperate lands. In a small proportion of infants, physiological jaundice is prolonged by breast feeding, but the condition is usually benign and seldom requires treatment other than reassurance (p. 188).

There is much ignorance about breast feeding

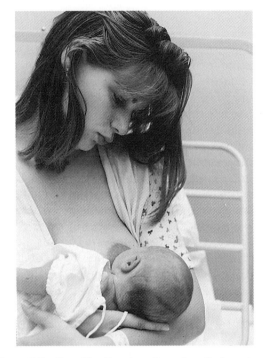

Figure 6.5 Breast feeding strengthens the attachment between mother and baby.

from which the nursing and medical professions are not exempt, although increasing research is beginning to provide a much greater understanding of it. Misconceptions concerning the effect on the mother's health and appearance, and the almost universal view of the breast as a sex symbol in Western culture, will only change gradually through altering cultural attitudes and with help from health education at home, in schools and in the media, and the recognition of a need to provide places in public buildings which enable mothers to feed their infants in a suitably discreet environment.

Reasons for not breast feeding

The size of the breast has no bearing on its potential for producing milk, although structural abnormalities such as non-protractile nipples may make breast feeding more difficult. Cosmetic breast surgery is usually compatible with successful breast feeding unless the nipple has been repositioned. Maternal ill health or some defect in the infant may account for a few failures. Some mothers have clear social reasons for choosing artificial feeding – for instance the return to a job. A few give up because they find breast feeding distasteful or painful. The majority do so because they are faced with a discontented baby in the third or fourth week resulting from an insufficient supply of milk which may be only temporary. If the mother feels that her baby is being starved, she may be ready to accept a suggestion that a change to the bottle would be wise. There are several possible causes for this reduction of milk secretion and, although prolonged engorgement of the breasts during the first week predisposes to it, improving the feeding technique or allowing more frequent suckling often improves the supply (p. 81). The worry of managing the home as well as the new baby also contributes.

The contraindications to breast feeding are few. Milk secretion adds a considerable load to the metabolic activity and for this reason any severe chronic maternal illness may be a contraindication; cardiac disease, chronic nephritis with hypertension and chronic respiratory infection are examples. Most acute infective maternal illnesses require only brief separation from the infant whilst breast milk production is maintained by expression.

Most drugs taken by the mother are secreted in the milk, but fortunately the concentration is often small and may not affect the baby adversely. It is advisable, however, to avoid breast feeding when the mother has to be on treatment with any of the drugs listed in Table 6.3 in full dosage. The list is not exhaustive and for further information the current edition of the British National Formulary (BNF) should be consulted. Some of the by-products of cigarette smoking, e.g. cotinine, are found in breast milk and may increase the risk of respiratory problems in the infant.

Although it is not an absolute contraindication, current recommendations suggest that mothers who are infected with HIV or who have AIDS should not normally breast feed, to reduce further the small risk of infecting the infant through the milk (p. 172). Hepatitis B carriers

Table 6.3 Maternal drugs and breast feeding; the baby should not breast feed if the mother is taking these drugs

Non-steroidal anti-inflammatory drugs	Indomethacin
	Phenylbutazone
Anticoagulants	Phenindione
	Dicoumarol
Anticonvulsants	Carbamazepine
	Primidone
Antithyroid drugs	Carbimazole
	Thiouracil
Antibiotics	Chloramphenicol
	Metronidazole
	Novobiocin
	Tetracyclines
	Trimethoprim
Cortisone	
Cytotoxic agents	Cyclophosphamide
Ergotamine	
Hypotensive agents	Propranolol
	Reserpine
Lithium	
Radioactive isotopes	Radio-iodine
Sedatives	Chloral hydrate
	Diazepam
	Phenothiazines
Tolbutamide	
Vitamins	A and D in high dose
Drugs of addiction	Heroin
	Methadone
	Cannabis

with the e antigen in the blood can transmit the infection to the infant through their milk and should not breast feed.

Pre-term birth or severe neonatal disease and some congenital abnormalities (e.g. cleft lip and palate) may render breast feeding impossible initially, although a mother who is very keen to breast feed can keep her milk flowing either by hand expression or by the use of a breast pump until the baby is able to feed from her, and in the meantime the milk is given to the baby by another means. Social contraindications can only be judged individually, but it must be recognized that there are mothers who feel such an antipathy to the idea of breast feeding that forcing the issue may only do harm. Finally, inadequate breast milk secretion may be a good reason for a change to artificial feeds, especially where an attempt at improving the feeding technique (p. 81) fails to increase the infant's weight gain after a reasonable trial period.

ANTENATAL EDUCATION FOR INFANT FEEDING

Infant feeding should be discussed in the antenatal period with the parents in 'education for parenthood' classes and in the antenatal clinic, and excellent visual aids are now available to assist in this task. It is important that the advantages and disadvantages of breast and formula of feeding are explained, so that the mother and her partner can make an educated decision about how to feed the infant if they are undecided. It should be explained to the parents that the first few weeks of caring for the new infant will be exacting and that some mothers do not find breast feeding easy and satisfying initially. Many mothers give up breast feeding early because they fear that the baby is not thriving on it (p. 82), and the attitude of mind in which discussion of feeding is approached by both the mother and the midwife has an important influence on its success. If the young mother realizes that breast feeding is not always straightforward, but learns that those who look after her understand these difficulties and can give continuing consistent guidance and practical help, she is the more likely to want to carry it through.

Nutrition

The extra intake of food in pregnancy, which is necessary for the developing fetus, should continue during lactation. The fatty acid pattern of the milk and its content of many vitamins and minerals is adversely affected if the maternal diet is deficient. In addition to her own normal diet, she should take an extra 15 g of protein per day and additional carbohydrate, calcium, vitamins and water. This can be supplied by at least one pint of milk a day together with a good mixed diet containing meat, fish or cheese and fresh fruit and vegetables. Extra vitamin A, C and D and folic acid should be added, and she should be encouraged to take fluids liberally.

Preparation of the breasts

The breasts should be examined before the sixth month of pregnancy with a view to evaluating certain minor variations from normal. The normal nipple protrudes when the breast is pinched between finger and thumb at the junction of areola with skin (the protractile nipple), but when there is anchoring to underlying structures the protrusion fails to occur. For these and the more obviously inverted nipples, the wearing of plastic nipple shields from the sixth month is advocated by some, although there is little evidence yet that they are effective. Some improvement occurs naturally as the pregnancy progresses and this problem is less likely in older mothers and those who have breast fed previous infants. Since the nipple plays little part in the release of milk from the ducts, successful breast feeding can often be achieved despite these anomalies.

The breasts should be washed carefully daily, although frequent use of soap on the nipple reduces the natural protective lubrication and should be avoided. The application of creams to toughen up the nipple and the routine antenatal expression of colostrum neither reduce the incidence of subsequent nipple soreness nor improve subsequent lactation and are unnecessary. Careful positioning of the infant on the breast seems more important than any antenatal preparation in increasing the success of breast feeding and reducing nipple problems and breast engorgement.

FEEDING IN THE IMMEDIATE POSTNATAL PERIOD

It is now common practice to put the baby to the breast within a few minutes of birth. There is good evidence that this both influences the success and duration of breast feeding and provides an early opportunity for the relationship between the mother and infant to develop. There is only a small nutritional content in the colostrum obtained, but even a few moments of suckling will provide the infant with a valuable amount of the substances which give some protection against infection (p. 158). Even if the baby does not suckle immediately after birth, feeding should begin at some time within the first 4 hours and for a healthy term infant the first feed should be at the breast. In some cultures there is an erroneous belief that the colostrum is not good for the infant, which may be a barrier to early breast feeding. The first feed should be supervised by a midwife skilled in the techniques of breast feeding to ensure that both mother and baby are comfortable, that the infant fixes correctly on the nipple, that the baby sucks well and that his colour remains healthy and pink throughout the feed. Correct positioning of the infant at the breast will help to prevent nipple damage and ensure that breast feeding is maintained. Subsequently the infant should be allowed to determine the frequency of feeds and, as long as a correct feeding technique is used, the suckling time should not be limited. One additional benefit of unrestricted suckling is that more bilirubin is excreted in the increased number of stools passed, which may reduce the severity of jaundice in the infant.

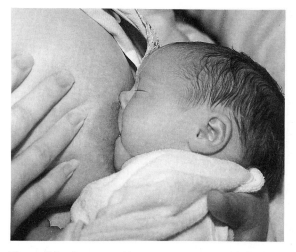

Figure 6.6 Correct positioning of the baby on the nipple prevents sore nipples and maximizes the effectiveness of breast feeding.

FURTHER MANAGEMENT OF BREAST FEEDING

Successful breast feeding depends upon the secretion of two maternal pituitary hormones: prolactin from the anterior pituitary gland acts upon the glandular tissue of the breast to promote milk production; and oxytocin from the posterior pituitary gland stimulates the ejection of milk from the breast during feeding. Oxytocin is released in response to the sucking of the baby at the breast but secretion may be inhibited by stress, anxiety and other emotional factors. Breast feeding should therefore take place in a relaxed atmosphere and the mother should be positively encouraged throughout feeding. This should promote adequate oxytocin secretion during suckling, a phenomenon known as the let-down reflex. This enables the milk in the alveoli of the breasts to be pushed forward through the duct system to the place where the mechanical rolling action of the baby's tongue can remove the milk from the breast.

For successful breast feeding the mother should be comfortable and the baby physically well supported. Either lying or sitting, she should support the baby's back and buttocks in the crook of her arm, allowing the nipple to touch

the cheek, thus stimulating the rooting reflex (p. 65). Correct attachment may be achieved by keeping the infant's lower jaw as low on the areola as possible so that the maximum amount of the nipple is taken into the mouth (Fig. 6.6). It may also be assisted by holding the breast underneath or behind the areola to aid protrusion of the nipple, but the mother should not push the nipple towards the baby.

Making breast feeding effective

The rigid code of 'schedules' with exact timing of feeds which seemed to be so important in the past has been abandoned in favour of an attitude that allows the baby to have more choice. This has happened largely because certain facts have been realized which, though not newly discovered, were apparently ignored. The quantity and constituents of breast milk taken at one feed are not the same as those of the next feed, but if the amount taken by the baby in the whole 24 hours is compared with that taken in the next 24 hours the difference is small. Individual babies differ in the amount they can take at one time, so that some need as many as eight or more feeds a day at first to keep them happy, although they usually change naturally to longer intervals within a week or two. Feeding a baby at relatively short intervals early in his life and giving one or more night feeds does not get him into bad habits. Moreover, unrestricted breast feeding is likely to increase the duration of successful breast feeding and to reduce the amount of nipple trauma and breast engorgement. Although 150 ml of milk per kg body weight per day (2.5 oz/lb) gives a rough guide to average requirements, it is not necessarily the right amount for every baby at every age. Some babies require more than this in the early months and less later on.

Making breast feeding more effective

Healthy full-term infants should be fed on demand and at least one breast should be emptied at every feed (Box 6.3). This may mean that a baby feeds from only one breast at each feed and this is adequate as long as he remains healthy, seems satisfied after the feed and is seen to be gaining weight. If the breast is not emptied, the infant will not obtain the hind-milk from the back of the breast which is higher in calories than the foremilk and may therefore not gain weight optimally. Also, stasis of milk in the breast may lead to engorgement and eventual infection. Babies will take different times to remove the available milk and therefore the length of the feed should not be rigidly timed. It had previously been thought that the duration of sucking would adversely affect the condition of the nipple, but if the baby is properly fixed the nipple should not be damaged. The length of time the baby is fixed on the breast should be determined by the infant and allowing this should ensure that he takes an adequate amount of milk, including the hind-milk with its high fat and calorie content.

It is imperative that those who give professional advice to a mother about breast feeding should avoid laying down dogmatic rules and regulations, but rather they should have a deep understanding of the principles underlying successful breast feeding so that they can provide personal support and give consistent advice based on sound knowledge (Box 6.3). In this way she can be helped to breast feed more effectively and be encouraged to continue it longer for the benefit of both the infant and herself.

It is often the practice to give some supplementary fluid by bottle at this time, especially at night. There is no objection to the use of small amounts of 5% dextrose or water for this purpose when the baby is obviously thirsty, but its routine use is neither necessary nor conducive to effective breast feeding. Supplementary and complementary feeds of formula milk have been shown not to be beneficial to full-term healthy infants and should be discouraged. Supplementary feeds may interfere with lactation and have the ability to change the bacterial flora of the gut and potentially encourage the growth of pathogenic bacteria.

Box 6.3 Effective breast feeding

Breast feeding can be made more effective by:

- Consistent advice from professionals
- Advice based upon sound knowledge
- Personal support for the mother
- Unrestricted breast feeding on demand
- Correct positioning of the baby at the breast
- Correct fixing on the nipple
- Fully emptying at least one breast at each feed
- Avoidance of formula feed supplementation
- Avoiding routine supplements of water
- Supplementation by cup feeding

Box 6.4 Initiatives which have improved breast feeding rates

- Breast feeding training for medical staff
- Introducing cup feeding for babies not able to go to the breast
- Information booklets for the mother
- Breast feeding counsellors on postnatal wards
- Introducing the baby friendly initiative
- Encouraging fathers to accept breast feeding
- Producing guidelines for postnatal wards
- Providing rooms for breast feeding
- Promoting study days on breast feeding
- Helplines accessible by mothers
- Encouraging mothers to attend breast feeding support groups

Care of the breasts

The breasts, if heavy, may need support during the process of a feed and therefore a nursing brassiere which supports the breast while the cup is open should be encouraged. Otherwise a nursing brassiere which opens at the front, giving adequate support without pressing on the nipple, should be worn. Breast pads may be used within the brassiere to absorb leakage of milk and protect clothing but they should be changed frequently to prevent the nipple from being constantly wet. Nipples and breasts should be washed daily as advised in the antenatal period. The use of soap and alcohol have been shown to increase nipple soreness and should be avoided. There are many protective creams and sprays available commercially but there is little firm evidence to show that their continued use prevents nipple damage or promotes healing if it occurs.

Breast engorgement and mastitis

The breasts are subject to two types of engorgement – 'vascular' and 'milk' – although there may be an overlap between them. Vascular engorgement occurs 2–4 days after delivery and is due to the increased blood flow to the breasts which normally occurs at this time. Milk engorgement occurs as a result of the increased milk production accompanied by only limited removal of the milk by the baby. If this continues, overdistension of the alveoli will lead to eventual suppression of milk production and may even cause rupture of the alveoli and the symptoms of non-infective mastitis. It results in a painful lump covered by a red flush with fever and reduction of secretion, but may often be dramatically cured within a few hours by emptying the breast from which no pus, but only milk, flows. If this is not done, however, staphylococcal infection may supervene and a true breast abscess develop. Treatment consists of early and repeated emptying of the breast, but if after 48 hours there is no improvement an antibiotic may be necessary.

Milk engorgement rarely occurs if the mother is encouraged to feed her baby on demand day and night and if the baby is properly fixed and is removing the milk adequately. It may occur when the baby becomes ill and is separated from the mother. In these circumstances, the mother should continue to remove milk for the baby's use either manually or through the use of a breast pump.

Infective mastitis may also result from organisms infecting a break in the skin, especially if the mother is in a debilitated condition due to anaemia or malnutrition. It is treated with antibiotics but is not an indication to discontinue breast feeding.

Cracked nipples may follow engorgement or prolonged vigorous sucking at a stage when secretion is not established. Non-protractile nipples (p. 80) are more likely to become cracked because they are not drawn properly into the baby's mouth and may be subject to more trauma. The use of a latex nipple shield is often successful in promoting healing but it may be unacceptable to the mother and may reduce the milk flow. Other treatments include resting the affected breast with expression of the milk or repositioning the infant at the breast for the feeds. In either case, breast feeding can usually be maintained and the use of bottle feeding in this phase should be avoided if at all possible, since the technique of feeding from a bottle is quite different from that required to take milk from the breast.

Cup feeding

This technique is an alternative to both bottle and tube feeding in breast-fed infants, particularly in some pre-term infants, if supplementary feeds are required or when breast feeding must be interrupted.

The baby should be wrapped securely and a bib placed under his chin. He should be awake and alert if possible and held upright on the mother's lap with her hands supporting the baby's back and neck. The cup should be half full and the rim gently placed against the baby's upper lip, leaving the lower lip and jaw to move freely. It is then tipped until the milk just touches the upper lip, but is not poured into the mouth (Fig. 8.3, p. 115). The baby is allowed to suck the milk from the cup at his own pace until he is satisfied.

The advantages of the method are that it encourages good eye contact with the baby, avoids the confusion between the techniques of sucking at the nipple and a teat, and others can do it if the mother needs a rest. It also stimulates jaw movements and maximizes the calorie intake.

FEEDING DIFFICULTIES

Underfeeding

Underfeeding is common and shows itself as excessive crying, poor weight gain, small stools and sometimes vomiting. The most common reason for this is that the feeding technique is not allowing the infant to take the feed adequately. Test feeding, even by weighing the infant before and after a feed with accurate electronic baby scales, has been shown to be an unreliable means of estimating the amount of feed the infant is taking and cannot be recommended. One important reason for this is the variation of volumes taken at different feeds at different times of the day. If underfeeding is suspected, the position of the infant at the breast should be modified as the first step, but if no increase in weight occurs with improving breast feeding technique after 2–3 weeks, complementary feeds may be given from a cup after each breast feed, stopping when the infant appears satisfied.

Overfeeding

Some hold the view that overfeeding from the breast never occurs. It is certainly uncommon and is never a cause of really serious trouble, but in the neonatal period babies do sometimes become fretful, pass large frequent stools producing sore buttocks, and vomit small amounts after each feed, all of which cease when a small amount of milk is expressed from the breast before feeding is started. It should be remembered that about 80% of the feed is taken within the first 3 minutes of a breast feed and reducing the available milk may also reduce the speed with which it is taken yet stimulate the breast adequately to produce enough milk for the next feed.

Problems related to sucking

An inability to suck may be caused by abnormalities in the infant such as cleft lip and cleft palate or underdevelopment of the lower jaw (micrognathia). Partial nasal obstruction can be a cause and is most commonly due to a temporary excessive secretion of mucus which may be reduced by using one drop of 0.25% ephedrine in normal saline to each nostril before feeds for 2–3 days only. Obstruction of breathing from compression of the nose by the breast during feeding is avoided if the mother holds the breast away from the baby's face with her hand. In the absence of such a mechanical difficulty, more general causes must be sought, including the presence of infection somewhere (p. 161).

Occasionally the unwillingness to suck may simply be due to tiredness from repeated fruitless attempts when the milk supply is inadequate or the baby too small to grasp the breast successfully. If alterations in feeding technique fail to improve matters, it is justifiable to feed the infant by either cup or bottle for a day or two, whilst maintaining breast milk production by expression, so that the baby may become strong enough to resume breast feeding.

Occasionally breast feeding is not successful despite every attempt to support it, or the mother may have other reasons for discontinuing it. In these circumstances she may need considerable reassurance that she has not personally failed the baby, and the benefits of changing to artificial feeding should be described.

ARTIFICIAL FEEDING BY THE BOTTLE

If the mother has decided not to breast feed her infant, or if it is medically recommended that she should not do so (p. 79), her lactation can, if necessary, be suppressed. Firm binding of the breasts using a firm brassiere together with the use of a mild analgesic is often all that is required and little discomfort ensues. Where this is not enough for control of the milk flow, administration of the prolactin suppressants cabergoline or bromocriptine is usually effective.

Alternatives to breast feeding

The majority of artificial baby feeds are based on cow's milk. Some specialized milks designed for people who wish their baby to have vegetarian feeds, for either religious or moral reasons, are available but they should only be used under the guidance of a dietitian. Certain medical conditions, such as cow's milk protein allergy, lactose intolerance, phenylketonuria and galactosaemia, require treatment with highly specialized dietetic products and the specific exclusion of cow's milk formula. These are not discussed further as they require careful medical and dietetic management and are beyond the scope of this book.

Cow's milk formulae

Most artificial infant feeds are derived from cow's milk, which in its natural state has numerous nutritional disadvantages compared with human milk (Table 6.4) and is not suitable for any baby until after the sixth month of life. The casein portion of the protein is relatively high and there is less lactalbumin which renders digestion somewhat more difficult; the high protein content produces more urea during its metabolism than the neonatal kidney can excrete effectively. The sugar (lactose) content is less and the mineral salts (particularly sodium chloride and phosphate) are present in much greater concentration, with the consequent risk of hypernatraemia and neonatal hypocalcaemic tetany, respectively. This has led to the substantial modification of cow's milk by manufacturers so that it resembles more closely the composition of human milk and is suitable for babies in their first few months. Modifications required by such bodies as the European Community Council, the World Health Organization and the Department of Health in Britain include changes in the amount, and in some cases the type, of proteins, fats, carbohydrates, minerals and vitamins (Table 6.4). It must be remembered, however, that even such greatly modified milk formulae have only a nutritional similarity to breast milk and cannot provide the immunological advantages, the psychological benefits or the value to the mother of breast feeding.

In the modified formulae, total protein levels are reduced since the kidneys of the newborn infant are not able to handle large solute loads, and in some milks (often referred to as whey-based milks) the proportion of the more digestible lactalbumin is increased and casein decreased. In

Table 6.4 Comparison of human milk and cow's milk, modified cow's milk formulae and pre-term formulae

Component	Human milk	Cow's milk	EEC and WHO recommendations[a]	Pre-term formulae	Pre-term follow-on formula
Energy (kcal)	69	66	65–69	80	72
Protein (g/100 ml)	1.0	3.3	1.5–1.9[b]	2.0–2.2	1.85
Fat (g/100 ml)	4.2	3.7	2.5–3.8[c]	4.0–4.9[e]	4.0
Carbohydrate (g/100 ml)	7.4	4.8	6.9–8.60[d]	7.0–8.5	7.3
Vitamin A (μg/100 ml)	53–60	27	40–150	60–100	100
Vitamin D (μg/100 ml)	0.01	0.1	0.7–1.3	1.2–2.4	1.3
Sodium (mg/100 ml)	15	75	15–35	30–42	22
Calcium (mg/100 ml)	35	137	30–120	70–108	70
Phosphate (mg/100 ml)	15	91	15–60	35–54	35
Iron (μg/100 ml)	0.01	0.1	0.7–1.3	1.2–2.4	0.65

[a] All reputable commercial baby milk formulae in the UK conform to these international standards.
[b] In some milks the curd:whey ratio is made similar to human milk.
[c] Some milks have only butterfat; most have added vegetable oil.
[d] Some milks have lactose and maltodextrin mixtures, others only lactose.
[e] Pre-term formulae contain long chain polyunsaturated fatty acids but their origins differ and they may vary in effectiveness.

others (sometimes called casein-based milks), the total protein content is reduced, although the ratio of casein to lactalbumin is nearer that found in cow's milk. Because of the slightly increased renal solute load from these latter milks, it is usually recommended that they are introduced at around 6 weeks of age. Fat is reduced and in most milks some polyunsaturated vegetable oils are added. Lactose or maltodextrins (derived from hydrolysis of starch) are added to approximate to human milk and to ensure adequate immediate energy for cerebral metabolism and growth. The phosphate concentration is reduced to decrease the risk of hypocalcaemia (p. 150) and the sodium level is lowered to prevent hypernatraemia. Although most babies can maintain normal serum sodium levels on these low-salt milks, the pre-term baby may lose excessive amounts because of immaturity of renal sodium handling mechanisms.

All the common baby milks suitable for home use are supplied in dried powder form to facilitate storage and transport without risk of deterioration. Manufacturers also supply these preparations sterilized and ready to give to the baby in disposable bottles to which disposable or re-sterilizable teats may be fitted. Although more expensive, they are eminently suitable for use in maternity units because of their safety, without the need for costly milk sterilizing equipment and the trained staff to use it. The specialized milks designed for the pre-term infant are described on page 116.

Preparing the feeds

Great care is needed in preparing the feeds to ensure that the equipment and milk are not contaminated by potentially pathogenic bacteria and that the milk is made up to the correct concentration as detailed on the container. Before handling any utensils or making up the feed the hands must be washed thoroughly. The bottles, teats and other utensils can be sterilized by immersion in boiling water for 10 minutes or more simply by placing them in a solution of a commercial sterilizing agent. There are many such preparations available which are added to a specified quantity of water. They take several forms – tablets, crystals and solutions – which should be made up exactly according to the manufacturer's instructions. Most of these will sterilize the equipment within 30–60 minutes. Dishwashers and microwave ovens do not achieve adequate sterilization of baby feeding equipment, but suitable specialized steamers are available for use with microwaves. Plastic liners in baby bottles cannot be adequately sterilized and should be used only once and then discarded.

The milks are reconstituted by adding scoops of powder to cooling boiled water in the feeding bottle which is then sealed and shaken to ensure the milk is mixed. Usually one levelled scoop is added to 30 ml (1 oz) of water, but the directions on the tin or packet must be followed exactly since the concentration of the feed will vary considerably if, for instance, the powder is packed into the scoop, heaped scoops are used, the water is added to the powder or the wrong number of scoops are added to the water. Such mistakes are commonly responsible for under- or overnutrition in the first few weeks of life. So long as the stored powder is quite dry, the milk itself is adequately sterilized by the use of boiling water in the reconstitution process and a full day's requirement may be made up at one time. To ensure that bacterial contamination does not occur, the extra bottles must be stored in a refrigerator at or below 4°C and any left over after 24 hours should be discarded.

The water used for making up the feeds should be fresh and drawn from a rising main, boiled and allowed to cool. Reboiling water increases its mineral content and its use may result in unacceptably high levels in the reconstituted milk. Water from softening equipment has a high salt content and should not be used, since babies are not able to excrete salt adequately and they may become seriously hypernatraemic. Both fixed and portable water filters can become contaminated with pathogenic bacteria, some of which produce toxins which are not destroyed by boiling, and water treated in this way is not recommended. Some bottled water has a low enough solute content to be safe, and it is suitable if it contains less than 35 mg/L of sodium,

20 mg/L of potassium and below 0.05 mg/L of both lead and nitrates. Carbonated water should not be used.

Giving the feeds

Warming of the bottled feed in a water bath has been common practice for many years, but it has been shown not to be essential and many people just prefer to bring it to room temperature if it has been in a refrigerator. Feeds should not be warmed in a microwave oven as they may continue to heat and produce a 'hot spot' in the milk. Once a feed has been rewarmed, any remaining milk after the baby has completed the feed should be discarded, since it may become contaminated by pathogenic bacteria during the feed.

It is important for both mother and baby that feeding times should be both relaxed, unhurried and deliberate – a time during which they can get to know each other (p. 69). The baby is held comfortably, either cradled in the mother's (or father's) arm allowing no more than 15 inches between their faces, so that the parent's face is within the infant's range of clear vision (p. 65) (Fig. 6.7), or sitting on her lap with her hand supporting the back and head. The baby's arms should be free and the infant should be in a flexed posture with the head supported. Before the bottle is offered to the infant the rate of milk flow through the teat should be tested. With the bottle inverted the milk should flow in a rapid succession of drops. The teat hole size can be enlarged by a heated needle if necessary to achieve this. The bottle should then be gently inserted into the mouth, ensuring that the teat passes above the tongue, and should be held at such an angle that the teat remains full of milk until the end of the feed to avoid swallowing of air. It is then held still to encourage the baby to work for the feed.

Sometimes a baby's lips have a weak grip on the teat which can be improved by gentle support under the chin. If the milk flows too slowly the teat hole size can be enlarged as described. An average time for a feed is 15–20 minutes and anything slower than this may mean that some modification of technique is required. The infant

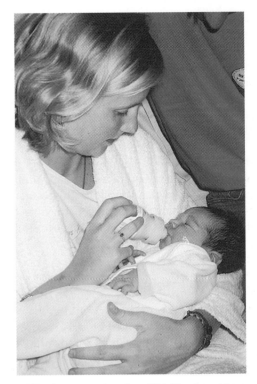

Figure 6.7   Correct posture for artificial feeding of the newborn infant.

should be winded halfway through the feed, or more often if he is feeding rapidly.

The amount and frequency of feeds

As with breast feeding, individual babies differ greatly in the volume and frequency of feeds that they seem to need to satisfy their appetite and to ensure growth at a normal rate. The amount taken at one feed may also vary throughout the day. Feeding on demand is not quite as easy to carry out successfully from the bottle as it is from the breast, and some planning as to how much and how often is necessary for practical purposes.

An average term baby takes about 60 ml/kg body weight on the first day, divided into four or five feeds. This amount gradually increases to 150–180 ml/kg per 24 hours, divided into six or seven feeds by the end of the first week, although the number of days taken to reach this varies considerably from baby to baby. This means offering 30–45 ml per feed to a newborn baby of an average birth weight, and by the end of the first week he will be taking about 75–90 ml at each feed.

Low birth weight babies require more food in relation to body weight to keep them thriving, particularly if they have suffered intrauterine growth retardation; this is discussed in more detail in Chapter 7.

Not all formula milks suit every baby and constipation is a common problem. This can sometimes be remedied by giving extra drinks of water, but if this is not effective medical advice should be sought.

Cow's milk intolerance

This problem can present as vomiting, diarrhoea or a skin rash but it is not commonly seen within the first week or two of life. Some milks have been produced using soya protein instead of cow's milk protein to prevent exposure of potentially allergic babies to bovine antigens, although there is also a similar risk of the baby developing antibodies to the soya protein. The milks are not recommended for the newborn baby in the first month of life as their high aluminium and low calcium content make tham unsuitable for routine use. They are, however, valuable for use under medical supervision in those babies who prove to have true cow's milk sensitivity.

COMMON PROBLEMS RELATED TO FEEDING

Wind, posseting and vomiting

The normal infant swallows a variable amount of air when feeding which is normally easily expelled by sitting the infant upright or holding him over the shoulder after a feed. It is not usually necessary to pat the infant's back to achieve this although some infants gain comfort from having the back gently rubbed. A teaspoonful or two of milk is often regurgitated within the first 10 minutes after a feed (posseting) and occasional larger vomits without serious cause are not uncommon

in healthy infants in the first 2 weeks. If swallowed during the process of birth, amniotic fluid and mucus can irritate the stomach and a simple stomach washout using a nasogastric tube and warmed normal saline will usually cure the problem.

Repeated small vomits, especially when they occur shortly after feeds, are often caused by gastro-oesophageal reflux which is particularly common in pre-term infants (p. 119). Rarely does this cause pain in the first weeks of life, but if the baby is failing to thrive from loss of calories in the vomit or if he has aspirated the milk into the lungs, treatment may be necessary. Food thickeners or antacids may help, but if they do not, cisapride, a drug which increases the tone of the lower oesophageal sphincter, is often useful. Occasionally reflux is associated with a hiatus hernia (p. 199). Feeding mismanagement is also a common cause. This can include underfeeding, mechanical problems with the breast such as engorgement, or an inappropriate hole size in the teat in bottle-fed infants.

Vomiting has many possible causes, most of which are simple and benign, and in general only *persistent vomiting* is likely to have a serious origin.

Vomited blood in the first day or two is almost always swallowed maternal blood and can be distinguished from the infant's blood by confirming that it contains no fetal haemoglobin. If the vomit contains *bile*, it must always be taken seriously and intestinal obstruction excluded with an erect plain abdominal X-ray. Obstruction can occur at many levels in the gut and all such infants require urgent attention from a specialist paediatric surgeon. Most lesions are readily amenable to corrective surgery within the first few days of life (p. 201). Bile-stained vomiting may also occur with a cerebral disorder such as intracranial bleeding (p. 144) or meningitis (p. 162).

Distension of the abdomen

Abdominal distension has many causes. If it is present at the time of birth, it usually indicates enlargement of one or more of the intra-abdominal organs such as the kidneys, liver or spleen, the presence of ascites, or rarely an abdominal tumour. Sometimes the cause of the distension can compress the diaphragm and cause additional respiratory distress, and this requires urgent attention.

Distension developing over the first few days of life will most commonly result from gaseous distension of the gut caused by obstruction at some level, although the higher in the gut the obstruction occurs, the more likely it is to present with vomiting rather than distension.

Unusual bowel actions and stools

Green stools are not necessarily abnormal in breast-fed infants and the stool often turns greener after being passed. An infant taking more breast milk than usual may pass looser and more frequent motions which are often frothy, but this need not be regarded as overfeeding unless there is an accompanying failure to gain weight. Underfeeding commonly results in stools which are not hard but are characteristically small and dark-coloured. Small streaks of blood are often present if the baby has to strain to pass a hard stool, e.g. when changing from breast to formula milk.

Failure to pass meconium within the first 24 hours is uncommon and the longer the delay the more likely it is to be associated with an abnormality. A plug of thick meconium in the rectum is the commonest cause and can be relieved by a small rectal washout or can be encouraged to pass by a gentle rectal examination.

In the condition known as meconium ileus, the whole large bowel may be full of thick and sticky meconium which the baby is unable to pass, which is the mode of presentation of a minority of patients with cystic fibrosis (p. 201).

FURTHER READING

Andersen E S, Wailoo M P, Petersen S A 1989 Keeping babies warm. Health Visitor 62: 372–373

Bennett V R, Brown L K (eds) 1989 Myles' textbook of midwifery, 11th edn. Churchill Livingstone, Edinburgh

Bindels J G 1992 Artificial feeds for infants – human milk substitutes: current composition and future trends. Current Paediatrics 2: 163–167

Bowlby J 1989 A secure base: clinical applications of attachment theory. Tavistock, London

Chalmers I, Enkin M, Keirse M 1992 Effective care in pregnancy and childbirth. Oxford University Press, Oxford

Dalzell A, Dodge J 1992 Enteral nutrition. Current Paediatrics 2: 168–171

David T J (ed) 1991 Recent advances in paediatrics 9. Churchill Livingstone, Edinburgh

Davies D P (ed) 1995 Nutrition in child health. Royal College of Physicians, London

Department of Health: Chief Medical Officers Expert Group 1994 The sleeping position of infants and cot death. HMSO, London

Franks S (ed) 1990 Physiology of lactation. Clinical endocrinology and metabolism. Baillière Tindall, London

Leaf A 1996 Essential fatty acids in neonatal nutrition. Seminars in neonatology. 1: 43–50

National Brestfeeding Working Group 1995. Brestfeeding: good practice guidance to the NHS. DOH, London

Office of Population Censuses and Surveys 1990 Feeding the newborn baby. HMSO, London

Orlando S 1995 The immunological significance of breast milk. Journal of Obstetric and Gynaecological Neonatal Nursing 24: 678–683

Poskitt E 1988 Practical paediatric nutrition. Butterworths, London

Royal College of Midwives 1991 Successful breastfeeding. Churchill Livingstone, Edinburgh

Ryan S W (ed) 1996 Seminars in neonatology – enteral nutrition. W B Saunders, London

Schaffer R 1977 Mothering. Fontana, London

Short R 1994 What the breast does for the baby and what the baby does for the breast. Australian and New Zealand Journal of Obstetrics and Gynaecology 34: 262–264

Sinclair J, Bracken M 1992 Effective care of the newborn infant. Oxford University Press, Oxford

Suskind R M, Lewinter-Suskind L 1993 Textbook of paediatric nutrition, 2nd edn. Raven Press, New York

Taylor J, Sanderson M 1995. A re-examination of the risk factors for Sudden Infant Death Syndrome. Journal of Paediatrics 126: 887–891

Taylor J A, Krieger J W, Reay D T, Davis R L, Harruf R, Cheney L K 1996. Prone sleeping position and the Sudden Infant Death Syndrome in King County Washington: a case control study. Journal of Paediatrics 128: 626–630

Thomas A 1992 Vitamins and trace minerals. Current Paediatrics 2: 172–174

Vandenplas Y, Ashkenazi A, Belli D et al 1993 A proposition for the diagnosis and treatment of gastro-oesophageal reflux disease in children: Working group of the European society of paediatric gastroenterology and nutrition (ESPGAN). European Journal of Paediatrics 152(9): 704–711

Wang Y, Wu S 1996 The effect of exclusive breast feeding on development and the incidence of infection in infants. Journal of Human Lactation 12: 27–30

Wells J 1996. Nutritional considerations in infant formula design. Seminars in Neonatology 1: 19–26

Common disorders of the newborn infant

DISORDERS OF INTRAUTERINE GROWTH

Approximately 80% of all babies grow normally during fetal life, are born within the range of 2500–3800 g birth weight and between 37 and 41 weeks of completed gestation, and are referred to as appropriately grown for their gestational age. Most of these infants will be entirely healthy and have an uncomplicated neonatal course. The rest are affected by one or more factors which prevent appropriate growth and leave the infant more vulnerable in the first few days of life to the consequences of the abnormal growth or its causes. The baby may be heavier or lighter than expected and may be assigned to one of several groups which are defined according to specific criteria. Each group has its own causes and problems which will be described.

Low birth weight babies

The birth weight of between 6 and 9% of babies born in Britain is below 2500 g and about 1% weigh less than 1500 g. Low birth weight is a major contributor to perinatal and neonatal mortality, around 60% of perinatal deaths occurring in this group of infants. Its incidence rises to 12–13% in UK babies of mothers of Afro-Caribbean and Asian origin, which partly explains the higher perinatal mortality figures in these groups. Approximately half of all low birth weight babies have grown well for their period of gestation but are born before term (pre-term babies), and in general the lower the birth weight

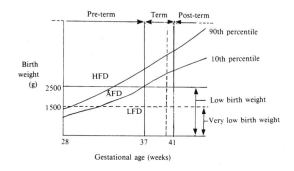

Abbreviations
HFD – Heavy for dates:
     – all babies above 90th percentile
AFD – Appropriate weight for dates:
     – babies between 10th and 90th percentiles
LFD – Light (or small) for dates:
     – all babies below 10th percentile

Figure 7.1 Categories of babies according to weight and maturity.

in this group, the more pre-term the infant is likely to be. The other half are more mature but have not grown as well as expected before birth. Although most perinatal statistics classify infants according to birth weight categories (Fig. 7.1), and the smaller the babies the higher the perinatal mortality and morbidity, the two groups have very different origins, problems and outcomes and thus are described separately. The effects of pre-term birth are described in Chapters 8 and 9, while those infants who have reached term but have suffered restricted intrauterine growth have the problems of 'light for dates' infants and are discussed here.

The light for dates infant

Those babies whose weight, when plotted on a growth chart, lies below the 10th percentile for their gestational age are called *light for dates* infants. Such a baby may also be pre-term (less than 37 weeks of gestation), term (37–41 weeks) or post-term (more than 41 weeks). It is therefore necessary to assess the gestational age of an infant in order to put her into one of these categories, and the way this is done is described on page 106. *Intrauterine growth retardation* is a clinical description of a state in which the infant at birth is malnourished or appears to have lost

weight during the latter stages of the pregnancy.

There are several reasons why an infant may be of unexpectedly low birth weight for the gestation period, including:

- placental insufficiency, often associated with pre-eclampsia
- maternal chronic illness
- extreme maternal malnutrition
- maternal heavy smoking
- excess alcohol consumption in pregnancy
- congenital abnormalities
- maternal drug abuse
- congenital infections
- normal small babies from small mothers.

As long as any congenital malformations or infections have been excluded by careful examination, the majority of these babies will be well and will behave and feed normally for their gestation, and many will require little special attention. However, those infants who are light for dates because of chronic intrauterine malnutrition and hypoxia are more prone to certain problems which may affect the baby in the neonatal period or diminish the child's developmental progress later and thus merit separate description.

The baby with restricted intrauterine growth caused by one of these predisposing disorders is more prone to suffer from fetal distress during labour because of a reduction of oxygen transfer across the placenta and to require resuscitation at birth. Birth asphyxia and meconium aspiration pneumonia are therefore relatively more common than in a well-grown infant and consequently the incidence of hypoxic-ischaemic encephalopathy is also raised (p. 144), although none of these complications occurs frequently. Because they are small, heat loss from the skin at birth in such babies is increased and this can result in hypothermia and hypoglycaemia (p. 97).

Some of these infants will also be pre-term and they may need additional treatment for any of the associated complications (p. 108). However, the stress of intrauterine growth retardation frequently accelerates the maturation of the lungs, and hyaline membrane disease is less severe as a result. These babies are often more polycythaemic than well-nourished infants since the mild chronic hypoxia which results from placental insufficiency causes a compensatory increase in red cell production before birth (p. 177). Occasionally the blood is so viscous from the excessive red cell numbers that the circulation becomes sluggish. In these circumstances, removal of some blood and replacement with human albumin improve the blood flow to vital organs (p. 177).

Clinical features

A mature light for dates infant is shown in Plate 7. There is an appearance of wasting of soft tissues and a lack of subcutaneous fat which are features of inadequate intrauterine nutrition. The skin is loose and rather dry, often peeling and discoloured, and there is little vernix. The ribs are easily seen and the abdomen may be hollowed, a feature sometimes identifiable by ultrasound examination before birth to demonstrate poor fetal growth. Scalp hair is sparse and the skull bones feel relatively hard. The head often appears large when compared with the size of the body, and the head circumference is on a higher percentile line on the growth chart than the weight. The umbilical cord is thin and often has a yellowish-brown colour.

When over 1800 g at birth, such infants are vigorous and active when awake and have a flexed posture during sleep indicating that they are mature. They are often particularly hungry feeders.

Management after birth

During the first day or two of life, the light for dates infant is particularly prone to the closely related problems of hypothermia and hypoglycaemia. A small thin baby will lose heat rapidly at birth, but to counteract the potential fall of body temperature the infant raises her heat production by increasing the rate of glucose metabolism. As the blood glucose is used up in this process, the diminished liver glycogen stores in these infants are insufficient to replenish it and the baby becomes hypoglycaemic. Particular attention should therefore be paid to keeping the baby

warm at birth and it may be necessary to nurse her in an incubator until the infant's temperature is stable and she is feeding well (p. 000). Breast feeding should start as soon as possible after birth, feeds being given at least every 3–4 hours initially. Regular measurement of capillary blood glucose using colorimetric strips should be done at 4 hour intervals for the first day, and then 8-hourly until 48 hours. A level below 2.5 mmol/L (35 mg/100 ml) at any time should be regarded as potentially hazardous and treated accordingly (see p. 98).

Feeding the light for dates infant

The malnourished light for dates infant requires a calorie intake above the normal quantities to enable her weight to catch up. If the infant is breast fed but does not seem satisfied with the quantities taken, she should be given formula milk by cup feeding, allowing her to determine the additional amount she needs. The fully formula-fed baby should be offered an amount appropriate for a baby whose weight is somewhere nearer the average for the gestational age rather than using her actual weight for the calculation. This will enable her to make up for the calorie deprivation suffered before birth. In most cases this results in a period of accelerated weight gain which levels off when the baby nears her genetic centile on the growth chart.

Despite these measures, blood glucose values commonly fall to levels of 2 mmol/L (35 mg/100 ml) or below in the first 2 days. If clinical signs of hypoglycaemia appear, such as apnoeic attacks, lethargy, jitteriness, cyanosis or fits, they must be treated vigorously to prevent brain damage (p. 98).

Prognosis

Whereas the mildly malnourished babies normally suffer no adverse long-term consequences, the very light for dates baby (less than the 5th percentile weight for gestation period) who has suffered significant malnutrition or hypoxia in the third trimester of pregnancy may grow slowly and remain small throughout childhood.

Although unlikely to suffer from severe neurological handicap or frank cerebral palsy unless also very immature, she has a bigger chance of having mild learning difficulties and of suffering from epilepsy. Minor neurological disorders like hyperactive behaviour and specific learning difficulties are also more common.

The post-term infant

Prolongation of pregnancy beyond the expected date of delivery can sometimes be due to a variation in the fetomaternal physiology and result in a perfectly normal baby. On the other hand, it is also clear that the impairment of placental function which tends to take place after 42 weeks' gestation in some cases causes intrauterine death or the delivery of a sick newborn infant. The baby presents a recognizable clinical picture. She is much thinner than normal; the skin is parchment-like, cracked and peeling; and in severe cases there is yellowish-green discoloration of the nails and umbilical stump. The thin face bears a worried expression and, if not ill, the baby appears unusually alert, restless and hungry for feeds. The haemoglobin content of the blood is relatively high, as a compensation for intrauterine hypoxia in the previous weeks. Intrapartum asphyxia and aspiration pneumonia are common hazards at birth.

Antenatal ultrasound measurements can sometimes identify these infants and the complications can be prevented by induction of labour at the optimal time. Where the gestation period is accurately known, induction of labour is usually undertaken before 42 weeks. More accurate methods for the assessment of fetal distress in the early stages have also helped to reduce the mortality from this cause (p. 35). Hypoglycaemia is the main immediate hazard and the baby should be treated along the same lines as the light for dates baby with intrauterine malnutrition. They require similarly increased nutrition and show catch-up growth also.

Infant of the diabetic mother

Although in the past the risk to the infant of the diabetic mother was high, the careful control of the condition before conception and during the pregnancy can bring down the risk to little more than that seen in normal infants of healthy mothers. When the mother has been able to keep her blood glucose values within the normal range throughout most of the pregnancy, the baby will look quite normal at birth, but with higher average blood glucose values the infant will develop a characteristic physical appearance. The baby is often larger and heavier than the period of gestation would suggest, the umbilical cord is thickened and the appearance of the baby with its bulging cheeks, plethoric complexion and hirsutism is reminiscent of Cushing's syndrome (Plate 8). The heaviness is, however, due to a real increase in growth and not just fat or oedema. It is sometimes possible to diagnose the pre-diabetic state in mothers who have borne babies of successively increasing birth weight.

The main hazards to the infant are as follows:

• Early hypoglycaemia; this results from overproduction of insulin from the islets of Langerhans which have hypertrophied because of maternal and fetal hyperglycaemia.

• Respiratory distress syndrome with all the clinical features seen in the pre-term baby (Plate 8).

• Trauma during delivery can occur, particularly if the baby is of large size. This can take the form of a fracture to the clavicle, which is often asymptomatic and found incidentally when a lump is noticed on the bone, or a more serious injury to the cervical nerve roots which can be damaged during delivery of the neck if shoulder dystocia occurs. The consequent Erb's palsy can take many months to recover and in some cases improvement is incomplete (p. 153).

• There is an increased incidence of congenital malformations, particularly of the heart (p. 207) and, much more rarely, sacral agenesis.

• Polycythaemia is common and a dilution exchange may be required if the haematocrit rises above 70% (p. 177).

• Occasionally hypocalcaemia may occur.

• Weight gain after birth is often less than normal and the infant's growth chart shows a falling weight centile. This is usually a natural adjustment to the child's genetic size, and as long as the infant is well and apparently feeding to her own satisfaction there is no reason to intervene.

Management to prevent hypoglycaemia

The blood glucose falls rapidly to its minimum value from 2 to 6 hours from the time of delivery, and during this time the baby should be nursed at the mother's bedside, as long as specialized neonatal care is immediately available. Breast or formula milk feeding is started before 2 hours of age and the blood glucose level checked every 2 hours in the first 12 hours to identify hypoglycaemia, and thereafter every 8 hours until the end of the second day. If the blood glucose value falls below 2.5 mmol/L (40 mg/dl), the treatment detailed on page 000 should be followed. Glucagon 100 μg/kg body weight intramuscularly may raise the blood glucose level rapidly if needed but an additional feed should be given also to prevent a further fall about 30 minutes later. The hyperinsulinism usually resolves within 48 hours and it is unusual for hypoglycaemia to persist after the second day of life.

Heavy for dates infants

Babies with a birth weight over the 90th percentile are termed *heavy for dates*. Most are simply well grown infants of larger mothers or the consequence of poor control of maternal diabetes during the pregnancy. Some, however, have features rather like the offspring of diabetic mothers and behave in the same way, developing hypoglycaemia in the first day or two of life. This should be treated similarly. These babies should be allowed to breast feed on demand unless the development of hypoglycaemia calls for additional feeding. Formula-fed infants should be offered the full amount for their weight but they will frequently take less than this. Commonly their weight gain over the first few months is less than expected and they fall towards their genetic centile on the growth chart, a feature which may occasionally be difficult to distinguish from failure to thrive due to genuine underfeeding. Other

rare causes of heavy for dates infants are Beckwith's syndrome, transposition of the great arteries and nesidioblastosis, a serious condition in which profound hypoglycaemia results from an abnormally increased secretion of insulin from excessive numbers of islet cells in the pancreas.

Twin births

Twinning happens about once every 80 births in the UK, although its incidence has increased recently as a result of the use of fertility treatments and ovulation-stimulating drugs. It can result from either the splitting of a single fertilized ovum in early pregnancy (monozygotic twins) or the fertilization of two separate ova (dizygotic twins). There are considerable extra risks for the infants of any multiple pregnancy. Over half of all twins are of low birth weight. Premature labour is common and each infant is subject to the complications of prematurity and breech position for one twin may add to its risk of asphyxia. As a result of these risks the perinatal mortality for twins, particularly the second-born baby, is about four times greater than that in singletons, and is even higher in higher order births. The incidence of congenital malformations is approximately double that in singleton births and birth trauma is more common, particularly to the second twin. One member of the pair commonly has a poorer share of available nutrition in utero as a result of placental insufficiency, is born with all the signs of fetal malnutrition (Plate 9), and is therefore at greater risk of asphyxia during labour (p. 35). As a result of this, there is a higher incidence of cerebral palsy in twins than in singleton births, although in contrast to the mortality statistics it occurs equally in both the first and second baby.

Occasionally there is a connection between the circulations of the two twins in the placenta. This can result in cross-transfusion of blood between the two fetuses, giving rise to a high haemoglobin level and polyhydramnios in one baby, and anaemia and growth retardation with a diminished liquor volume in the other. In severe cases repeated aspiration of excess amniotic fluid may prolong the pregnancy and thus reduce the risks from premature delivery. After birth the poly-cythaemic twin runs into more difficulty from the increased blood volume and consequent cardiac strain than the anaemic one. If the poly-cythaemic twin has a packed cell volume of over 70%, a dilution exchange transfusion using 20 ml/kg body weight of plasma is often advisable to reduce the blood viscosity and improve blood flow (p. 177). The anaemic twin may occasionally need a top-up blood transfusion if she becomes symptomatic from the physiological fall of haemoglobin which occurs in all infants over the first few weeks of life (p. 177).

Feeding of twins

There is no reason why both twins should not be breast fed as long as the mother is producing enough milk to maintain adequate growth of the babies. The mother may wish to feed one from one breast and then the second baby on the other side, or feed both of them at the same time (Fig. 7.2). Sometimes there may not be enough milk for both infants, and supplements of formula milk must then be given. The babies may be

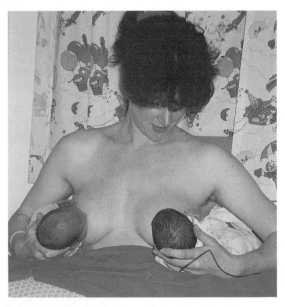

Figure 7.2 Tandem feeding of twins.

given the breast and a formula feed alternately or a part breast and part cup feed on each occasion. As long as the infants are contented and growing, the method of coping with the feeding is not crucial. The principles of good breast feeding are, however, more important, since inevitably there is unlikely to be much excess milk when two infants are partaking.

If the infants are pre-term, either or both may have any of the usual perinatal complications and they may recover at different rates. Cerebral palsy occurs much more frequently in twins than in singleton babies and may only affect one twin. On the whole it is probably better to keep the twins together until they are both ready to be discharged, since it is inevitably more difficult to visit the twin who remains in hospital. However, since one of the pair may need additional treatment for a congenital abnormality this is not always possible and it can cause the parents to have a difference of approach to the two infants. It can also be particularly difficult for them if one of the twins dies, since they will then have to cope with both the joy of having the surviving infant and at the same time the grief over the one who has died. Each set of parents will handle this difficult situation differently and it requires a particular sensitivity on the part of the professionals involved to recognize and help the parents with these dual emotions. Many parents find help and assistance from joining a local twins club and in the UK there is a national organization which can also give advice.

Triplets and more

The problems encountered in these higher order births are similar to those of twins, although the greater the number of babies, the more likely they are to be pre-term and the more immature they will be. There is, of course, a much higher risk of such infants dying and the family may be faced with a multiple bereavement, perhaps with one or more surviving infants with a risk of permanent handicap. For example, the risk of cerebral palsy in triplet survivors is about 7%. In many instances such pregnancies are the result of in vitro fertilization and thus are conceived after a period of infertility, which adds to the confused emotions such families suffer. Fortunately, improved techniques have reduced the risk of such large numbers of fetuses growing and this problem may diminish as further experience is gained.

HYPOGLYCAEMIA

Glucose is the major source of energy for the baby's brain without which its function may be affected or its later growth and development impaired. It is therefore of the greatest importance to be aware of the clinical features of hypoglycaemia, the situations in which it may occur and the methods of preventing and treating it.

Hypoglycaemia is common in infants in the first 48 hours of life. In normal babies the blood glucose falls from the normal maternal levels before birth to levels around 3 mmol/L in the first 2 days, rising again towards more normal levels after the third day, as long as the baby is receiving an adequate calorie intake. Although it is difficult to define what constitutes an abnormal blood glucose level, any value below 2.5 mmol/L (40 mg/dl) should be regarded as hypoglycaemia regardless of whether the infant has symptoms or not. Although no baby is immune from the problem, certain groups of babies are more at risk of developing low blood glucose levels than others. These include:

- infants of diabetic mothers
- babies of mothers with gestational diabetes
- babies with intrauterine growth retardation
- pre-term infants who are unable to feed adequately
- infants with serious infections
- babies deprived of enteral feeds (e.g. when the breast milk supply is inadequate)
- hypothermic infants.

In all such infants, regular measurement of capillary blood glucose should be carried out and treatment given if the blood glucose falls below 2.5 mmol/L. If clinical signs appear at all they will consist of jitteriness, apnoea, lethargy, sleepiness, cyanosis or fits, but even if these are not present low blood glucose levels may cause brain damage and the risk is greater if the baby has suffered asphyxia or is infected, or if the hypoglycaemia is prolonged. Since there may be no clinical indication that the infant has a low blood glucose, it is necessary to bear it in mind and measure the blood level whenever an infant is in one of the risk groups or is behaving in any unusual way.

Prevention and treatment

Prevention of hypoglycaemia should be the aim in all babies. In the higher risk infants, a feed should be given within an hour of birth, by nasogastric tube if necessary, or an intravenous infusion of 10% dextrose should be established. Giving the first feed to the normal infant within the first 4 hours and leaving no more than 4 hours between feeds will usually maintain a normal blood glucose level unless she is under an additional physiological stress such as hypothermia or infection. From Table 7.1 it can be seen that if a baby develops asymptomatic hypoglycaemia for any reason she should be given a feed of 15–20 ml/kg of breast or formula milk and the blood glucose measured again in 1 hour. If the level has risen above 2.5 mmol/L, a further check should be made before the next feed; if it has not, the infant must be assumed to be suffering from persistent hypoglycaemia and be given an intravenous infusion of 10% dextrose at a rate of 60–90 ml/kg per day or more until a level above 2.5 mmol/L can be maintained by feeds alone. If a baby has a fit or other symptoms clearly related to a low blood glucose value, an intravenous bolus of 10 ml/kg of 10% dextrose must be given urgently and followed by a dextrose infusion. Glucagon and steroids are not usually effective in raising the blood glucose level.

BABIES WITH RESPIRATORY DISTRESS

Many respiratory conditions present in the same way in the newborn infant and they cannot often be distinguished clinically. Respiratory symptoms such as dyspnoea, tachypnoea, grunting respirations, and costal or subcostal recession

Table 7.1 Management of neonatal hypoglycaemia

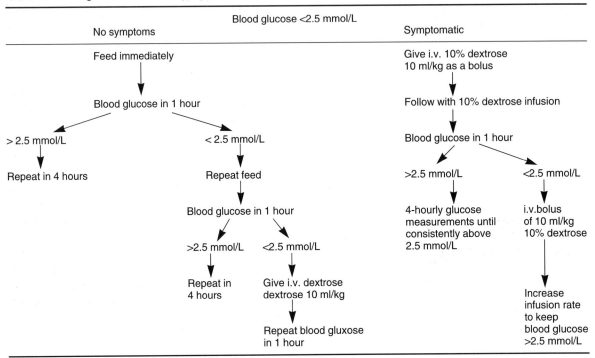

should always be investigated by a chest X-ray. Grunting alone can be a feature of hypothermia or septicaemia which should be urgently investigated and treated (p. 162). Persistent cyanosis suggests complex congenital heart disease or a very serious pulmonary disorder. Box 7.1 shows causes of neonatal respiratory distress.

Box 7.1 Causes of neonatal respiratory distress

- Atelectasis
- Aspiration of:
  — liquor
  — meconium
- Pneumonia
- Pneumothorax
- Diaphragmatic hernia
- Hypoplastic lungs
- Respiratory distress syndrome
- Choanal atresia
- Heart failure
- Persistent metabolic acidosis
- Transient tachypnoea of the newborn

Atelectasis, the aspiration syndrome and pneumonia

Atelectasis

The failure of portions of the lungs to expand with the first few breaths or the collapse of part of the lung secondary to inhalation of fluid or mucus is described as atelectasis. In this situation the respiratory distress is at its maximum immediately after delivery and in the case of primary atelectasis it eases off over the first 24 hours. Fine crepitations and diminished air entry may be detectable clinically, but the collapse is difficult to localize accurately.

The meconium aspiration syndrome

The inhalation of meconium occurs when the fetus has passed meconium into the liquor before birth. This usually follows fetal asphyxia and is commoner in the baby who has suffered intrauterine malnutrition. There may be evidence of inhaled meconium when suction from the pharynx is undertaken at birth. The symptoms vary from mild to very severe and may progress rapidly over the first day. X-rays show scattered opacities in both lungs with intervening areas of overinflation and depression of the diaphragms caused by airways obstruction. A pneumothorax may result from the rupture of an emphysematous bulla.

Pneumonia

When infection has been acquired either before or during passage through the birth canal, pneumonia may ensue and it is difficult to distinguish clinically. It is most commonly due to the group B streptococcus or *E. coli* and the subject is discussed in Chapter 11 (p. 164).

Management

In each case the baby should be nursed in an incubator to control body temperature and allow observation of colour and breathing. The airway should be cleared by pharyngeal suction as required, oxygen given if any cyanosis is present and antibiotics administered to control infection. A combination of penicillin and an aminoglycoside antibiotic, e.g. gentamicin, is usually chosen since it covers the predominant organisms encountered (p. 167). Physiotherapy with gentle percussion to the chest can help to re-expand collapsed lung lobes. In severe cases, intermittent positive pressure ventilation becomes necessary (p. 131).

Respiratory distress syndrome

This is mainly confined to the pre-term infant and is described in detail in Chapter 9.

Upper airway obstruction

Obstruction to the upper airway should be excluded whenever a baby seems to be in respiratory difficulty immediately after birth. Choanal atresia is a congenital abnormality in which there is bony or cartilaginous obstruction in the posterior nasal passages. Since a newborn baby has the greatest difficulty breathing through the mouth when the nasal airway is obstructed, repeated vigorous inspiratory efforts are made before a small intake of air passes the tongue, momentarily relieving the shortage of oxygen which may be severe enough to cause cyanosis. When seen immediately after birth this struggle for effective respiration can be mistakenly attributed to a disorder of lung function until it becomes clear that no air is passing the nose. Thick stringy mucus usually occupies the nasal space. The diagnosis is likely if a nasogastric tube cannot be passed beyond the posterior part of the nose, and confirmed by the absence of airflow past a wisp of cotton wool held under the nostril. Feeding from the breast or bottle is impossible for any length of time and orogastric tube feeding is necessary until the condition can be relieved surgically.

Treatment

Breathing may be eased temporarily by pulling the tongue forward to allow air to pass through the mouth into the pharynx and nursing the baby in the prone position. A small oral airway strapped into position can be very effective as a temporary measure. The next step involves surgical treatment in a specialized unit, and the methods of relieving the obstruction vary. Good results have been obtained by using a trochar and cannula to make a new opening through the solid occlusion in the posterior nasal passages, followed by the insertion of polythene tubing as an airway to keep the passage from closing until epithelium has formed.

Oesophageal atresia

Oesophageal atresia with or without a tracheo-oesophageal fistula may also present as obstructed breathing, due to the accumulation of fluid secretion in the upper respiratory tract. The diagnosis and management of this condition are described in Chapter 13.

Pneumothorax

Pneumothorax is not uncommon. It may be idiopathic but mainly occurs after meconium aspiration, positive pressure resuscitation, or as a complication of artificial ventilation or continuous positive airway pressure (p. 135). Respiration is shallow and rapid and the chest may be overexpanded in severe cases. Breath sounds are diminished, and if the pneumothorax is on the left side the heart sounds are noticeably faint. Milder degrees of the condition are, however, impossible to detect clinically and an X-ray or transillumination using a cold-light source will be needed to confirm the diagnosis. Fortunately, the lung usually re-expands spontaneously within 3–4 days. However, when the hole in the pleura is valvular, air continues to accumulate, causing a shift of the mediastinum to the opposite side and increased respiratory distress (Fig. 7.3). The insertion of a needle or cannula into the pleural cavity allows the pleural air to escape

and thus relieves the respiratory distress rapidly, but it is normally also necessary to insert an indwelling pleural cannula to drain the air through an underwater seal to prevent its reaccumulation until the perforation has healed (p. 135).

Diaphragmatic hernia

In this congenital malformation, part of the diaphragm fails to develop, allowing the abdominal organs to occupy the left side of the chest, and displacing the heart and mediastinum to the right. The presence of polyhydramnios may suggest the possibility of the condition, and ultrasound scanning can often confirm the diagnosis before birth. If it is identified antenatally, it is important that the infant is resuscitated by endotracheal intubation at birth and that positive pressure by mask is avoided since it may cause distension of the stomach which will further embarrass respiration. Severe respiratory distress and cyanosis are present from birth, and if not previously diagnosed, the condition may be suspected when the maximum area of intensity of the heart sounds is over the right side of the chest and the abdomen is noticeably hollowed.

An X-ray (Fig. 7.4) immediately confirms the condition and it must be regarded as a surgical emergency, for early operation may be life-saving. Sometimes, however, the lungs are hypoplastic and are unable to sustain adequate oxygenation despite maximal endotracheal ventilation, and the respiratory failure may be compounded by persistence of fetal pulmonary hypertension. The resulting hypoxia accounts for the high mortality of the condition, particularly in the pre-term infant.

Heart failure

Heart failure due either to congenital heart disease or to an arrhythmia frequently shows itself first as laboured breathing or tachypnoea. The diagnosis and treatment are described on page 206, but the clinical features which should give rise to suspicion are:

* rapid respiration with marked indrawing of the lower ribs on inspiration

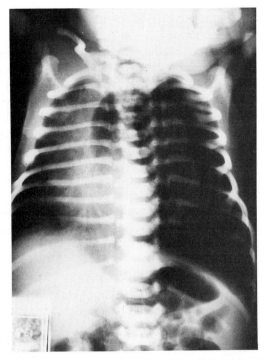

Figure 7.3   Tension pneumothorax of the left lung, showing displacement of the heart to the right.

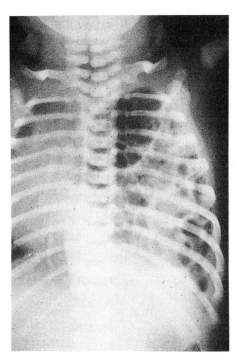

Figure 7.4 Diaphragmatic hernia in the left side of the chest.

- tachycardia
- enlargement of the liver
- cyanosis
- oedema with unexpected weight gain
- heart murmurs, which may or may not be present at this stage.

Persistent metabolic acidosis

If an infant develops a persistent metabolic acidosis, a compensatory increase in respiration rate and depth occurs to reduce the CO_2 level and thus restore the pH of the blood. This overbreathing may occasionally be mistaken for cardiac or pulmonary disease, but it can be distinguished by a low P_{CO_2} in the arterial blood gas values. Further investigation of the cause of the acidosis is required before deciding on treatment.

Transient neonatal tachypnoea

Transient neonatal tachypnoea occurs in about 2% of babies and presents as respiratory distress on the first day. It is normally mild and resolves without treatment in a few days. It is usually attributed to delayed absorption of the fetal lung fluid and in the first day or two it mimics respiratory distress syndrome. It occurs more frequently in male infants born at term, particularly after fetal asphyxia, and occurs in around 9% of infants born by elective caesarean section. X-rays show no atelectasis or pneumonia and, as long as sepsis can be confidently excluded, no specific treatment is needed, although oxygen supplementation may be required if the oxygen saturation is low.

Apnoeic attacks

Brief apnoeic attacks are common in the pre-term infant, reflecting the immaturity of the baby's respiratory centre in the brain, but in a full-term infant they are often associated with disorders such as hypoglycaemia, infection or fits and they should always be taken seriously and investigated accordingly.

Intrapulmonary haemorrhage

Intrapulmonary haemorrhage, a usually fatal event, is a rare sequel to infection or to hypothermia. Respiratory difficulty is usually already present and the bleeding is manifested by the appearance of bright red blood in the mouth and upper airways or suction of bright red blood from an indwelling endotracheal tube.

JAUNDICE

A golden yellow coloration of the skin and sclerae is common and has many possible causes which are described fully in Chapter 12. Since it can result in death or severe brain damage in extreme cases, it should never be ignored, but it becomes evident in about a third of all term babies and is so familiar in its mild form that it has been labelled 'physiological'.

No case of neonatal jaundice should be dismissed as normal without consideration of its possible cause. As a general guide, a serum bilirubin of more than 200 μmol/L (12 mg/100 ml) in a term infant on or before the third day should lead to further examination and investigation (p. 180).

SKIN CONDITIONS

Haemangiomas

Since the 'strawberry mark' (naevus vasculosus) (Plate 10) is rarely present at birth, it cannot strictly be called a birthmark; it develops in the first week or two as a small bright red spot which enlarges to a variable extent during the first 3–6 months, forming a raised purplish-red mottled area occasionally with underlying sub-cutaneous thickening extending beyond its margins. The natural history of its development is cessation of further spread by 6 months with gradual regression thereafter by flattening and the formation of paler patches of skin on the surface. Most are scarcely detectable by the age of 8 years. In pre-term infants these naevi are more commonly multiple. The usual advice given about treatment is to leave them strictly alone because of the good eventual outcome, but in certain situations where they are a cause of real handicap in childhood (e.g. around the eye or on the nose) there may be good grounds for dealing with them surgically or by using laser therapy whilst still only a minute lesion and before the characteristic enlargement has begun.

Nappy rash

Rashes in the nappy area at this early period of infancy are most commonly around the anus and are often attributable to irritation of the skin by faeces rather than urine. This perianal excoriation often accompanies a change from breast to artificial feeding and can usually be treated successfully by exposure to air in warm surroundings or by the use of a silicone barrier cream.

Monilial dermatitis

Monilial dermatitis (thrush) in the perineum is also common and may occur even in the absence of visible thrush in the mouth. It typically affects the moist areas and flexures as a localized shiny redness with superficial desquamation of skin (Plate 17). Such a rash here is most unlikely to have any other cause and treatment with local application of nystatin cream, together with oral nystatin suspension (p. 161), is usually successful. A number of other antifungal preparations are available as alternatives. Sometimes a sensitization reaction of the skin to the *Monilia* requires a short period of local steroid application as additional treatment.

Ammoniacal dermatitis

Ammoniacal dermatitis is commoner after the first month and consists of erythema, peeling or ulcerating eruptions over the projecting parts of the nappy area, sparing the flexures. Treatment is by reducing the duration of contact of the skin with urine, by frequent washing with a moisturizing soap, drying and putting on a dry nappy. Secondary monilial infection is common and should be treated with topical nystatin cream. Towelling nappies must be washed thoroughly and used with a water-repelling nappy liner to keep the skin as dry as possible, but the use of highly absorbent paper-based disposable nappies significantly reduces the frequency of this condition.

SUPERFICIAL MINOR DISORDERS

Breast engorgement

Breast engorgement due to changes in hormonal balance is a common phenomenon in both female and male babies after the third day of life, and although it generally subsides within a week or two, persistence for several months is occasionally seen.

The secretion of small amounts of colostrum sometimes occurs. No treatment is needed for the engorgement and expression of the breasts should be avoided for it predisposes to the development of infective mastitis which requires antibiotic treatment (p. 160).

Male genitalia

Hydroceles, undescended testes and malformations of the male genitalia are discussed on page 62.

Inguinal hernia occurs more commonly in preterm than in term infants. Since it is liable to become incarcerated in the neonatal period, necessitating emergency surgery, elective operation should be undertaken as soon as the hernia is identified.

Female genitalia

Most female infants have a mucoid discharge from the vagina and occasionally it becomes bloodstained from shedding of the endometrium as a result of the hormonal changes after birth. It is a normal feature and resolves without intervention within about a week.

Umbilicus

The umbilical cord normally contains two arteries and one vein. A single umbilical artery is associated with an increased incidence of other congenital malformations (p. 196). The cord dries and sloughs off between the sixth and 10th days, the time being influenced to some extent by the method of care. Some moistness of the stump remains for a day or two and although this does not mean that there is sepsis, the area is a ready culture medium for bacteria, particularly the staphylococcus. Excessive granulation tissue sometimes accumulates and delays the healing of the stump, which then discharges and forms a small granuloma. Treatment with one or two applications of a silver nitrate stick usually effects a cure within a week, but it is important to distinguish it from the much rarer umbilical polyp. This is a remnant of the mesenteric duct consisting of intestinal mucosa and has a bright red smooth shining surface. A persistent urachus may present a similar appearance or show itself as a sinus discharging urine. Both require surgical exploration but are fully remediable.

The cord stump occasionally protrudes 1–3 cm from the abdominal wall, being covered by abdominal skin – the cutis navel – and differs from an umbilical hernia in feeling solid on palpation. No treatment is required as it becomes flatter with time.

An umbilical hernia developing in the first month of life is very common (especially in preterm infants) and it generally requires no treatment. Spontaneous cure by the age of 2 years is the rule. However, a supraumbilical hernia, which protrudes from a defect just above the umbilicus, will require surgical correction since it never closes spontaneously.

Sternomastoid tumour

This is a diffuse or localized hard rounded swelling in the substance of the sternomastoid muscle about its middle third arising some days or weeks after birth (Fig 7.5). There is sometimes an association with a difficult delivery and manipulations which involve traction to the head, but this is not always the case and the swelling is probably due to interference with the circulation in the muscle. The lump resolves after a variable

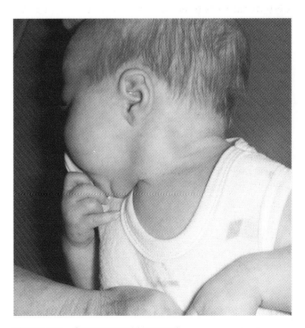

Figure 7.5 Sternomastoid 'tumour'.

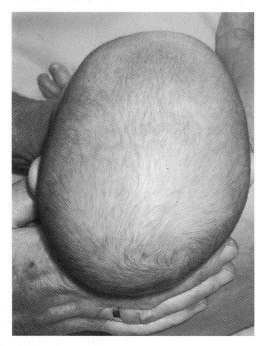

Figure 7.6 Asymmetrical head shape known as plagiocephaly.

period of 2–4 months, but it may be accompanied by a degree of torticollis which seldom persists after the age of 1 year. Physiotherapy is often used in treatment, with stretching of the involved muscle, but its efficacy is doubtful. Only when shortening remains after a year may surgical correction be required.

Plagiocephaly

After moulding of the skull has disappeared, only minor asymmetry of the cranial vault usually remains, but it is not uncommon to see asymmetry of the chin and mandible so that the alveolar margin is not quite parallel to that of the maxilla. This appears to be the effect of posture in utero, the flexed head having been also tilted sideways. It usually resolves but may occasionally persist as malocclusion into later childhood.

There is an unexplained tendency for some infants to prefer lying with their head slightly rotated towards one side, and this may lead to postural deformity descriptively termed 'parallelogram skull' or plagiocephaly, with flattening of one side of the occiput and the opposite frontal region and face (Fig. 7.6). It becomes more noticeable towards the end of the first month and increases to a maximum towards the ninth month, after which symmetry returns over the next 2 years. This can clearly be distinguished from unilateral craniosynostosis – the much rarer asymmetry resulting from premature fusion of one of the coronal sutures in the first few weeks with consequent lack of growth on that side. In this condition, the whole of the side of the vault appears to be shorter from back to front than the other side and the diagnosis can be confirmed radiologically. Early surgical treatment may be necessary to prevent further deformity.

FURTHER READING

David T J (ed) 1992 Recent advances in paediatrics 10. Churchill Livingstone, Edinburgh, ch 3

Heine R G, Jaquiery A, Lubitz L, Cameron D J, Catto-Smith A G 1995 Role of gastro-oesophageal reflux in infant irritability Archives of Disease in Childhood 73: 121–125

Roberton N R C (ed) 1992 Textbook of neonatology. Churchill Livingstone, Edinburgh

Sinclair J, Bracken M 1992 Effective care of the newborn infant. Oxford University Press, Oxford

Sommerfelt K, Ellertsen B, Markestad T 1995 Parental factors in cognitive outcome of non-handicapped low birthweight infants. Archives of Disease in Childhood 73: F135–F 142

The Scottish Low Birthweight Study Group 1992: The Scottish low birthweight study 1. Survival, growth, neuromotor and sensory impairment. Archives of Disease in Childhood 67: 675–681

The Scottish Low Birthweight Study Group 1992: The Scottish low birthweight study 2. Language attainment, cognitive status and behavioural problems. Archives of Disease in Childhood 67: 682–686

Wilson D, McClure G 1992 Respiratory problems in the newborn. British Journal of Intensive Care 2: 287–294

8

Pre-term infants

Of all babies, 3–4% are born before 37 weeks' gestation and are called pre-term infants. Almost all of them weigh less than 2500 g and are therefore low birth weight babies. They provide the great majority of work in neonatal units and it is in this group that 60% of all neonatal deaths occur. The incidence of pre-term birth and low birth weight varies from one part of the country to another and according to ethnic group, and this contributes significantly to the difference in neonatal mortality rates in different places (p. 6).

Pre-term infants may either have grown well for their gestation or be light for dates and show the characteristics and problems of this group of babies in addition to their prematurity (p. 92). It is important to remember that pre-term infants account for only half of all low birth weight babies, the others being mature but light for dates infants who, despite their size, behave more like term infants. They are described in Chapter 7.

Gradually the gestational age at which an infant has been regarded as viable has been falling, and current technology and medical care can offer considerable hope to those down to 25 weeks. Even some babies at 23–24 weeks can now be enabled to survive by using the whole range of neonatal intensive care facilities that are available.

The lower the gestational age at birth, the greater the risk of neurological handicap in the survivors, yet 90% or more of surviving infants from 26–28 week infants, and higher proportions of more mature infants, will develop into healthy children.

CAUSATIVE FACTORS OF PRE-TERM BIRTH

Pre-term delivery is about equally distributed between those that follow spontaneous early onset of labour and those in which the early labour is elective. Although we are ignorant of the direct cause of most spontaneous pre-term births, some predisposing factors are known which have much in common with those that lead to low birth weight, from impairment of intrauterine growth. They include:

- poor socioeconomic status
- pre-eclampsia
- smoking and alcoholism in pregnancy
- antepartum haemorrhage
- multiple pregnancy
- fetal developmental abnormalities
- primiparity
- short maternal stature
- maternal age below 18 years.

THE ASSESSMENT OF GESTATIONAL AGE

Apart from distinguishing between the pre-term and the light for dates mature infant, the value in assessing the gestational age of the newborn baby lies in helping the staff on the neonatal unit to plan his care and giving the parents some idea of when he will be ready for discharge. The more mature pre-term infant at, say, 35 weeks may be active, able to maintain his body temperature well, and able to feed from the breast from the beginning, whereas a 28 week infant will almost invariably require artificial ventilation to maintain adequate respiration, nasogastric or even parenteral feeding and the full range of intensive care.

In about 80% of cases a careful history of the date of the mother's last menstrual period is the best guide to the length of gestation within a week either way, although the use of oral contraceptives can cause confusion. The size of the uterus and measurement of the biparietal diameter of the fetal head using ultrasound in early pregnancy increase the accuracy of the assessment (p. 17). After birth it is possible to estimate

maturity with reasonable accuracy by examination of the baby. However, this requires a well-defined method and a fair amount of practice. The criteria used are based on neurological development and a set of physical characteristics which alter with increasing gestational age.

In one system of assessment the changes of four physical features (skin texture, skin colour, breast size and ear firmness) with increasing maturity put the infants into four general categories: very premature, premature, transitional and mature. Another method employs the progression of some neurological reflexes (pupil response to light, glabella tap, traction response and neck righting) to give similar general guidance about the degree of prematurity of the infant. For babies between 28 and 34 weeks of gestation, the progressive reduction in the number of surface blood vessels on the lens of the eye is probably the most accurate method of estimating maturity, but the technique requires considerable skill and experience with an ophthalmoscope.

In the more elaborate system devised by Dubowitz and its modification by Ballard, a score is given to each of a series of neurological and physical features, the total score being converted on a rating scale to the baby's gestational age. Although useful in research work it is more complicated than is needed for most routine care in neonatal units when the method used should primarily be to confirm the accuracy of the antenatal assessment of maturity. For most practical purposes, Table 8.1 gives enough information to make a reasonable estimate from relatively few selected characteristics which are easy to assess and have been found to correlate closely with gestational age.

GENERAL CHARACTERISTICS OF THE PRE-TERM INFANT

Figure 8.1 is a chart for pre-term infants showing the range of dimensions of infants from 24 weeks to term, and it can be seen that the weights of individual pre-term babies at the same maturity vary widely. Length is more closely related to maturity than is weight, but is not easy to mea-

Table 8.1 Chart for the assessment of gestational age, showing selected characteristics which have been foun[...] if the examination is to be kept brief and simple

Feature	Weeks of gestation							
	28	30	32	34	36	38	40	42
Colour and texture of skin	Uniformly red Smooth, thin 'transparent'			Pink, not completely smooth		Pale pink varying; slight superficial peeling		Pale thick with widespread peeling
Ear firmness and response to folding of pinna	No resistance to folding; stays folded		Very pliable but does not quite stay folded		Returns after folding; cartilage palpable to edge		Springs back rapidly; cartilage palpable throughout	
Diameter of breast tissue	Not palpable		Nodule 2 mm		Nodule 4 mm		Nodule 7 mm or more	
External genitalia, male	Testes not palpable		Testes palpable above scrotum, few scrotal rugae			Testes in scrotum, obvious scrotal rugae		
External genitalia, female	Labia majora widely separated, labia minora very prominent			Labia minora nearly covered by labia majora		Labia minora covered by labia majora		
Scarf sign	No resistance		Slight resistance		Elbow reaches midline of body	Elbow reaches only to nipple line or less		
Heel brought towards ear	No resistance	Slight resistance	Heel reaches ear with difficulty			Impossible to get heel to ear		
Arm recoil after extension at elbow		None		Partial flexion		Full flexion		
Dorsiflexion of foot (angle with tibial surface)	40°			20°		Dorsum of foot will just touch tibial surface		

sure accurately and is not by itself a reliable indicator of gestational age. The head circumference exceeds that of the chest, which tends to be relatively small and narrow. The length of the trunk in proportion to the limbs is greater than that of the term infant. Figure 8.2 illustrates some of the clinical features of the pre-term infant at birth. Fine hair on the face and trunk (lanugo) is more plentiful, especially if less than 30 weeks' gestation. The nails are soft but not necessarily short. There is a rather shiny unwrinkled appearance to the skin which is a darker pink colour than at

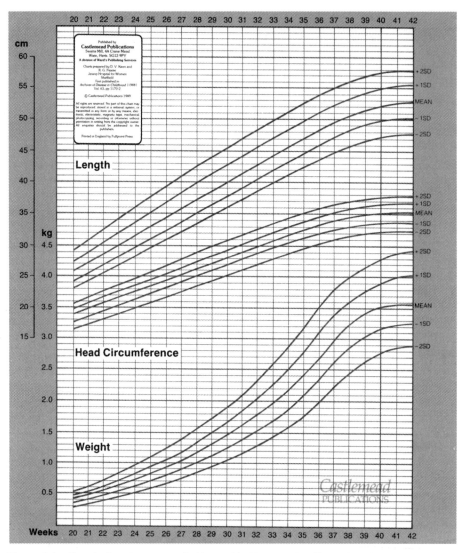

Figure 8.1 Growth chart for pre-term babies – girls 20-42 weeks. (Reproduced with permission from Castlemead Publications.)

term. The labia minora in the girl are protuberant and gaping, whilst in the boy the testes are usually incompletely descended. Below 34 weeks, the creases on the soles of the feet are almost absent except for a single one anteriorly. Ears are floppy and, lacking formed cartilage, tend to remain folded after the infant has lain on them. The palpable nodule of breast tissue at the nipple is absent before 34 weeks, 1–2 mm across from 34 to 36 weeks, about 4 mm from 36 to 38 weeks and about 8 mm at term. The skull is soft and easily indented around the fontanelles before 36 weeks, but becomes much harder towards term.

Effects of immaturity on the baby

The major problems faced by pre-term infants relate to the level of maturity of their organ systems and the greater the immaturity, the more

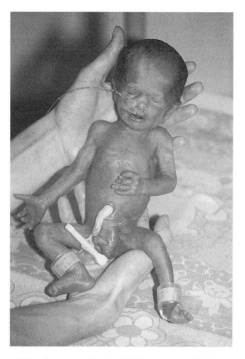

Figure 8.2 A pre-term baby of 29 weeks' gestation.

serious they are. Immaturity is shown most clearly by differences in the baby's physical activity and neurological responses. The shorter the gestation period, the less muscular activity is shown by the baby. In a pre-term infant born before 34 weeks, the eyes remain closed for most of the time and the cry, if any, is weak. The movements of body and limbs, when they occur, tend to be in little bursts of activity and are often jerky and frog-like. The posture of the pre-term baby is generally extended, becoming more flexed towards term and muscle tone is low but gradually increases as gestational age advances. Some of these features are summarized in Table 8.1. It must be remembered that even these neurological responses are suppressed if the baby is sick.

Temperature control

Heat production is low because of limited physical activity and heat loss is high because the baby's surface area is large in proportion to his weight and there is little insulation from subcu-

taneous fat. 'Brown fat', which is a specific source of heat production in normal term babies, is deficient in pre-term infants.

The baby's thermostatic mechanism is also poor, as he has only limited development of the cutaneous vascular responses and practically no ability to sweat. Heat production by shivering or muscle activity is minimal. Great care is thus necessary both to clothe the baby properly and to maintain a surrounding temperature and humidity which suits the individual infant (p. 112).

Blood

Capillary walls are weak and this, combined with reduced clotting factors in the blood, leads to a greater tendency to bleed and bruise easily. Pre-term infants, whether born vaginally or by caesarean section, are often born with bruising even after the most gentle handling. The haemoglobin is as high in cord blood as in a term infant and there is no clear correlation between its level and maturity. The blood volume is around 80 ml/kg body weight, which limits the amount of blood which can safely be taken for testing.

Heart and circulation

After birth the adaptations of the circulation occur more slowly and are less complete than in the term infant. The tone in the pulmonary arterioles is high, reduces more slowly and remains labile in pre-term infants. Thus the pulmonary blood pressure is high and varies widely. The systemic blood pressure is, by contrast, relatively low. The ductus arteriosus does not close firmly and is capable of opening again to allow shunting of blood between the circulations. This instability may result in significant variation of the oxygen saturation in the peripheral circulation if an excessive elevation in the pulmonary blood pressure shunts desaturated blood across either the foramen ovale or the ductus arteriosus.

Respiration

The nasal airway is narrow and easily obstructed. The thoracic cage is soft, so that it is sucked in by a small rise in negative pressure, and the respiratory passages are narrow, giving greater resistance to air flow (Fig. 9.2, p. 129). The infant breathes irregularly using the diaphragm more than the chest. The cough reflex is poorly developed. Gaseous exchange is relatively inefficient in very immature babies because the alveoli are lined by thick cuboidal epithelium in contrast to the flattened thin cells in the mature lungs and are surrounded by a meagre supply of capillaries which only start to increase significantly after the 28th week. Production of pulmonary surfactant by the alveolar cells is also minimal, causing the alveoli to collapse progressively (p. 128). The mechanisms that regulate depth and rate of breathing by stimulating the respiratory centre in the brain stem are not fully developed and the baby is thus liable to periods of apnoea when he seems to 'forget' to breathe altogether (p. 135). The result is an unstable respiratory system.

Gastrointestinal tract function

The mechanism of sucking and swallowing is poorly developed in the smallest pre-term babies, the mechanisms only becoming sufficiently coordinated for the infant to begin to feed from the breast at about 32–34 weeks and becoming fully effective around 36–37 weeks. On the whole, the function of digestion itself matures early and only in babies of less than 25 weeks is a deficiency of enzymes of functional importance. The lack of mucosal folds in the small bowel reduces the surface area for absorption of digested food. Sugar is well assimilated while protein is less so, and fat is least well tolerated. Immaturity of liver function is seen mainly as a reduced ability to conjugate bilirubin, which results in an increased incidence of jaundice in pre-term infants (p. 119), although reduced liver glycogen stores limit the baby's production of glucose in response to hypoglycaemia, and reduced bile secretion diminishes fat absorption from the gut. Immaturity of other liver enzyme systems may affect the rate of metabolism of many drugs and influence both the dose to be given and the frequency of administration (p. 233).

Renal function

Although the kidneys are usually able to excrete urea and water adequately, even in the very premature baby, they are unable to excrete large fluid loads and oedema may result. Metabolic acidosis can occur from excessive loss of bicarbonate from the renal tubules and an inability to secrete enough hydrogen ions into the urine. They are also less able to retain sodium than in the more mature baby and the sodium intake may need to be increased to overcome the resulting hyponatraemia. The immature kidneys may be unable to excrete some potentially toxic drugs rapidly, e.g. gentamicin, so they should be given less frequently in pre-term infants to avoid accumulation in the blood (p. 168).

Poor resistance to infection

Transfer of maternal immunoglobulin (IgG) across the placenta starts slowly at about 28 weeks, the fetal blood levels only increasing rapidly after 34 weeks. The most immature infants therefore have limited passive immunity and their own ability to produce antibodies in response to infection is poorly developed, as are the cellular immune responses (p. 158).

MANAGEMENT OF THE PRE-TERM INFANT
Prevention

The obstetrician is sometimes able to foretell a premature labour from the maternal history and clinical signs, in which case bed rest is the mainstay of treatment, possibly combined with the use of a uterine muscle-relaxing drug such as ritodrine. Once labour has started, provided that no complications develop which make early delivery necessary, it can sometimes be delayed for at least 24 hours by giving the same group of drugs intravenously or by giving a prostaglandin inhibitor. This delay gives time for administration of a corticosteroid such as dexamethasone for 1–2 days which reduces the risk of hyaline membrane disease in the baby after birth by about 50%.

Delivery and care in the delivery room

It should be possible in most cases to diagnose the onset of premature labour sufficiently early to arrange for delivery to take place where full paediatric back-up and a neonatal intensive care unit with appropriate facilities are at hand, thus avoiding the extra hazard of transfer after birth. The paediatric staff should be fully informed in advance of the history of the pregnancy and someone experienced in resuscitation of very immature infants must be present at delivery.

In pre-term labour, it is wise to minimize narcotic analgesia and provide pain relief by either epidural or light nitrous oxide anaesthesia.

All equipment for resuscitation (including the extra small endotracheal tubes of 2.5 and 3 mm width) and for maintenance of normal body temperature must be checked and made ready.

At birth the baby must be handled very gently. If possible the umbilical cord is allowed to pulsate for at least 1 minute before clamping (p. 32) and the baby is placed in a pre-warmed towel under a correctly adjusted source of radiant heat. He should be gently wiped dry to minimize evaporative heat loss.

A small number of pre-term infants cry vigorously at delivery and in these cases additional respiratory support is unnecessary. However, prompt resuscitation with elective endotracheal intubation and ventilation is advisable for most pre-term babies of less than 30 weeks' gestation and also for some infants of greater maturity, to provide maximal initial expansion of the alveoli and thus reduce the severity of any subsequent respiratory distress syndrome. Details of resuscitation procedures are as described on page 38. A single dose of vitamin K 0.5 mg should be given by intramuscular injection once breathing is established to improve blood coagulation by stimulating hepatic production of clotting factors.

Anxiety over the baby's physical welfare should not be allowed to obscure the emotional needs of the parents in their relationship with him at this time. Unless there is clearly a need for immediate intensive treatment elsewhere, it should be possible to allow the parents to hold their infant at least briefly before tran... neonatal unit. The infant should then be ... ferred in a transport incubator at 34–35°C (93–95°F) or in a specially warmed cot. Time must be set aside for a well informed talk with the parents about the management of the baby and his outlook, and questions about the future answered as honestly and sensitively as possible.

If transfer to a distant intensive care unit is necessary, it is best to undertake the initial assessment and treatment in the hospital of birth and make unhurried preparation for the journey when the infant's condition has been stabilized. In ideal circumstances, an experienced team from the receiving neonatal intensive care unit should travel to the hospital of birth and provide the necessary treatment during the transfer. In some areas, ambulances have been equipped specially to undertake full intensive care during transfer of very sick pre-term infants.

The baby should travel in a continuously warmed portable incubator, but extra insulation is often necessary to prevent excess heat loss, and some favour the use of a plastic bubble wrap or a silver foil swaddler completely enclosing the trunk and limbs.

Care of the pre-term infant in the neonatal unit

Pre-term infants require care which is adapted to take account of the immaturity of their organ systems and homoeostatic mechanisms. However, it must not be forgotten that they have similar human needs to babies born at term. They need sleep, feeding, to be kept clean, to feel secure, to be comfortable and to be subjected to as little stress as possible. Their sight, hearing, senses of touch and smell are well developed. They can feel pain, both physical and emotional. They can respond to pleasant and unpleasant stimuli in appropriate ways. They can communicate their feelings. The ways in which pre-term infants convey distress is through subtle changes of movement, alterations of body functions such as heart rate and blood pressure, or as periods of apnoea rather than crying. Inappropriate methods of care can delay the baby's progress, but providing a suitable environment and sensitive handling can promote a more normal pattern of physiological and emotional development.

Environment

The ambient light in the neonatal unit should only be as bright as is needed to carry out normal care procedures and it is good practice to dim the light at night. There is some evidence that persistent exposure to intense light may damage the retina of the very pre-term infant. Several studies have demonstrated the adverse effects on the baby's physiology of noise generated by the equipment used for care and more particulary by the activities of members of the unit staff. Reducing the volume of equipment alarms and telephones, opening and closing doors and incubator ports gently and speaking quietly all avoid such disturbance. The importance of the environmental temperature is discussed on page 113.

Emotional and developmental needs

So long as their condition permits, pre-term infants should be disturbed as little as possible since they tolerate handling poorly. They should be allowed adequate sleep and rest so that energy is conserved and to ensure the development of a proper sleep pattern. Some nursing and medical interventions are inevitable and the observations and investigations necessary to ensure the baby's safety must be carried out. However, it should be recognized that such procedures as venepuncture, chest physiotherapy and endotracheal suction are particularly uncomfortable for the baby and should be performed only when they are essential. Gentle handling, stroking and talking, particularly from the baby's parents, can settle a distressed infant and induce sleep and should be encouraged. It is also found that maintaining the infant being nursed in an incubator in a flexed position, using supporting towelling rolls, bean bags or sheepskins for example, can relax the baby, prevents his tendency to develop an extended posture in his back, arms and legs, and encourages more normal motor development later.

Care of the skin

The skin of the term infant provides an effective barrier against water loss through evaporation by rapidly developing a thick stratum corneum (p. 47). This process is much slower in the pre-term infant and it may be 2 weeks before its permeability resembles that of a term infant. Insensible water loss through the skin is thus greatly increased until it is fully cornified. Those who care for very pre-term babies will recognize how poorly adhesive monitoring pads stick to their moist skin and how readily it can become sore. Toxic substances applied to the skin may be absorbed rapidly, and adhesive tapes, monitoring pads and urine collecting bags can all traumatize the skin surface as they are removed. The use of only small amounts of tape to secure, for instance, intravenous cannulae or splints safely, and collection of urine into a cotton wool ball placed at the urethral opening are examples of how skin trauma can be limited. Pressure marks occur readily if the position of the infant is not changed at least every 6 hours, and lying the baby on a sheepskin or specialized mattress can also minimize skin damage.

The skin should normally only be cleaned if it is significantly soiled using warm water and cotton wool. Only removal of excessive vernix is necessary initially and full bathing is unnecessary until the baby is ready to go home. Creams, lotions and soaps should not be used routinely as they may all affect the pH of the skin and alter its natural harmless bacterial flora. If a procedure requiring sterilization of an area of skin is performed, only the smallest suitable amount of antiseptic solution should be used to reduce the risk of absorption into the circulation.

Maintenance of body temperature

The importance of providing a sufficiently high ambient temperature to minimize the need for the pre-term baby to produce extra heat and maintain his body temperature has been described on page 32. The smaller the baby, the higher the surrounding air temperature needs to be to keep the body from cooling. Although nursing pre-term infants naked in incubators has the great advantage of easy observation, those of very low birth weight may require extra insulation which is most conveniently provided by baby clothes. The design of current monitoring equipment is such that it can be attached to a clothed infant so that observation of a naked infant is needed only in exceptional circumstances. A perspex heat shield inside the incubator helps if the infant is not covered, but it interferes with access to the baby. Alternatively the baby can wear a bonnet to eliminate excessive heat loss from the head whilst a semi-transparent insulating sheet of bubble plastic which can easily be removed for access covers the rest of the body. A constant room temperature of 24–27°C (75–80°F) surrounding the incubator greatly increases its efficiency. Body temperatures may be monitored either from axillary readings or from an electronic probe on the skin of the abdomen, depending upon equipment available.

Incubators are the traditional means of providing a controlled micro-environment for pre-term infants while allowing ready access to them. The simplest type consists of a perspex hood with access ports in which the temperature and oxygen content can be varied manually. Servo-controlled incubators, which automatically vary their temperature with the changes of the baby's skin temperature, are not a substitute for nursing observation and are generally not adequate to maintain a steady body temperature in the very low birth weight baby. In general, if nursed naked, a 2000 g infant will need an incubator temperature of 34–35°C (93–95°F), reducing to about 32°C (90°F) after 10–14 days. Smaller

babies need even higher surrounding temperatures but the danger of overheating is also considerable. Clothed infants require temperatures about 6–7°C lower than this. For this reason, most incubators are made with a safety device which automatically prevents air temperatures reaching more that 35°C (95°F). Calculations have been made to estimate the ambient temperature at which oxygen consumption, and therefore energy requirement of the naked infant to maintain body temperature, is at a minimum and this has been termed the 'neutral thermal environment'. The environmental temperature needed to achieve this is higher for the small pre-term infant than for his larger full-term counterpart. Such figures are used to set incubator temperatures to minimize the thermal stress to the infant (Table 8.2).

Humidity

To reduce the loss of water through the skin, the relative humidity in the incubator is best kept at about 55–60%. There is no proven advantage in increasing it to very high levels, except for the extremely small infants under 1000 g birth weight in whom losses are often considerable but can be reduced by covering the infant with a polythene sheet. It is, however, essential to humidify oxygen when given in high concentration in order to avoid excessive drying of the respiratory tract.

Precautions against cross-infection

No nurse or doctor with an infection (particular-

Table 8.2 Average incubator temperatures for babies nursed naked

| Birth weight (kg) | Incubator temperature (°C) | | | | | |
	37	36	35	34	33	32
Less than 1.0	l d*	2–14 d	14–21 d	Over 21 d		
1.0–1.5			1–10 d	Over 10 d	Over 21 d	
1.5–2.0				1–10 d	Over 10 d	
2.0–2.5				1–2 d	Over 2 d	Over 21 d
Over 2.5					1–2 d	Over 2 d

* d = days.

ly of skin or bowel) should be allowed to work in a special care unit until clear. However, rigorous barrier nursing of well pre-term infants by healthy attendants is generally unnecessary (p. 72). Meticulous attention to hand washing or the use of an alcohol-based antiseptic lotion before and after handling babies is the greatest practical safeguard against transmitting infection. The wearing of individual gowns or polythene aprons for dealing with any possibly infected babies helps to reduce the contamination of the care giver's clothing, but their routine use and wearing of masks does not reduce cross-infection.

Observation and recording of changes

During the first 24 hours, especially careful observation and frequent recording of the baby's general state is necessary, for it is then that most problems begin. Skin colour, type and rate of respiration, heart rate, core temperature and any abnormal movements must all be included.

Weighing

It is useful to know of changes in body weight, especially as a guide to the regulation of food intake, because, unlike term infants, immature babies do not readily show their need for more food by crying. In an ill baby with respiratory difficulties, the disturbance of weighing should be avoided, but otherwise it should be done at least twice a week. The accumulation of oedema from renal or cardiac failure (p. 206) may cause an excessive weight gain and there is a relatively big drop in weight when it diminishes, so these changes must be allowed for. The rate of weight gain which was taking place before birth can only rarely be maintained in the first week, and although early feeding and the use of specialized premature baby formula milks help to minimize this fall-off, it is often 2 or 3 weeks before adequate weight gain begins, particularly if the baby is sick.

Feeding

Recent advances in our understanding of the nutritional needs of pre-term infants have signif-

icantly improved the prognosis for these infants, although there is as yet no clear consensus on the most appropriate feed to give them. Gastric feeding from the first day or two carries a slightly increased risk of regurgitation and inhalation of milk, but this is outweighed by the benefits of preventing hypoglycaemia, dehydration and undernutrition, all of which can have adverse effects on the developing brain. Even providing very small quantities of gastric feed enhances the functional maturation of the gut and reduces the severity of both jaundice and metabolic bone disease. So long as the baby is well, gastric feeds are usually tolerated and the first one may be given 2–3 hours after birth. Subsequently, the frequency will depend upon the maturity of the baby and the method used. It may be given as a continuous infusion, as hourly or 2-hourly bolus feeds in the smaller infants, or 3-hourly for the larger babies. The mother's colostrum provides some protection against infection and should be given to the infant wherever possible. However, most very small immature babies need their fluid and calorie requirements intravenously for at least the first 48 hours.

Parenteral nutrition

Intravascular administration of 5–10% dextrose solution is required routinely initially for babies under 30 weeks' gestation, those with respiratory distress, seriously growth-retarded infants and any ill babies for the first 48 hours. If enteral feeding beyond this period is inappropriate, adequate nutrition can be achieved by giving a balanced mixture of amino acids, glucose, fats, electrolytes, minerals and vitamins in solution intravenously. The merits and risks of this method of feeding and details of its practical application are described in Chapter 9 (p. 126) but this section will focus on enteral feeding.

Methods of enteral feeding

The method for giving feeds also depends upon the size, maturity and vigour of the individual baby. Infants of more than 35 weeks' gestation are usually able to feed from the *breast* or *bottle*.

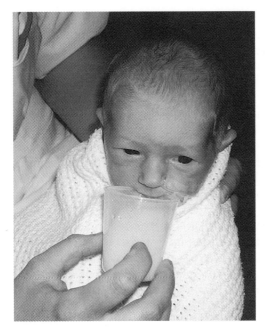

Figure 8.3   Cup feeding with breast milk in a pre-term infant.

is the distance between the nares and the left hypochondrium. Its situation can be checked either by aspirating acid from the stomach or by blowing air down the tube and listening with a stethoscope over the stomach.

Nasojejunal feeding in which a longer tube with a weighted end is passed through the stomach into the jejunum is used for infants of very low birth weight in some units, although its popularity is diminishing as it can be a difficult and prolonged task to site the tube correctly. The method is probably less hazardous than prolonged intravenous feeding if it can be tolerated, but the risk of aspiration of feeds is comparable to nasogastric feeding. Intestinal hurry and diarrhoea may result from such an infusion of milk into the upper small bowel and prevent its continued use.

Types of oral feed

While it is generally agreed that breast milk is best for most pre-term infants, the decision is less clear-cut for the very pre-term baby. Breast milk has the merit of being well tolerated, better absorbed in the gut and, if not heat-treated, it provides some protection against infection and necrotizing enterocolitis (p. 136). It also contains some long chain polyunsaturated fatty acids (such as arachidonic and decosahexanoic acids) which are essential for optimal brain development but are not present in some formula milks.

The mother's early breast milk usually provides between 3 and 5 g protein/kg per day, which is adequate for growth for all but the most growth-retarded infants, but it is very variable in its other constituents. Milk collected by hand or mechanical expression and drip milk are largely composed of fore milk which contains little fat and the calorie content is often inadequate for the pre-term baby. The low sodium and calcium content of breast milk may lead to hyponatraemia and hypocalcaemia in very pre-term infants, and rickets of prematurity may result from too low a supply of phosphate. The total calorie content of human milk is closely related to its fat content and heat treatment may reduce it below the baby's energy needs. Consequently, the baby's

Even if the baby takes no milk, the act of putting him to the breast enhances milk production and increases the chance of successful breast feeding later. Some less mature babies may also manage to take part of a feed which may be supplemented by *cup feeding* (p. 83) (Fig. 8.3). This method has the advantage that the parents can learn the technique rapidly and become more involved in the care of their infant at an early stage.

Oro- or nasogastric feeding using a small-bore disposable polythene tube passed via the mouth or nose into the stomach are alternative methods for the smaller babies who are unable to suck adequately. They have the merit of avoiding disturbance, since the tube can usually be left in place for 2 or 3 days, and demand minimal expenditure of the baby's energy. Provided that experienced nurses are available, it is safer to give a few tube feeds than to allow a pre-term baby to tire himself out by prolonged periods of ineffective sucking. As long as they are trained and supervised, parents can rapidly become adept at tube and cup feeding and should be encouraged to become involved if they so wish. The length of tube required to reach the stomach growth rate may be diminished and the reduced fat intake may provide an inadequate supply of fatty acids for optimal brain growth. Some indication of the calorie intake can be obtained by measuring the percentage of cream in centrifuged milk samples as a 'creamatocrit'. In general, samples with less than 5% fat will supply inadequate calories.

Contamination of breast milk with normal skin flora and pathogenic bacteria frequently prevents consistent supplies and the fear of transmission of HIV infection in pooled breast milk has diminished confidence in its safety, even though heating the milk adequately should abolish any infection risk. In some neonatal units it has become possible to maintain a supply of donated breast milk for the babies by careful selection and informed testing of donors for HIV infection and pasteurization of the milk.

Pasteurization denatures some of the antibacterial substances in breast milk and is probably not necessary for prevention of bacterial infection provided that strict sterile precautions are taken in the collection of the milk and regular microbiological monitoring is carried out.

It can be seen, therefore, that unmodified breast milk does not reliably provide for all the pre-term infant's needs. In addition, standard formula milks which have similar nutrient content to breast milk are also unsuitable for the very pre-term baby, although their more reliable calorie content may be adequate for those nearing term.

Supplementation of breast milk with a commercial 'fortifier' containing additional protein, carbohydrate, sodium, calcium and phosphate may overcome these apparent deficiencies and experience so far suggests they improve the nutritional suitability of breast milk for the very pre-term infant. However, since individual babies have differing requirements, the blood levels of these minerals need to be measured regularly and the amounts of supplements adjusted accordingly.

With these potential problems, it is not surprising that some favour the use of artificial feeds specially adapted for the nutritional needs of the very low birth weight infants using the guide-lines for composition laid down by the European Society for Paediatric Gastroenterology and Nutrition. A number of such preparations are available for use in the first few weeks of life, each 100 ml providing about 75 kcal for energy purposes and containing approximately 1.8 g protein, 7.5 g carbohydrate in mixed form, and 4.5 g fat – mainly as polyunsaturated fatty acids (Table 6.4, p. 85). The sodium content is also increased over the levels occurring in breast milk. The initial growth rate of well pre-term infants is greater when they are fed on these special milks than on unmodified breast milk, although it is comparable when fortifier is added. Comparative studies of the later developmental progress of infants have not shown a clear-cut advantage for pre-term formula milk and some even favour the breast milk groups. Some concern currently exists that the absence of long chain polyunsaturated fatty acids (LCPs) from some formula milks may have an adverse long-term effect on retinal and brain structure and function. Attempts are being made to modify all specialized pre-term baby milks to include LCPs to rectify these deficiencies.

Despite these uncertainties, there is real value in allowing the mother to contribute her milk to her baby as at least part of his feeds, supplementing this with fortifier or pre-term formula to ensure an adequate calorie intake. This should make her feel more involved in his care, that she is contributing to his well-being, and will increase the chance of successfully breast feeding him later on (Fig. 8.4).

The amount of feed necessary is dependent upon the baby's size, maturity and age, modified by individual variation in requirement which can only be judged by experience. When no initial period of intravascular feeding is necessary, the first feed should be the mother's expressed colostrum, supplemented, if the blood glucose is low, by some formula milk. Pre-term infants need more per unit of body weight than those who are fully mature and an energy value of between 105 and 150 kcal/kg is required to maintain weight gain. It will be seen, therefore, that requirements will vary considerably from one infant to another, but the figures in Table 8.3

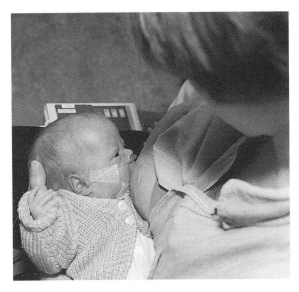

Figure 8.4   Early experience enables mothers to breast feed their pre-term infant.

Table 8.3   A guide to average volumes of milk needed by babies under 2000 g birth weight

Day	Volume (ml/kg body weight per day)	Calories (per kg body weight per day)
1	60	50
2	90	70
3	110	90
4	150	120
5	180	130
6	180–210	140

give a guide to average volumes of milk needed by babies under 2000 g birth weight.

Feeds may be given either as hourly boluses infused over 10–20 minutes or as a continuous infusion, but if a syringe pump is used for breast milk it must be sited below the baby to allow the fat to rise and thus reach the infant.

Although little gain in weight will occur in the first week to 10 days, thereafter an increase of 15 g/kg body weight per day, in the absence of oedema, indicates an adequate calorie intake and the volume of feeds should be adjusted, within the limits of the baby's tolerance, to achieve at least this rate of growth.

Complications of enteral feeding in pre-term infants

Not all pre-term infants tolerate gastric feeding initially. If vomiting, large aspirates before bolus feeds or abdominal distension occur, the feed should either be discontinued or reduced in volume and only gradually be increased again. Very rarely, a mass of milk curd may obstruct the stomach or small bowel and require surgical removal.

Other feeds

Soya milks are not suitable for pre-term infants and should not be used. Elemental feeds, where the constituents of milk have been broken down to basic elements which can be absorbed directly without digestion, are occasionally needed during recovery from necrotizing enterocolitis or following surgery for meconium ileus.

Food supplements

The pre-term infant below about 32 weeks' gestation has an increased liability to develop rickets after about 3 months of age, and this is related to an inadequate phosphate intake. The blood phosphate level should be measured weekly and breast-fed babies with low values should receive a phosphate supplement of 30–40 mg/day and 800 IU/day of vitamin D to ensure good bone mineralization. Pre-term milk formulae are supplemented with adequate amounts for initial feeding but their mineral content is too high for use after the baby has reached 1800 g. Pre-term baby follow-on milks (p. 85) have a reduced mineral content while supplying the phosphate and vitamin D the baby needs and an enhanced protein and calorie content. Studies have shown an increase in growth of pre-term infants fed on this formula.

All growing pre-term infants should also receive vitamin A 500 IU and vitamin C 50 mg daily. Vitamin B supplements are probably not essential but the evidence for this is conflicting, so for convenience and ease of administration a multivitamin preparation is usually given from the third week. Vitamin E deficiency may, rarely, cause a haemolytic anaemia and some authorities recommend supplements of 10 mg daily to prevent it. The doses of vitamins given must be adjusted according to the amounts already incorporated in the milk preparation used and this varies from one brand to another.

Iron. The second phase of anaemia of prematurity (p. 120) is prevented by giving an iron supplement from 4–6 weeks of age onwards. Ferrous sulphate 2.5 mg/kg daily is generally satisfactory, although if it causes constipation, some babies may tolerate another preparation of iron better. Some authorities suggest that giving iron reduces the anti-infective properties of unsaturated iron-binding proteins in breast milk but the risk from this effect is small. Pre-term babies of very low birth weight require a small folic acid supplement of 100 mcg daily to prevent a later macrocytic anaemia.

The important parental link

In spite of what has been said about the need for specialized nursing care for these small infants, the role of the baby's parents as part of the caring team must be recognized. The initial separation which is often necessary is liable to strain any parent–child relationship and much can be done to reduce this by encouraging them to become involved in the baby's care at every opportunity – what happens at this early stage will increase their confidence in their parenting skills and thus affect the child's future development.

THE COMMON DISORDERS OF THE PRE-TERM INFANT

Most of the conditions described in other sections of this book may affect these babies. When illness occurs, the many disadvantages from immaturity of his organ systems diminish the infant's ability to deal with it, and the diagnosis may be delayed since the clinical signs are often non-specific and can be difficult to interpret. The immaturity of the central nervous system, gastrointestinal tract, lungs, liver and immune system lies behind many of the disorders encountered.

Respiratory problems

Periodic respiration

Periodic respiration with repeated short spells of very shallow breathing or complete cessation lasting 3–10 seconds is a commonly observed phenomenon which is almost normal for small pre-term babies. The pattern reflects diminished responsiveness of the respiratory centre in the brain stem to changes in the oxygen and carbon dioxide levels in the blood which varies with the state of consciousness and is therefore more common during sleep. More regular respiration may be achieved by slightly raising the oxygen content of the surrounding air, although it is important to avoid high oxygen levels in the blood by careful saturation monitoring.

Apnoeic attacks

True apnoeic attacks are different and potentially more serious. Breathing stops suddenly, the apnoea usually lasts for more than 20 seconds and may be accompanied by bradycardia and cyanosis. The attacks may not always have a clear predisposing cause, but they are often associated with the respiratory distress syndrome (p. 135), hypoglycaemia (p. 97), cerebral haemorrhage, electrolyte imbalance or the presence of sepsis.

Treatment of the underlying cause may be effective, but if it is not, the possibility that the apnoeic attacks may be fits should be investigated (p. 149). The accompanying cyanosis should be treated by stimulating the baby to breathe and giving additional oxygen if the colour does not return promptly.

Apnoea alarm devices are useful in alerting nursing staff to the need for action. The baby lies on a pressure-sensitive pad or has a similar sensor attached to the skin which automatically activates a buzzer after breathing has ceased for more than a selected period. Stimulation of the baby by touch or movement may be successful when apnoea is not prolonged and the attacks will gradually diminish.

Raising the oxygen content of the inspired air is ineffective in more prolonged apnoeic attacks and may be dangerous if the baby is left in a high oxygen environment after breathing restarts (p. 138). Administration of caffeine is an effective treatment where the infant has no treatable cause for the attacks. It is reliably absorbed after oral administration and blood level monitoring is not often needed. It is given as an initial dose of 50 mg/kg intravenously over 1 hour, or as two oral doses of 25 mg/kg 1 hour apart, followed by 12 mg/kg orally as a daily maintenance dose. Alternatively, aminophylline can be given intravenously or as a suppository of 2.5–5 mg at 6-hourly intervals but the blood level should be measured to confirm that a therapeutic dose is being given. When simple measures fail to maintain adequate respiratory function, continuous positive airways pressure (CPAP) is often successful. Only rarely is continued artificial ventilation needed.

The respiratory distress syndrome

Difficulty with breathing soon after birth is very common in pre-term infants. An increased respiratory rate, grunting or recession of the sternum or rib margins may indicate one of a number of possible conditions, amongst which are pneumothorax, congenital heart disease with cardiac failure, septicaemia and pneumonia (especially from group B β-haemolytic streptococcal infection), meconium aspiration and cerebral birth injury. However, by far the commonest cause in the pre-term infant is hyaline membrane disease, the familiar clinical picture of which led to the use of the term 'respiratory distress syndrome' (RDS). It occurs in almost all infants under 30 weeks' gestation but is less frequent in more mature babies. This is the main condition requiring artificial ventilation in the newborn period and is described in detail in Chapter 9.

Alimentary tract problems

Gastro-oesophageal reflux

Regurgitation of gastric contents into the lower oesophagus between feeds occurs in most pre-term infants. Occasionally, more major degrees of this reflux result in vomiting or posseting, which may be associated with aspiration of milk or acid into the lungs and a consequent respiratory infection. This gastro-oesophageal reflux can be confirmed by a barium swallow X-ray, by ultrasound or by measuring the pH (acidity) of the lower oesophagus continuously using an indwelling naso-oesophageal electrode. It is treated by keeping the infant tilted head-up and using an antacid and alginate mixture to thicken the feed.

Abdominal distension

Distension of the abdomen caused by gaseous dilatation of the immature gut is often troublesome, especially in the second week, and may be severe enough to interfere with respiration by restricting diaphragmatic movement. Whilst it is often benign and relieved by a modification of the feeding schedule, it can also be a manifestation of more serious disorders such as septicaemia or due to a congenital malformation of the intestine. Intestinal obstruction from inspissated milk curd is a rare cause when formula milk is used for feeding and can sometimes necessitate surgical intervention (p. 203). Hard faeces in the lower colon and rectum may also be a problem but can often be relieved by the use of small rectal suppositories or saline washouts.

Jaundice

Immature liver function renders the baby slow to deal with bilirubin by conjugation and excretion (p. 187). Kernicterus, with its later consequences of nerve deafness, athetoid cerebral palsy and learning difficulties, is more likely to follow in a pre-term infant with a lower level of serum bilirubin than in a term baby. Opinions differ about the level of serum bilirubin at which the pigment is likely to pass the blood-brain barrier, but in the smallest infants, more than 250 (μmol/L (15 mg/100 ml) may be a danger, whilst 300–340 μmol/L (18–20 mg/100 ml) can be regarded as a hazard for those over 34 weeks' gestation. Phototherapy (p. 187) has reduced the need for exchange transfusion, but it must be employed at an early stage to be effective, and charts indicating the levels at which it should be applied are available (Fig.12.1).

Oedema

The shiny 'full' appearance of the skin of the pre-term infant at birth is due to water retention and is lost within a few days, but it should not be regarded as pathological. True oedema with pitting on pressure, due probably to increased capillary permeability, is, however, a common finding in the first week and usually affects the feet, hands, face and external genitalia, subsiding gradually without apparent harm. More serious generalized oedema is seen in conjunction with the respiratory distress syndrome, congestive cardiac failure or severe haemolytic disease. The use of a diuretic such as frusemide may be justifiable, although fluid restriction is the treatment of choice if the baby is hyponatraemic.

Sclerema

Sclerema is now rare and affects mainly pre-term or debilitated infants, particularly those who have suffered either prolonged asphyxia, septicaemia or chilling. There is hardening of the skin and subcutaneous tissue, often starting over the buttocks and spreading to the whole body, but no pitting oedema. The tightness of the skin upon the underlying parts with the accompanying stiffness of the joints has given rise to the apt description 'skin-bound'. It is generally a sign of serious import but exchange transfusion using fresh blood has been found to be occasionally effective when the condition has resulted from severe infection. Systemic steroids are usually ineffective.

Anaemia

There are two phases of anaemia following pre-term birth. In the first, the initial high haemoglobin slowly falls over the first few weeks, reaching an average of 9 g/dl by 2 months of age (compared with 11 g/dl in a term infant). This early anaemia is normochromic and in healthy pre-term infants is largely due to a reduced rate of red cell production in the bone marrow, which is common to all babies and is caused by the diminished erythropoietin production from the immature infant's kidneys. Taking blood samples for laboratory testing adds to the decline in haemoglobin level, and in babies requiring frequent tests, such as those undergoing intensive care, it may also reduce the blood volume. Treatment with iron or folic acid does not alter its progress. As the haemoglobin falls towards a figure of 10 g/dl, a high reticulocyte count (p. 178) in the peripheral blood indicates that the bone marrow is actively producing red cells again and no action is needed as long as the baby is well. If, on the other hand, the infant is unwell, or unable to fully breast or bottle feed because of breathlessness from the anaemia, a small blood transfusion of about 25 ml/kg body weight may be beneficial to keep the haemoglobin level above 12 g/dl. Treatment with a combination of intramuscular erythropoietin and oral iron can restore the haemoglobin level, but it is expensive and is not yet in common use.

Some 4–6 weeks after the expected birth date, the haemoglobin level begins to rise, but there may be a second fall at 3–4 months of age which is characterized by hypochromia of the red cells. This phase is related to iron deficiency and responds well to oral iron supplements. Macrocytic anaemia is occasionally seen in the second or third month and routine administration of folic acid (50–100 mcg daily) to babies of less than 34 weeks' gestation is advised.

Haemolytic anaemia in the second month due to vitamin E deficiency has also been reported.

Infections

Minor infections found in term infants are described in Chapter 11. These may all occur in the pre-term infant but are less easily detected because of the immature infant's poorer immune responses.

Severe infections are even less easy to recognize. The body temperature is more likely to drop than to rise and the other signs are often entirely non-specific – a general lethargy, refusal to feed, vomiting, pallor and persistent mild jaundice. In any baby showing such signs, full septic screening and treatment with intravenous antibiotics should be started while awaiting the results of the bacterial cultures. Intravascular long lines and endotracheal tubes may become infected with normally harmless bacteria such as *Staph. epidermidis*. Such infections will not respond to antibiotics and the tubes must be removed.

Other minor disorders related to pre-term birth

Umbilical hernias, undescended testes and multiple strawberry marks (Plate 8.11) are all more common in babies born prematurely. None requires treatment in the newborn period, although orchidopexy may be needed in infancy. On the other hand a third of inguinal hernias (Fig. 8.5) will strangulate and require emergency surgery if untreated and therefore early elective surgical correction should be carried out.

Routine immunizations in pre-term infants

Pre-term babies should receive the recommended schedule of immunisations at 2, 3 and

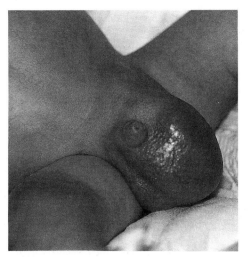

Figure 8.5   Inguinal hernia is common in pre-term babies.

4 months after the birth date, irrespective of the extent of prematurity. They are able to produce adequate antibody responses at this time and adverse reactions are no more common than in term infants.

THE OUTLOOK FOR SURVIVING PRE-TERM BABIES

All the evidence shows a big improvement in the quality of life to be expected for these babies due to improvements in obstetric and perinatal care in the last few years. Because changes are taking place continuously, it is impossible to give accurate statistics applicable to the present time. The outlook for development depends upon the cause of the prematurity, and it is often more affected by factors operating during intrauterine life than by complications in the neonatal period. The addition of any major congenital malformation will influence developmental progress. Poor maternal fertility and low socioeconomic status also greatly influence the outcome.

The prospects for survival and normal development in pre-term infants are now good, especially if they are more than 1500 g at birth and do not have any associated congenital abnormalities. Reviews of progress over the past 10 years show that the marked rise in the number of surviving infants below 1500 g birth weight has been accompanied by a small increase in the number of children with cerebral palsy, particularly the survivors of extreme prematurity although there is no increase in those with serious developmental impairment. Those most at risk have a gestation period of well under 28 weeks or are less than 750 g birth weight, especially if they are also undernourished in utero. The outcome for babies under 1000 g is that about one baby in 10 who survives will have a measurable and lasting disability, including impaired growth or retinopathy of prematurity (p. 138), and a smaller number will have a more severe handicap. With good obstetrics and the best neonatal care, well over 80% of all babies under 1500 g can now be expected to survive and only some 5% will suffer a handicap sufficient to interfere seriously with their lives. A rather greater number will be found to have some degree of learning difficulties or disorders of behaviour, but perinatal events may have less bearing on this than socioeconomic and genetic factors.

Cerebral palsy in the form of spastic diplegia, which used to be the predominant handicap to be feared in babies born very prematurely, is now relatively uncommon; but the incidence of other forms such as quadriplegia and athetosis has not significantly diminished and has shown a slight rise in recent years, particularly in babies of over 1500 g birth weight.

As methods of care improve, there is every reason to expect the complications of both prematurity and its management to diminish. However, even for intact survivors there is an increased risk of sudden infant death syndrome during the first year of life and this is greater still if the baby has bronchopulmonary dysplasia (p. 139). It should not be forgotten that the emotional stress suffered by the parents during the initial illness may result in continued anxiety about the baby and this is the probable reason for the increased rates of admission to hospital in the first year of life. In general it seems likely that whilst better facilities for neonatal intensive care for low birth weight infants over 750 g will have some further beneficial effect on the quality of their lives, greater benefits overall will result from improvement in the supporting health services and in providing better antenatal education for those families who are at a socioeconomic disadvantage.

FURTHER READING

Ballard J, Novak K, Driver M 1979 a simplified score for assessment of fetal maturation of newly born infants. Journal of Paediatries 95: 769–774

Balmer S, Wharton B 1992 Human milk banking at Sorrento maternity hospital Birmingham. Archives of Disease in Childhood 67: 556–559

Chalmers I, Enkin M, Keirse M 1992 Effective care in pregnancy and childbirth. Oxford University Press, Oxford

Davies D P (ed) 1995 Nutrition in child health. Royal College of Physicians, London

Decsi T, Koletzko B 1994 Polyunsaturated fatty acids in infant nutrition. Acta Paediatrica Supplement 83(395): 31–37

Gray P, Burns Y, Mohay H, O'Callaghan M, Tudehope D 1995 Neurodevelopmental outcome of preterm infants with bronchopulmonary dysplasia. Archives of Disease in Childhood 73: F128–F134

Levene M, Dowling S, Graham M, Fogelman K, Galton M, Philips M 1992 Impaired motor function (clumsiness) in 5-year old children: correlation with neonatal ultrasound scans. Archives of Disease in Childhood 67: 687–690

Levene M, Liford R (eds) 1995 Fetal and neonatal neurology and neurosurgery. Churchill Livingstone, Edinburgh

Lucas A, Bishop N J, King F J, Cole T J 1992 Randomised trial of nutrition for preterm infants after discharge. Archives of Disease in Childhood 67: 324–327

Powls A, Botting N, Cooke R W, Marlow N 1995 Motor impairment in children 12–13 years old with a birthweight of less than 1250g. Archives of Disease in Childhood 73: F62–F66

Roberton N R C (ed) 1992 Textbook of neonatology. Churchill Livingstone, Edinburgh

Ryan S W (ed) 1996 Seminars in neonatology – Enteral nutrition. W B Saunders, London

Salisbury D M, Begg N T 1996 Immunisation against infectious disease. HMSO, London

Sinclair J, Bracken M 1992 Effective care of the newborn infant. Oxford University Press, Oxford

Stanley F, Watson L 1992 Trends in perinatal mortality and cerebral palsy in Western Australia 1967–1985. British Medical Journal 304: 1658–1662

Steer P 1991 Premature labour. Archives of Disease in Childhood 66: 1167–1170

The Scottish Low Birthweight Study 1992 1. Survival, growth, neuromotor and sensory impairment. Archives of Disease in Childhood 67: 675–681

The Scottish Low Birthweight Study 1992 2. Language attainment, cognitive status and behavioural problems. Archives of Disease in Childhood 67: 682–686

The Victorian Infant Collaborative Study Group 1995 Neurosensory outcome at 5 years and extremely low birthweight. Archives of Disease in Childhood 73: F143–F146

Tsang R C, Lucas A, Uauy R, Zlotkin S (eds) 1993 Nutritional needs of the preterm infant. Williams and Wilkins, Baltimore

9

Intensive neonatal care

The large reduction in the overall perinatal mortality rate over the last 25 years is due to many factors, including better antenatal care, improved management of labour and the development of skilled intensive care for sick babies, particularly those of very low birth weight. Although they amount to only about 1% of births, babies under 2500 g birth weight take up a relatively large proportion of skilled medical and nursing resources. Not only has there been an increase in survival of these infants, but also the risk of serious handicap in the survivors is small, except for the minority with a birth weight below 750 g.

Excellent texts have been written which describe intensive care in detail, but it is the intention here to introduce the subject, outlining the main requirements for its provision and the general principles involved.

CATEGORIES OF CARE FOR NEWBORN BABIES

The degree of nursing and medical expertise required to provide newborn babies with the care they need varies markedly from one infant to the next. Normal care can be defined as that given by the mother with access to medical and nursing advice at her request. Special care exceeds normal care but can be provided at the mother's bedside or in a separate unit. It requires qualified neonatal nursing skills and involves teaching and supporting the baby's parents. High dependency care needs continuous skilled neonatal nursing and rapidly available paediatric medical care. Maximal intensive care requires a fully equipped unit with specially trained medical and nursing staff on hand at all times.

Babies requiring intensive care are for the most part those who need prolonged assistance with ventilation, continued monitoring by access to the arterial circulation or total parenteral nutrition.

They include the following categories:

- Extremely immature babies of very low birth weight (under 1000 g or less than 30 weeks' gestation)
- Respiratory disorders – pre-term babies with severe respiratory distress syndrome, severe pneumonia, meconium aspiration or pneumothorax
- Cerebral disorders – severe or persistent fits, severe hypoxic-ischaemic encephalopathy
- Certain severe infections – meningitis, septicaemia
- After major neonatal surgery, e.g. for congenital heart disease, intestinal atresias, gastroschisis, neural tube defects, diaphragmatic hernia
- Haemolytic disease of the newborn requiring exchange transfusion.

REQUIREMENTS FOR NEONATAL INTENSIVE CARE

In Britain the facilities for long-term intensive respiratory care are mainly situated in major regional hospitals, often many miles from the parents' home. Such care is complex and requires a full range of support for it to be safe and effective. It cannot be provided in every maternity hospital and ideally all infants requiring intensive care should be born in a hospital which can provide it, if necessary by transferring the mother to that hospital before she delivers. However, it is not always possible to achieve this goal and all maternity units in district general hospitals need to provide the facilities to support an infant requiring ventilation until she can be safely transferred to an intensive care unit.

The intensive care unit itself should be sited as near as possible to the delivery suite or operating theatre where the babies are delivered to minimize the hazards during transfer. It should be provided with facilities to vary the temperature of each section to suit the needs of the infants being nursed there, hand washing facilities in each room, good lighting and piped oxygen, air and suction outlets for each baby. There should be a section in which babies may be isolated if they have an infectious disease and a place where parents may be reasonably private if, for instance, their baby is dying. The parents should have access to facilities to enable them to stay with their baby for as much of the time as possible, including being able to sleep alongside her at critical times, although in practice this is rarely possible because of the intensive nature of the nursing care.

The unit must have support from the full range of laboratory services to provide rapid and accurate results throughout the day and night. They should be able to work with very small blood samples for biochemical and haematological investigations. Arterial blood gas analysis is preferably done on the ward itself so that the results are immediately available. It must be possible to X-ray the baby with minimum disturbance and undertake ultrasound examination of the brain or heart within an incubator and without disrupting ventilation. Pharmacy services must be able to provide emergency supplies of drugs and materials for intravenous nutrition at all times, and a dietitian should be able to advise on the nutritional requirements of the infant. Since many such infants develop cardiac or surgical complications, there must be rapid access to the relevant departments for advice, investigation and intervention when needed. Much of the equipment used in intensive care is complicated and highly technical and requires maintenance for which expert advice and support must be available.

Medical and nursing staff

The best survival rates of very immature babies without serious handicap are reported from units where there is an adequate number of nursing and medical staff who have had training and experience in treating the conditions and illnesses encountered and who understand and are familiar with the complex equipment and techniques involved. The intensive care of newborn babies is rewarding but also very demanding, requiring a high degree of skill, understanding and an ability to respond rapidly to the emergencies which are common in such infants. The emotional costs are also high – parents, other relatives and staff all being likely to feel stressed at times. Some units have a system to ensure that this is recognized so that those feeling the strain can be counselled and supported.

PRINCIPLES OF INTENSIVE CARE

Monitoring

Whatever the underlying condition for which a baby requires intensive care, there are certain general principles which govern how she is supported and treated. In general, since she is unable to maintain her normal physiological activities adequately, each needs to be evaluated regularly, deviations from normal detected and corrective measures applied. Routine nursing observations of the infant are the basis of such an evaluation, but for a more continuous assessment specific electronic apparatus is needed.

The best equipment is able to monitor several body functions simultaneously and to give an alarm signal when one function strays outside the limits of the normal range, in order to warn the staff immediately that action is needed to remedy it. It can also retain the information gained in its memory and display graphically the variation in the baby's progress over a specified period of time. (Fig. 9.1)

The apparatus should be able to give continuous monitoring of the following items:

- heart rate and ECG pattern
- central (abdominal skin) and peripheral (toe) temperature
- respiration rate
- blood pressure – invasive and non-invasive
- oxygen and carbon dioxide levels in the blood
- oxygen content in the inspired air in the incubator

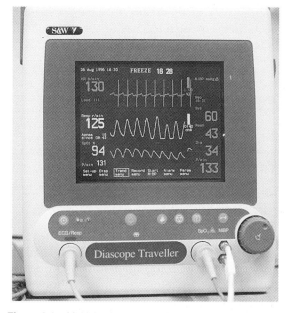

Figure 9.1 Multiple physiological functions monitoring apparatus using both numerical and graphical displays.

All this can be achieved using electrodes or apparatus attached to the skin of the infant or by sensing equipment placed in the incubator. Other information can be obtained only by testing the baby's blood directly, taking samples from catheters placed in an artery or vein, or by collecting capillary blood from a heel prick.

Direct measurement of the blood gases on arterial blood samples must be immediately available to monitor the infant's lung function, and regular measurements of the blood glucose and bilirubin should be possible on the ward.

All information obtained must be recorded on an intensive care chart designed to show it in such a way as to demonstrate the changes which occur and when they do so. If the infant is being artificially ventilated, all ventilator settings should also be recorded. The nurse should chart the environmental factors, such as the incubator temperature, humidity, oxygen concentration of the inspired gas and any other feature which might affect the infant. The type and volume of fluids administered and whether they are given parenterally or enterally should be recorded with times at which the infant passes urine or faeces.

Attention to small details of changes in such observations is often the key to a successful outcome for the infant and the importance of careful recording cannot be overstated.

Temperature control

The very small infant loses heat rapidly through the usual mechanisms of conduction of heat to the objects she is touching, convection through heating the surrounding air, radiation and evaporation of fluid from the skin. The immaturity of response in the extremely pre-term infant's skin blood vessels limits severely her ability to retain heat, and the increased permeability of her skin to water results in excessive fluid losses. To minimize these problems the infant must be nursed in a surrounding temperature which reduces energy expenditure to a minimum (p. 112) and high humidity to diminish fluid loss. For many larger infants an open cot with an overhead radiant heater is suitable, although excess water loss from the skin may occur. For babies under 1000 g it is difficult to prevent excessive loss of heat and fluid when nursed on an open cot and a closed incubator is preferable. In incubators, heat losses are minimized by maintaining a high temperature, controlling the flow of air, and by keeping the humidity high, thus limiting losses from convection, conduction and evaporation. In addition the walls of the incubator reduce radiant heat losses by reflecting the heat back towards the infant. However, it is sometimes more difficult to nurse babies in closed incubators, particularly if several practical procedures are required, and the choice of apparatus used must take into account all these factors.

Fluids and nutrition

Correct management of fluid and electrolyte balance is vital for very small infants and in general more harm is done by giving too much fluid than too little, for it can cause pulmonary and cerebral oedema, cardiac failure and persistent shunting of blood through a patent ductus arteriosus. Sodium depletion or overloading easily occurs. Hypocalcaemia commonly requires correction with a 10% calcium gluconate supplement during the first few days. The plasma albumin level may fall due to impaired synthesis and can contribute to hypotension and oedema. This can be treated by an infusion of plasma or human albumin. Daily measurements of blood electrolytes and protein levels are essential to enable adjustments to be made to the infant's fluid regime.

In view of the almost inevitable respiratory disorders, oral or nasogastric fluids are seldom tolerated well at first. The baby's fluid requirements in the first 2 days can be satisfied by giving 10% dextrose intravenously, starting at a rate of 50–60 ml/kg per day for the first 2 or 3 days, gradually increasing to 180 ml/kg per day over 5–7 days. Sodium and potassium additions are necessary after the first 24 hours. When the baby is well enough to start nasogastric or nasojejunal feeding (p. 115), feeds can be given hourly either as bolus feeds of 2 ml/kg body weight of expressed breast milk or, in similar amounts, as a continuous intragastric infusion. This amount can be increased every 6–12 hours depending on how well the feeds are absorbed, which is assessed by measuring how much milk remains in the stomach before the next feed is given. Intravenous fluids should be reduced by an equivalent amount until the whole of the fluid requirement is being administered into the gastrointestinal tract.

Total parenteral nutrition

In cases where the infant is unable to tolerate enteral feeding, total parenteral nutrition will become necessary sooner or later depending on the degree of prematurity and the nutritional status of the infant. The solution given will consist of an amino acid mixture, to enable the infant to make proteins; calories, in the form of 10% dextrose; lipid, to provide the essential fatty acids for brain development; and minerals, vitamins and electrolytes.

The minerals will include phosphate, calcium, magnesium, zinc and copper. In most units the infusions are prescribed according to written protocols and made up for use in the pharmacy. The lipid, amino acid and dextrose contents are increased each day at standard rates to allow for metabolic compensation and are adjusted according to the results of regular blood tests. It is essential to monitor lipid levels in the serum since high values may result in pulmonary, hepatic and possibly retinal damage. Appropriate water-soluble and fat-soluble vitamins are added each day to the aqueous and lipid solutions, respectively. If parenteral nutrition is prolonged, additional vitamin K and B_{12} may need to be given as intramuscular injections. Occasionally, a small blood transfusion may be needed to replace the blood taken for monitoring purposes.

Accurate monitoring of blood for electrolytes, calcium, glucose, albumin, lipids and packed cell volume is essential at least daily and other investigations such as serum bilirubin, transaminases and triglycerides at longer intervals. Adjustments to the various constituents are made daily according to the results of these tests.

Complications are not infrequent and these include electrolyte imbalance, phosphate depletion and cholestatic jaundice. Thrombosis at the site of the indwelling catheter and septicaemia (especially *Candida albicans*) also occur but can be minimized by extreme care in inserting the catheter and preparation of fluids.

It can be appreciated from this very brief account that total parenteral nutrition should not be undertaken lightly and requires both experience and close cooperation among medical, nursing, laboratory and pharmacy personnel to be safe and successful.

Technique of venepuncture, insertion of intravenous cannulae and central venous catheters

Suitable veins for setting up intravenous infusions are found in the antecubital fossae, the back of the hand, the dorsum of the feet and on the side of the scalp. Sometimes in a thin baby the saphenous vein at the ankle can be used. If time allows, the topical application of local anaesthetic cream for an hour beforehand may reduce the pain of cannulation. Full aseptic technique is required to avoid introducing infection. After preparing the skin with an antiseptic lotion, the limb is squeezed gently above the intended site and secured below it. For scalp veins, compression below the entry site makes the vein prominent. In each procedure the cannula is gently advanced into the vein until the blood flows well and samples are collected if needed. The outer cannula is then pushed further up the vein as the stilette is withdrawn. Either an infusion is set up or, if not required, the patency of the cannula may be maintained by intermittent flushing with a weak heparin solution or normal saline.

If a long intravenous line is required, either a fine silastic catheter can be threaded through a larger needle placed in the vein or a fine guide wire can be inserted into the vein and the catheter passed over it. When the tip of the catheter is near the central veins, the guide wire is withdrawn and the tube secured with tape. Such long lines often last many days and are suitable for prolonged parenteral feeding.

Prevention and management of infection

Natural protection against infection is limited in the newborn infant and especially so if the baby is born prematurely (p. 157). Intensive care inevitably involves invasive procedures, such as insertion of cannulae and endotracheal intubation, which give increased opportunity for organisms to gain entry, so that all the methods of prevention described on page 72 must be employed all the more rigorously. When these precautions fail and there are general signs of infection, samples of blood, urine and usually cerebrospinal fluid (CSF) should be sent for bacterial cultures, together with swabs from suspected infected sites, and broad-spectrum intravenous antibiotics should be started while awaiting the results of the investigations. A combination of gentamicin and flucloxacillin or cefotaxime alone would be suitable initial antibiotics.

In many situations, such as the respiratory distress syndrome, infection enters the differential diagnosis of the baby's symptoms. In such cases, antibiotics should always be given until infection has been excluded by a combination of an improvement in the baby's condition and the results of the initial investigations.

Respiratory care

Many very pre-term infants and some sick but more mature babies either cannot breathe adequately or their lungs are unable to maintain normal gaseous exchange. Oxygenation and removal of carbon dioxide from the blood are impaired, which results in abnormal blood gas values and acidaemia. In these circumstances, it is often necessary to provide artificial mechanical ventilation for the baby.

Although it is not the only disease for which ventilation is needed, the respiratory distress syndrome is by far the commonest disorder in pre-term infants to require it, and thus it is described in detail as one example of neonatal intensive respiratory care.

RESPIRATORY DISTRESS SYNDROME (RDS, HYALINE MEMBRANE DISEASE)

Difficulty with breathing is a very common problem for the newborn baby. In the term infant, the possible causes include pneumothorax, congenital heart disease, pneumonia (especially with group B β-haemolytic streptococci), meconium aspiration, cerebral birth injury and transient tachypnoea of the newborn. Although any of these can occur in the pre-term baby, by far the commonest cause in this group is hyaline membrane disease, which is often called respiratory distress syndrome (RDS). This title describes the clinical picture seen in the first few hours of life. It is the major underlying cause of death in the pre-term infant and constitutes the largest group requiring intensive care. It occurs occasionally in mature neonates, particularly in the infants of diabetic mothers, those born after caesarean section or in the case of any illness causing hypotension in the mother in labour. The condition varies greatly in intensity, causing severe problems in some infants, yet, surprisingly, some extremely immature babies do not develop it at all, particularly if there has been prolonged stress or poor nutrition in utero. Pre-eclampsia, maternal hypertension, retroplacental bleeding and prolonged rupture of the membranes all reduce the risk or severity of RDS, as, curiously, does narcotic addiction. The incidence of RDS can be halved by the administration of intramuscular corticosteroids to the mother in the 48 hours prior to delivery. Conversely, acute stress just prior to delivery or placental abruption may increase the severity of RDS.

Pathogenesis of RDS

The pathogenesis of the condition is complex but relates to both the immaturity of the cells lining the alveoli and the inadequate amount of surfactant they produce. Although the bronchi have been completely formed by about the midtrimester, the cells lining the alveoli are cuboidal rather than the thin flattened cells of the mature lung. This thickening of the alveolar walls reduces the rate both of oxygen transfer from the air in the alveoli to the blood in the pulmonary circulation and of the loss of carbon dioxide from it. As they mature, some of the cells lining the alveoli, known as type II alveolar cells, produce surfactant, a phospholipid substance which reduces the surface tension in the alveoli. This prevents the air sacs from collapsing when the baby exhales and enables them to expand during the phase of negative intrathoracic pressure which occurs in inspiration. In the absence of surfactant, the surface of the lung available for gas exchange progressively diminishes as more and more alveoli collapse, oxygenation of the blood becomes impaired and carbon dioxide cannot be exhaled adequately. If untreated, the lungs become unable to sustain adequate function, and in the most severe cases death may result. In this situation the postmortem histology of the lungs shows an exudate of hyaline material in the collapsed alveoli and the terminal bronchi.

Before birth, an indication of the amount of surfactant and thus the maturity of the lungs can be obtained by measuring the lecithin–sphingomyelin ratio in the amniotic fluid. If the level is greater than 1.5:1 then severe RDS is unlikely to occur. The production of surfactant can be increased by giving the mother a 48 hour course of oral steroids before delivery. The effect is only temporary, but it is known that it reduces the mortality from RDS substantially. Further courses can be given, if necessary, if labour is delayed by more than a week.

As well as the immaturity of the lungs, the pulmonary arterioles do not dilate as rapidly after birth as they do in the mature baby. As a result the pulmonary vascular resistance remains high, causing shunting of blood through the foramen ovale in the heart, the open ductus arteriosus and through the intrapulmonary capillaries in unventilated portions of the lungs.

Clinical features

Respiratory distress is the major symptom of the condition. It may be present from birth or may develop slowly over the next few hours. The respiration rate increases and, if the disease is severe, an increasing concentration of inspired oxygen is needed to prevent cyanosis. There is retraction of the sternum and the lower ribs on inspiration (Fig. 9.2) and a marked expiratory grunt. Auscultation is often unhelpful but occasionally fine râles are heard and breath sounds are always reduced and often inaudible. The baby usually lies still, although she sometimes develops cerebral irritation from birth asphyxia. Although present in almost all cases of RDS, these features are common to many respiratory conditions and a chest X-ray may establish which, if any, of the other causes of respiratory distress is present. In hyaline membrane disease, the X-ray shows diffuse 'ground glass' mottling of the lung fields against which the bronchial tree shows up prominently as an air bronchogram (Fig. 9.3). Even this appearance is not specific to RDS, since the same pattern is seen in congenital group B β-haemolytic streptococcal pneumonia. Thus, initially the diagnosis must be provisional. Infection is excluded by negative blood cultures and transient tachypnoea of the newborn (p. 101) by observing rapid resolution within 48 hours. Hyaline membrane disease itself persists for much longer, being at its

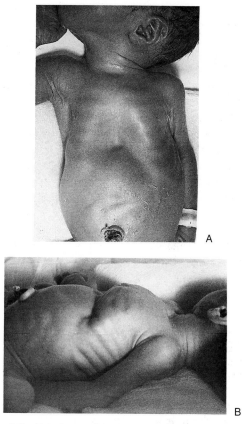

Figure 9.2   Respiratory distress syndrome in pre-term infants. A: Sternal recession B: Subcostal recession.

worst between 24 and 72 hours with gradual resolution thereafter.

Management

The course of RDS in any individual baby is difficult to predict, being mild and resolving rapidly in some but becoming profound and life-threatening in others. In general, babies of less than 32 weeks' gestation will often require assisted ventilation at some point. For those infants below 28 weeks, it is usual to assume the condition will be severe and to apply assisted ventilation from the start.

Treatment starts in the labour ward where any infant who may develop RDS should be effectively resuscitated at birth by giving active respiratory support to those infants who do not

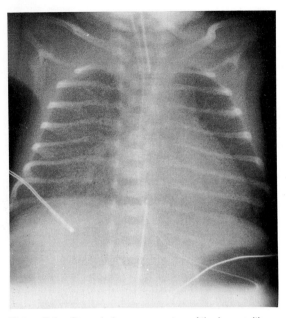

Figure 9.3 Ground glass appearance of the lungs with a superimposed air bronchgram in a chest X-ray in respiratory distress syndrome.

breathe adequately. Ensuring rapid initial oxygenation and expansion of the alveoli, preventing hypothermia and maintaining a normal blood glucose level all reduce the severity of the subsequent RDS.

The object of treatment thereafter is:

- to maintain the oxygenation of the blood at a safe level
- to ensure the elimination of carbon dioxide from the blood
- to maintain a normal body temperature
- to keep the baby's biochemical status within normal limits
- to provide adequate nutrition to ensure optimal growth.

This should be achieved with the minimum of handling and disturbance consistent with obtaining the necessary observations from the infant. It will continue until the lungs are able to function normally as natural surfactant begins to be formed in the alveoli.

Increasing respiratory distress is an indication for continuous monitoring and recording of clinical signs. Enteral feeds should be stopped and replaced by an infusion of 10% dextrose through a venous cannula inserted into a peripheral vein. The insertion of an umbilical or peripheral arterial catheter enables arterial blood to be taken as necessary for blood gas analysis and glucose and electrolyte estimation. It also allows the direct measurement of arterial blood pressure.

Oxygen therapy

The objective of oxygen therapy is to prevent both hypoxia and hyperoxaemia. This can be achieved by varying the concentration of oxygen in the humidified inspired air to maintain an oxygen saturation of between 92 and 95% or an arterial Po_2 between 6 and 9 kPa. Too much oxygen is as dangerous as too little and may cause not only a deterioration in lung function but also permanent eye damage in the form of retinopathy of prematurity. Skin colour is a misleading indicator of significant hypoxia. If a concentration of greater than 30% oxygen is needed, it indicates significant lung dysfunction, and both oxygen and carbon dioxide levels should be measured. Transcutaneous oxygen saturation and Po_2 recorders are useful in showing trends in the levels of blood oxygen, but regular arterial blood gas measurements should be undertaken to obtain accurate figures. It is occasionally impossible to site an indwelling arterial line and in this situation radial artery puncture or even arterialized capillary blood samples should be used. Unfortunately, any disturbance to such immature infants is likely to alter the blood gases, so the results obtained from such samples must be interpreted with care. Some neonatologists use indwelling aortic oxygen electrodes for continuous recording.

Blood gases

The maintenance of acid–base balance in a baby involves both respiratory and renal function, each adjusting constantly to keep the pH of the arterial blood within the narrow range of 7.33–7.47. If the lungs are normal, the amount of CO_2 exhaled will be adjusted to keep the arterial

Pco_2 between 4.4 and 6.0 kPa. A Pco_2 which rises above this level reduces the blood pH. The mature kidney will excrete hydrogen ion (acid) and bicarbonate (alkali) to maintain the pH within the normal values. Since renal function is limited in immature infants and respiratory function is diminished by RDS, a reduced pH (acidosis) is common and may be partly respiratory and partly metabolic in origin. A high Pco_2 suggests inadequate lung function and a low bicarbonate, or an increased base deficit (more than -5 mmol/L) indicates a metabolic cause especially if the Pco_2 is normal. Persistent hypoxia also results in increasing metabolic acidosis. The most common reason for this is poor perfusion of peripheral organs and muscles and the anaerobic metabolism which results from inadequate oxygen availability.

An arterial pH of less than 7.25, whether respiratory or metabolic, is harmful and requires correction. If the acidosis is metabolic, an infusion of 20 ml/kg body weight of plasma or human albumin over 30 minutes will improve peripheral perfusion by increasing the blood volume and blood pressure, and usually corrects it. Rapid infusion of bicarbonate has been shown to lower the intracellular and CSF pH which may be harmful. For this reason the use of bicarbonate has reduced considerably over the years and is only occasionally needed. Trometamol (THAM) can be used when all other methods fail to correct a serious metabolic acidosis.

A respiratory acidaemia can only be rectified by reducing the carbon dioxide level in the arterial blood by increasing the efficiency of breathing, if necessary by mechanical ventilation.

If it is clear from blood gas results that increasing inspired oxygen concentrations are required to maintain adequate oxygenation of the arterial blood or that carbon dioxide is being retained, mechanical support of breathing is needed using intermittent positive pressure ventilation through an endotracheal tube.

Surfactant therapy

Several natural and manufactured surfactant mixtures have been produced commercially to be administered to the lungs in RDS. They incorporate a substance to ensure dispersion of the phospholipid mixture throughout the bronchi and alveoli. It has been shown conclusively that the use of surfactant substantially reduces the mortality and morbidity of respiratory distress syndrome in babies between 24 and 34 weeks' gestation who require mechanical ventilation for the condition. It should be given as early as possible after RDS is diagnosed with one or two further doses over the next 24 hours. It is usually administered as a suspension in water and involves injecting up to 5 ml/kg of liquid down the endotracheal tube during active ventilation as rapidly as the baby will tolerate it. It may take only a few minutes to achieve this and surprisingly little distress is caused to the infant from instillation of this quantity of liquid into the lungs. The response to the drug can be rapid and it is often necessary to reduce the ventilator pressures shortly after it is given. Administration of surfactant also shortens the duration of artificial ventilation in many cases.

Principles of neonatal ventilation

There are several makes of neonatal ventilators with different ways of functioning, but most rely on sophisticated electronic devices to provide rapid and precise control of the delivery of gases to the baby while allowing for the monitoring of all aspects of the machine's function. Until recently all ventilators were designed so that the duration of inspiratory and expiratory air flow could be altered and maximum and minimum pressures set (Fig. 9.4). The volume of air delivered at each breath was determined by the settings chosen and the degree of compliance of the lungs. New ventilators are now being tested which deliver a specified volume of gas, varying the other parameters breath by breath. Most machines allow for several different methods of ventilation including intermittent mandatory and patient-triggered ventilation. Other modes enable varying degrees of synchronization of mandatory ventilation with the baby's own respiratory efforts, or simply produce a continuous positive airway pressure (CPAP) without positive pres-

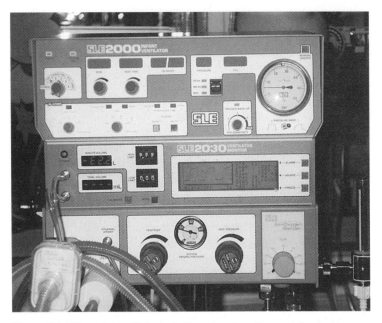

Figure 9.4 Neonatal ventilator including a breath pattern monitor.

sure ventilation. Since different modes of ventilation may be needed at different times in a baby's treatment, the ventilator must be able to alter many functions independently without disturbing the infant too much. The methods of ventilation most widely used are:

- intermittent mandatory ventilation (IMV) at rates which can be continuously varied between 0 and 80 per minute and, in high frequency ventilation, using much higher rates
- positive end-expiratory pressure (PEEP) of up to 7–8 cmH$_2$O; this is used in conjunction with IMV
- continuous positive airways pressure (CPAP; or continuous distending pressure, CDP) without IMV
- patient-triggered ventilation with variable mandatory back-up ventilation.

Intermittent mandatory ventilation (IMV)

This technique involves automatic mechanical ventilation at a rate and pressure determined by the ventilator settings irrespective of the baby's breathing efforts. The principle of IMV is to deliver oxygen to the alveoli in sufficient concentration to allow adequate transfer to the blood in the pulmonary capillaries and to wash out the carbon dioxide which accumulates in the alveoli when the respiratory efforts of the infant alone, or with the help of CPAP, are unable to do so. It is used if there is an increase in the oxygen requirement of the infant or if retention of carbon dioxide is causing a progressive respiratory acidosis.

IMV is applied through an endotracheal tube passed either through the nose or the mouth and fixed to prevent accidental displacement and to minimize laryngeal trauma. The method of fixation involves putting the tube through a modified tracheostomy tube holder which is then tied to a close-fitting bonnet to limit its movement. It is possible to fix the tube with sticky tape to the skin of the face but this method should be avoided to minimize the trauma to the skin (Fig. 9.5).

CPAP and PEEP

CPAP is used particularly in the infant with

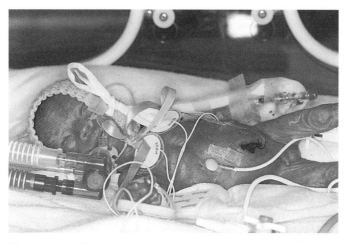

Figure 9.5   Full intensive care including endotracheal ventilation in a 25 week gestation pre-term infant of 720 g birth weight.

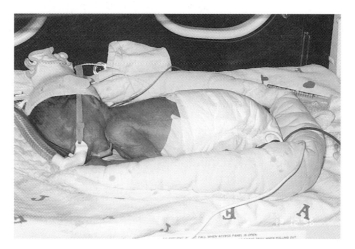

Figure 9.6   Nasal continuous positive airways pressure for mild RDS. Note the flexed posture of the infant in the restraining nest.

moderate RDS to prevent the alveoli from collapsing further while awaiting resolution of the condition from increasing production of natural surfactant. In this technique a continuous stable low pressure is applied to the baby's respiratory tract through close-fitting cannulae which are placed within the nasal airway (Fig. 9.6). During the process of weaning a baby from full ventilation, this same mode can be applied through the endotracheal tube. CPAP is usually applied at about 5 cmH$_2$O and it is rarely necessary to go above 7–8 cmH$_2$O. Since the continuous pressure

may limit the volume of air expelled from the lung during expiration, carbon dioxide retention may be observed on the regular blood gas measurements and either the pressure must be reduced or the baby fully ventilated to reduce it. PEEP is the equivalent of CPAP during full endotracheal mechanical ventilation, and is almost always applied in the early stages of ventilation for RDS, the minimum airway pressure being kept elevated throughout the expiratory phase of the ventilation cycle. It is normally kept at a pressure of about 3–5 cmH$_2$O.

Patient-triggered ventilation

Some neonatologists favour the use of the infant's own respiratory drive and rhythm to determine the rate of ventilation, allowing the response of her respiratory centre to modify the rate of breathing to keep her blood gases normal. The baby's own inspiratory effort is detected within milliseconds by sensing the change of pressure in the endotracheal tube. This signal is sent to activate the ventilator, which is thus coordinated with the infant's own respiration. This method of ventilation has enthusiastic proponents but larger studies comparing it with conventional ventilation are underway to determine its real value. It is, however, certainly useful while weaning the baby from the ventilator.

Other methods of respiratory support

In some centres, oscillatory ventilation is increasingly being used. In this technique less than the tidal volume is moved in and out of the lungs up to 2000 times a minute. Another method of providing gaseous exchange which shows promise in some specific conditions is extracorporeal membrane oxygenation (ECMO) in which blood is diverted from the body through a membrane oxygenator and back to the circulation again in a manner similar to bypass oxygenation circuits used in cardiac surgery.

Ventilator settings

Although neonatologists vary in their practices, the following figures give an indication of the range of settings commonly used for IMV at the start of ventilation:

- ventilator rate: 30–80/min
- peak inspiratory pressure: 18–24 cmH$_2$O
- PEEP: 3–5 cmH$_2$O
- inspiration/expiration ratio: between 1:1 and 1:1.5
- oxygen concentration: 40%.

The air/oxygen mixture must be fully humidified and warmed to prevent drying of the bronchial tree and cooling the infant.

The settings of the ventilator and oxygen concentration of the inspired gas mixture will be altered from time to time to maintain normal blood gas values, but the following guidelines are worth noting:

- Arterial oxygen saturation is largely maintained by the concentration of oxygen in the inspired gas, although areas of pulmonary atelectasis may also contribute to poor oxygenation. It can be improved by increasing PEEP pressures, prolonging the inspiratory time and by setting higher mean airways pressure from the ventilator.
- Carbon dioxide levels are affected by the volume of gas exchanged each minute (the minute volume) which relate closely to the rate and pressure of the ventilator. The greater the minute volume, the lower the CO$_2$ will fall.
- PEEP associated with slow ventilation can result in CO$_2$ retention.
- If the baby is fighting the ventilator despite changing the settings, it can cause pulmonary hypertension and consequently cyanosis from right to left shunting of blood. Sedation using an opiate analgesic or paralysing the baby with pancuronium can sometimes improve the effectiveness of ventilation.
- Keeping the inspiratory time to less than half of the respiratory cycle reduces the risk of pneumothorax.
- Every ventilated infant must be monitored by frequent blood gas measurements and the settings altered accordingly.

Complications of ventilator care

If the infant fails to respond to, or deteriorates during, ventilation, one or more of the following complications should be suspected and urgent treatment given if found:

- blocked endotracheal tube
- pneumothorax
- pulmonary interstitial emphysema
- intraventricular haemorrhage
- hypoglycaemia
- hypotension
- metabolic acidosis

Box 9.1 Common complications of respiratory distress syndrome

Early
Pneumothorax, pneumomediastinum
Pulmonary interstitial emphysema
Persistent pulmonary hypertension
Necrotizing enterocolitis
Periventricular leucomalacia
Intraventricular haemorrhage
Patent ductus arteriosus

Later
Bronchopulmonary dysplasia
Oxygen dependency
Cerebral palsy and learning difficulties
Retinopathy of prematurity
Growth failure
Repeated minor infections
Rickets of prematurity

- shunting through a patent ductus arteriosus
- persistent pulmonary hypertension.

Other complications of RDS

Other complications associated with RDS are outlined in Box 9.1.

Apnoeic spells

Apnoeic spells, when the infant stops breathing for more than 15–20 seconds, are a common accompaniment of RDS and normally result simply from immaturity of the respiratory centre in the brain stem which fails to stimulate breathing as the CO_2 level rises. They occur more frequently if the RDS is treated with surfactant, because the baby becomes independent of artificial ventilation at a lower gestational age. To counteract this, it is helpful to give the baby an intravenous loading dose of caffeine as the infant is weaned from the ventilator and to continue it orally until the spells cease (p. 119). As the baby matures, these episodes become less frequent, briefer and eventually disappear. However, they can also be caused by hypoglycaemia, infection, metabolic disturbances, gastro-oesophageal reflux, intracranial bleeding and fits. Each of these should be investigated and treated as necessary.

Pulmonary air leaks

Pneumothorax, pneumomediastinum and pulmonary interstitial emphysema are caused by the leakage of air from the alveoli into the pleural space or the interstitium of the lung. They are particularly common where high inflation pressures have been required or the infant has been fighting the ventilator. Pneumothorax results in a partial collapse of the lung and, in more severe cases, the mediastinum is shifted across to the opposite side of the chest. Rapid deterioration of the infant, hypotension and cyanosis may occur requiring urgent attention. The diagnosis can be made either by cold-light transillumination or by a chest X-ray. A tension pneumothorax will often respond initially to the insertion of a butterfly cannula into the affected pleural space, which allows the escape of the air and re-inflation of the lung, but it is usually necessary to insert an indwelling pleural drain connected to a one-way valve or underwater seal to prevent its recurrence until it is clear the air is not reaccumulating.

Technique of insertion of an indwelling pleural drain. After localization of the pneumothorax, the baby is placed with the affected side uppermost and the arm fully abducted. The skin is sterilized with an antiseptic lotion and a point in the mid-axillary line in a suitable intercostal space infiltrated with 1% lignocaine. An incision of about 3–4 mm is made in the anaesthetized area and the pleural catheter bored gently between the ribs. Resistance to the pressure suddenly reduces as the pleural space is entered. The tip is then pointed towards the head and advanced until it reaches the apex of the pleural space. The trochar is withdrawn, the cannula attached to an underwater seal and the tube is fastened in place with a purse-string suture, which also prevents air from leaking in, and taped to the skin.

Circulatory problems

Persistent pulmonary hypertension. The pulmonary vascular resistance remains labile in any baby with RDS and rises whenever she is disturbed. This results in increased resistance to blood flow through the pulmonary arteries and a rise in right ventricular and pulmonary artery pressure. If this pulmonary hypertension persists and the pressure rises above the aortic blood pressure, cyanosis results from shunting of deoxygenated blood from the pulmonary artery to the aorta through the ductus arteriosus. A similar shunt may occur through the foramen ovale from the right atrium to the left. Management of this condition depends on improving the effectiveness of the ventilation, increasing the concentration of the inspired oxygen, and infusion of plasma to correct the acidosis caused by hypotension. However, if this does not correct the hypoxia, a continuous infusion of tolazoline may be used to dilate the pulmonary vessels and increase oxygenation. Addition of nitric oxide (NO) to the inspired gases can improve oxygenation in some cases but its use is not yet fully evaluated. Epoprostenol, a prostaglandin drug, may be a highly effective treatment in this condition but its major drawback is that it can cause serious systemic hypotension and diminish platelet function.

Hypotension. A mean arterial blood pressure equivalent to the baby's gestational age in weeks can be regarded as a minimum value for pre-term infants. Thus, for example, 30 mmHg is the lowest acceptable figure in a 30 week infant. Hypotension commonly occurs and often results from a low blood volume, which may be revealed by finding a low peripheral (toe) temperature compared with the central (rectal) temperature. The initial treatment should be to restore this with a volume expander such as plasma, but cardiac stimulant drugs may be needed if this is not sufficient.

Renal failure and electrolyte disturbances. Renal failure and electrolyte disturbances are common. Fetal bradycardia, especially during labour, can cause acute tubular necrosis in the neonate which results in a diminished urine output, a high blood urea and abnormal electrolyte levels. An excess production of antidiuretic hormone, causing water retention and hyponatraemia, occurs occasionally, particularly where there has been a significant degree of birth asphyxia.

Metabolic abnormalities. Conditions such as hypoglycaemia, hypocalcaemia and hypophosphataemia will be identified by frequent bio-chemical analyses and their intake by the infant regulated to prevent them.

Anaemia. Anaemia commonly results in the first week or so from the need to take blood samples for analysis, and corrective transfusions of blood are almost always required in the smallest infants. After a few weeks a second phase of anaemia emerges from a failure of the bone marrow to produce enough red cells (p. 120). This can also be treated with blood transfusions until the infant begins to make enough red cells herself at around 8 weeks of age, although the introduction of synthetic erythropoietin injections may reduce the need for these in future.

Gastrointestinal problems

Abdominal distension. Abdominal distension caused by gaseous dilatation of the gut often occurs and may be severe enough to interfere with respiration or ventilation by restricting diaphragmatic movement.

Nutritional deficiencies. Nutritional deficiency has been shown to be closely related to short- and long-term outcomes. The aim is to achieve a growth rate similar to that in the healthy fetus but this is not often possible. Some of the smaller pre-term babies with RDS are unable to tolerate full enteral feeding and total parenteral nutrition becomes necessary (p. 126). Less severely ill infants can tolerate gastric feeds administered through an indwelling oro- or nasogastric tube, and giving the mother's breast milk affords some protection against necrotizing enterocolitis. However, although the amount of gastric feed the baby can tolerate often provides too small a calorie intake for adequate growth, it can accelerate the maturation of the gastrointestinal tract and improve its function. Increasing the baby's calorie intake can be achieved by adding carbohydrate or commercial fortifier supplements to breast milk (p. 116) or using specialized pre-term formula milk which is higher in calories, protein, sodium, phosphate and calcium (p. 85).

Necrotizing enterocolitis. The cause of this serious complication is still poorly understood but established predisposing factors include the presence of umbilical catheters, sepsis and low blood pressure. Part of the gut becomes necrotic, allowing bowel organisms entry to the circulation, and it is frequently fatal. It is mainly seen in pre-term infants fed on cow's milk formulae but human milk does not protect the infant completely. The baby appears pale and ill with bile-stained vomiting or gastric aspirate, rectal bleeding, loose stools and abdominal distension. An X-ray of the abdomen reveals distended loops of gut, sometimes with air in the bowel wall, and there may be evidence of bowel perforation with gas in the peritoneal cavity. Treatment is by gastric aspiration, intravenous fluid and antibiotic therapy, operation for resection of bowel being required if there is a perforation of the gut or failure to respond rapidly to conservative management.

Infections

The pre-term infant is particularly susceptible to infection (p. 127) and the risk is even greater when the baby has an endotracheal tube and intravascular catheters in place. The organisms responsible for such infections in the very immature infant include *Staphylococcus epidermidis* and *Streptococcus viridans* spp. which are not pathogenic in the older child. Intravenous antibiotics should be given to cover these as well as the more usual coliforms and group B streptococci. If indwelling intravenous catheters become infected they must be removed. Parenteral nutrition is commonly complicated by bacterial or fungal septicaemia and may need to be interrupted until the infection is controlled.

Periventricular ischaemia and haemorrhage

Major intracranial bleeding occurs less frequently than in the past in babies with RDS but it is not an uncommon occurence. Hypoxia and hypotension are two treatable factors contributing to the development of intracranial bleeding, but the risk is diminished by preventing wide variations of heart rate, blood pressure and blood biochemistry. Bleeding limited to the immediate periventricular germinal matrix region (grade 1) or confined to the ventricle (grade 2) usually has a good prognosis, although symptomatic haemor-

rhage associated with ventricular dilatation or extension of the bleed into the brain substance (grade 3) has a high chance of producing permanent brain damage (Fig. 9.7). Periventricular leucomalacia (Fig. 9.8), which results from ischaemic damage during episodes of perinatal hypotension, is particularly associated with later brain

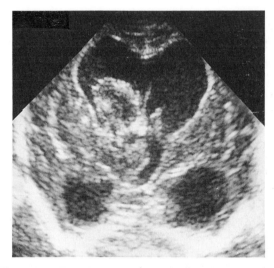

Figure 9.7 Transfontanelle coronal cerebral ultrasound scan showing intraventricular haemorrhage and ventricular dilatation. (By kind permission of Dr Stephen Chapman.)

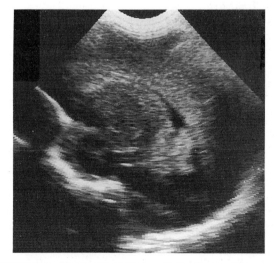

Figure 9.8 Periventricular leucomalacia. Parasagittal ultrasound scan shows increased periventricular echoes. (By kind permission of Dr Stephen Chapman.)

damage (p. 148). It is seen on the ultrasound scan as an area of echodensity around the lateral ventricles, and in the more advanced cases cystic areas can develop. Repeated ultrasound scans performed through the anterior fontanelle can accurately show the extent of the lesions and follow their progress and are thus useful in assessing the outlook for the baby's subsequent development (p. 148).

Persistent ductus arteriosus

Delay in closure of the ductus arteriosus is common in pre-term infants and often causes no symptoms, although it may make it difficult to wean a baby with hyaline membrane disease from a ventilator. As the pressure in the pulmonary artery slowly falls below the aortic pressure, blood flows from the aorta through the ductus into the pulmonary vessels, increasing the amount of blood in the pulmonary circulation. The lungs become stiffer, leading to increasing dyspnoea and CO_2 retention. The signs of an open ductus are a tachycardia and an audible systolic murmur in the second left intercostal space. Peripheral pulses are unusually prominent as a result of the high pulse pressure. A chest X-ray may show an enlarged heart and pulmonary plethora. Echocardiography can demonstrate the size of the ductus (Fig. 9.9) and Doppler colour flow mapping readily demonstrates blood flowing through it from the aorta to the pulmonary artery.

It is often possible to improve the situation by diuretic treatment, fluid restriction and alterations to management of ventilation until functional closure of the ductus occurs. If these measures are ineffective, indomethacin 0.1 mg/kg body weight given intravenously once daily for 6 days is often effective and can be repeated if the first course fails to close the duct. Very occasionally surgical closure is needed.

Later complications and prognosis

Retinopathy of prematurity (retrolental fibroplasia)

In the 1950s and 1960s, the survival of pre-term

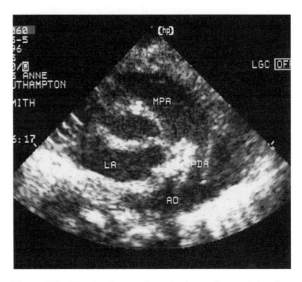

Figure 9.9 Short axis parasternal echocardiogram showing a persistent ductus arteriosus (PDA) between the aorta (Ao) and the main pulmonary artery (MPA) in a ventilated pre-term infant. (By kind permission of Dr Elspeth Brown.)

infants was improving yet a minority became blind from an unexplained progressive fibrosis of the retina. Since the discovery of its association with excessive oxygen administration, the incidence has dropped and the disease is now rare, although as greater numbers of increasingly premature babies are now surviving, there has been a recent increase in incidence of the disorder. It is a condition affecting the retinal blood vessels (Plate 12A and B). In the early stage, proliferative changes in the retinal vessels are seen, followed by haemorrhages and peripheral separation of the retina. Most cases do not progress beyond this stage and in these cases there is little effect on the child's eyesight. In more severe cases, the changes progress to fibrosis and opacity behind the lens, but treatment with cryotherapy can often halt the disease and prevent the progression to blindness. Although the condition is mostly seen in babies below 28 weeks of gestation, at birth the routine careful examination of the retina of all pre-term babies less than 1500 g birth weight or of less than 31 weeks of gestation should be carried out between 32 and 40 weeks, the age at which the condition appears, in order to allow timely intervention if it is needed. In general, retinopathy of prematurity is unlikely to occur if the oxygen content of the inspired air is kept below 40%. However, this should not prevent the use of higher concentrations to correct the effect of respiratory insufficiency since it is high blood oxygen levels that cause the damage. Arterial blood oxygen levels (P_aO_2) should not be allowed to rise above 10 kPa (80 mmHg).

Chronic pulmonary insufficiency of prematurity (Bronchopulmonary dysplasia)

This condition is characterized by progressive destruction of lung tissue and subsequent fibrosis. It is being seen more often now as survival of very immature infants after assisted ventilation becomes more commonplace. It is probably partly due to lung immaturity, and high oxygen concentrations may play a part, but positive pressure ventilation itself seems to be an important causative factor, although it may occur after only a brief period of ventilation.

The disorder should be suspected when there is difficulty in weaning a baby off the ventilator and X-rays show widespread opacities with patchy translucent areas (Fig. 9.10), followed later by fibrous scarring. Treatment of the condition consists in reducing as much as possible the peak pressure of ventilation, while maintaining some PEEP, and measures to close a persistent ductus arteriosus if it is present. A course of dexamethasone may accelerate the recovery. If the baby can be weaned from assisted ventilation, there may be a prolonged period of dependence on increased inspired oxygen concentrations but the eventual outlook is often surprisingly good. Almost complete recovery of lung function can occur after several months. However, there is a much higher incidence of sudden infant death syndrome in the first year of life and the infants have an increased susceptibility to respiratory infections.

Handicap following RDS

The outlook for pre-term babies is described on

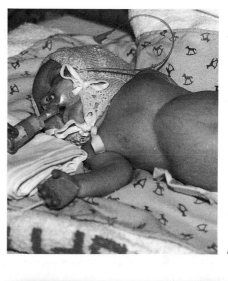

A

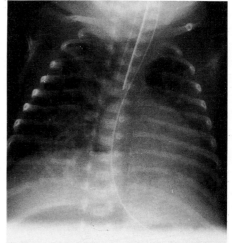

B

Figure 9.10 Chest X-ray in chronic lung disease (bronchopulmonary dysplasia) following respiratory distress syndrome. Bilateral patchy shadows are interspersed with areas of hyperinflated lung.

page 000 and in general this applies to the survivors of RDS. Neurological handicap occurs in less than 10% of such babies. It occurs largely, though not exclusively, in those in whom periventricular leucomalacia or intracerebral bleeding or ventricular dilatation is seen on ultrasound scans and babies who have fits or signs of severe cerebral irritability (p. 148). Ventilation for RDS alone and without complications does not cause persisting neurological handicap.

SURGICAL PROBLEMS AND INTENSIVE CARE

Some of the more serious congenital malformations require urgent neonatal surgery (Ch. 13). Intensive care is necessary for many, especially when they are born prematurely or are of low birth weight. The complex problems associated with most of these cases make it imperative that only a paediatric surgical team experienced with neonates should undertake this work. Special techniques in radiology, anaesthetics and laboratory back-up are often required.

Respiratory support in the form of assisted ventilation is frequently needed, e.g. in the case of diaphragmatic hernia with its associated pulmonary hypoplasia. After surgery for gastroschisis, exomphalos and gut atresia, there is often respiratory difficulty and a prolonged period of parenteral nutrition may have to follow. The surgery of congenital heart disease is another field in which intensive care facilities and specialized medical support are mandatory.

SOME WIDER IMPLICATIONS OF NEONATAL INTENSIVE CARE

Pain control

It has been thought that newborn infants do not suffer pain, discomfort and distress, but it is clear from both observational studies and investigation of metabolic responses in stressful situations in pre-term infants that they do. Many procedures used during intensive care are painful, and preventing or relieving such discomfort should be a high priority. The following methods can be recommended for painful procedures:

- Using a spring-loaded mechanical lancet considerably reduces the pain of heel pricks.
- Giving the baby oral sucrose before painful procedures seems to have an analgesic effect.
- Lignocaine 1% should be infiltrated into the skin and subcutaneous tissues before chest drain insertion.
- Gentle massage significantly reduces stress reactions in pre-term infants.

Drugs can be used for more prolonged pain relief and control. Paracetamol 15 mg/kg may be given up to four times a day either rectally or orally for moderate pain. Opiates are widely used to relieve the distress of endotracheal ventilation. Morphine is given as a loading dose of 50–100 μg/kg over 30 minutes followed by a continuous i.v. infusion of between 10 and 30 μg/kg per hour. The equivalent doses of intravenous diamorphine are 50 μg/kg over 30 minutes followed by 15 μg/kg per hour.

Respiratory depression from an acute overdose of opiates can be reversed by giving i.v. naloxone 30 μg/kg, but if they have been used over a prolonged period, naloxone may cause a severe withdrawal reaction (p. 15) and it should not be given. Doses should be slowly decreased over several days.

The application of specially formulated local anaesthetic creams to the skin reduces the pain of venepuncture and other painful procedures in babies and children and are used in some neonatal units, although their efficacy in pre-term infants is not yet proven. However, at the present time the drugs are not licensed for use in newborn babies in the UK.

Local anaesthetic creams

The value of topical local anaesthetic creams in reducing the pain of skin puncture is well established in older children and term infants. Their use in pre-term infants may not create adequate skin anaesthesia, and absorption of the drug could result in harmful systemic side-effects. At present they cannot be recommended and are not licensed for use in this age group in the UK.

Emotional care

The provision of intensive neonatal care can generate much emotional tension for parents and for caring staff. Physical stress during exceptionally busy periods and emergencies also takes its toll. Those who organize intensive neonatal care should take this into account and be ready to understand why staffing levels and standards of training have to be very high for it to succeed.

However, it is not enough that medical and

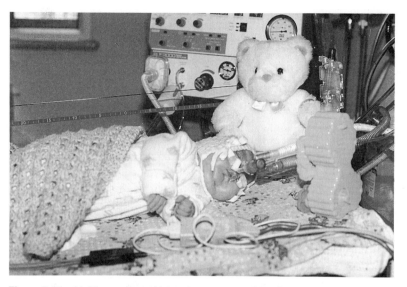

Figure 9.11 Making prolonged intensive care more friendly.

nursing staff should be efficient technicians. The baby's survival is important but the measure of real success is the quality of her future life with her parents and the period of hospital care can jeopardize this. Quite apart from the possible physical sequelae, the incidence of emotional family problems such as non-accidental injury and overanxiety leading to frequent hospital admissions and behaviour disturbance is known to be increased.

Much can be done towards preventing such ill-effects by ensuring that full involvement of the family, especially the baby's mother, is recognized as being vitally important from the start. There are numerous practical ways in which parents can be assured that they matter. An instant photograph can be given to the mother who is too unwell at first to see her baby. An unhurried discussion of anxieties between senior staff and the parents may be reassuring, especially when changes in treatment or big decisions are to be made. The parents should be encouraged to have as much physical contact with the sick infant as is compatible with the principle of minimal handling. At first, this may only amount to touching the baby's hand in the incubator, but later parents should be involved in almost all aspects of care.

It may be possible also to make the environment of the baby in special or intensive care look less forbidding by means of a friendly decor, but a good understanding of the family's needs can achieve more than any number of teddy bears (Fig. 9.11).

The death of a baby undergoing intensive care is not a rare event and giving effective help to parents at this time and afterwards is another difficult responsibility for senior medical and nursing staff to carry. The opportunity has to be given for expression of grief and fulfilment of any religious or ceremonial custom that may be important to the particular family, and at the right time interviews to discuss the medical aspects of the situation must be arranged (p. 229).

FURTHER READING

Aynsley-Green A, Ward-Platt M, Lloyd-Thomas A (eds) 1995 Stress and pain in infancy and childhood. Baillière Tindall, London.

Barker D P, Rutter N 1995 Lignocaine ointment and local anaesthesia in preterm infants. Archives of Disease in Childhood 72: F203–F204

Beeby P, Jeffery H 1992 Risk factors for necrotising enterocolitis: the influence of gestational age. Archives of Disease in Childhood 67: 432–435

Bevilacqua G, Halliday H, Parmigiani S, Robertson B 1993 Randomised multicentre trial of treatment with porcine natural surfactant for moderately severe respiratory syndrome. The collaborative European multicentre study group. Journal of Perinatal Medicine: 21(5): 329–340

British Association of Perinatal Medicine 1992 Development of audit measures and guidelines for good practice in the management of neonatal respiratory distress syndrome. Archives of Disease in Childhood 67: 1221–1227

Brutocao D P, O'Rourke P P 1992 Extracorporeal membrane oxygenation. In: David T J (ed) Recent advances in paediatrics 10. Churchill Livingstone, Edinburgh, ch 6

David T J (ed) 1994 Recent advances in paediatrics 13. Retinopathy of prematurity. Churchill Livingstone, Edinburgh, ch 12

Durand M, Sardesai S, McEvoy C 1995 Effects of early dexamethasone on pulmonary mechanics and chronic lung disease in very low birth weight infants: a randomised controlled trial. Paediatrics 95(4): 584–590

Fielder A, Levene M 1992 Screening for retinopathy of prematurity. Archives of Disease in Childhood 67: 860–867

Greenough A, Milner A, Roberton N 1995. Neonatal respiratory disorders. Edward Arnold, London

Hack M, Friedman H, Fanaroff A A 1996 Outcome of extremely low birth weight infants. Paediatrics 98: 931–937

Halliday H 1995 Overview of clinical trials comparing natural and synthethic surfactants. Biology of the Neonate 67(suppl 1): 32–47

Jaimovich D, Vidyasagara D 1995 Handbook of paediatric and neonatal transport medicine. Mosby, London

Keith C, Doyle L 1995 Retinopathy of prematurity in infants weighing 1000–1499 g at birth. Journal of Paediatrics and Child Health 31(2): 134–136

Levene M, Liford R (eds) 1995 Fetal and neonatal neurology and neurosurgery. Churchill Livingstone, Edinburgh

Paulson T E, Spear R M, Peterson B M 1995 New concepts in the treatment of respiratory distress syndrome. Journal of Paediatrics 127(2): 163–175

Pearson G A, Firmin R K, Sosnowski A, Field D 1992 Neonatal extracorporeal membrane oxygenation. British Journal of Hospital Medicine 47: 646–654

Phelps D 1995 Retinopathy of prematurity. Paediatric Review 16(2): 50–56

Puntis J 1992 Parenteral nutrition – practical considerations. Current Paediatrics 2: 175–177

Report of working group of the British Association of Perinatal Medicine and Neonatal Nurses Association on categories of babies requiring neonatal care 1992 Archives of Disease in Childhood 67: 868–869

Roberton N R C (ed) 1992 Textbook of neonatology. Churchill Livingstone, Edinburgh

Saugstad O D 1992 Neonatal oxygen radical disease. In: David T J (ed) Recent advances in paediatrics 10. Churchill Livingstone, Edinburgh, ch 11

Sinclair J, Bracken M 1992 Effective care of the newborn infant. Oxford University Press, Oxford

Sinha S, Donne S, 1996 Advances in neonatal conventional ventilation. Archives of Disease in Childhood, 75: F135–140

Speer C P, Gefeller O, Groneck P et al 1995 Randomised controlled trial of two treatment regimes of natural surfactant preparations in neonatal respiratory distress syndrome. Archives of Disease in Childhood Fetal and Neonatal Edition 72(1): F8–F13

Tin W, Wariyar U, Hey E 1997 Changing prognosis for babies of less than 28 weeks gestation in the north of England between 1983 and 1994. British Medical Journal 314: 107–111

Verma R 1995 Respiratory distress syndrome of the newborn infant. Obstetrics and Gynaecology Survey 50(7): 542–555

Wilson D, McClure G 1992 Respiratory problems in the newborn. British Journal of Intensive Care 2: 287–294

10

Birth injury and neurological disorders

There is often anxiety in the minds of new parents about the effects of injury to their baby during birth – particularly damage to the brain. Gross injury and intracranial bleeding of traumatic origin are now uncommon and in most cases complete recovery with normal development follows. Permanent ill-effects are more likely to result from a period of severe cerebral asphyxia or ischaemia related to inadequate placental function. This chapter describes the range of neurological problems which are encountered in the neonatal period and attempts to distinguish the more serious ones from those with a good outlook so that some of the unnecessary parental anxiety can be avoided.

INJURIES TO THE HEAD

Superficial injuries

Abrasions, superficial bruises (Plate 13) from forceps and 'traumatic cyanosis' (p. 57) from small petechial haemorrhages are usually not serious. The circular area of oedema and intracutaneous haemorrhage from the application of the Ventouse is not serious (Plate 14), but significant blood loss occasionally occurs into an underlying sub-aponeurotic haematoma which feels like a superficial bag of fluid.

Cephalhaematoma

This localized subperiosteal collection of blood is a common occurrence and often follows a normal delivery with no apparent trauma. It takes a few days to show itself as a soft fluctuant swelling overlying one of the skull bones, usually the parietal. It is strictly limited in extent to the area of the bone involved and within a few days a hard rim can be felt at its edge, giving a false impression that the base of the swelling is depressed. It is gradually absorbed and becomes firmer and smaller until it disappears entirely by the age of 3 months. In very exceptional cases the whole swelling becomes calcified and forms a hard, bony protuberance which takes over a year to absorb. No treatment is required and on no account should aspiration be attempted. In a small proportion of cases a fracture of the underlying skull can be found on X-ray.

Fractured skull

Linear fracture occasionally occurs after a difficult forceps delivery but is rarely diagnosed without X-ray. In itself, it is not of clinical importance but it may occasionally be associated with underlying brain injury. A depressed fracture is even less common and is seen as a localized hollowing, usually in the parietal region, but surgical treatment is seldom necessary.

CEREBRAL INJURY FROM BIRTH TRAUMA AND ASPHYXIA

As a result of advances in obstetrics, damage of traumatic origin has become uncommon, and only in a minority of babies dying from cerebral dysfunction is there macroscopical evidence of trauma to the brain.

Nevertheless, symptoms resulting from an injury to the brain before, during or after birth are common in newborn infants, and in most cases the cause is a period of asphyxia. Imaging techniques can identify such causes of these symptoms as haemorrhage, cerebral oedema, cerebral infarction and occasionally other more subtle changes in the brain substance, yet it is often difficult to correlate the site and degree of these abnormalities with the clinical picture. More recently, complex imaging techniques and biochemical investigations have demonstrated biochemical changes which occur in the brain cells following asphyxia and it is probably these which cause the greatest damage.

Intracranial haemorrhage

Intracranial bleeding is not uncommon. Birth injury may cause bleeding into the cerebrospinal fluid in the subarachnoid space from torn veins communicating with the sagittal sinus, or subdural haemorrhage from a tear in the tentorium or falx, in the edge of which are situated the straight sinus and the great vein of Galen, or from rupture of the small veins which bridge the subdural space. Both types of haemorrhage may follow a delivery in which marked deformation of the skull has resulted from head compression. More commonly it may result from perinatal asphyxia, be a complication of hyaline membrane disease in the pre-term infant (p. 137) or relate to a disorder of the blood-clotting mechanisms.

Intraventricular haemorrhage

In the majority of cases, this type of haemorrhage arises after birth in pre-term babies with complications of respiratory distress syndrome. There may be intracerebral extension of the bleed in more severe cases which often results in a poor neurological outcome for the baby (p. 148).

Hypoxic-ischaemic encephalopathy

In the majority of cases, injury to the brain is caused by asphyxia, ischaemia or severe cerebral oedema. During labour, each uterine contraction reduces placental blood flow, resulting in temporary fetal hypoxia. As long as placental function is normal, this does no harm since oxygenation resumes as the contraction ceases. If, however, the fetus has suffered prolonged mild asphyxia and malnutrition as a result of placental insufficiency then the risk of cerebral damage from these repeated bouts of hypoxia is increased. Identification of poor fetal growth is often possible by ultrasound examination, and prenatal Doppler ultrasound studies of the fetal arterial

Table 10.1 Predisposing causes of cerebral trauma and intrapartum asphyxia

Trauma	Asphyxia
Primiparity	Fetal growth retardation
Disproportion	Pre-eclampsia
Malpresentation (e.g. breech)	Retroplacental haemorrhage
Rapid second stage of labour	Post-term birth
Pre-term birth	Pre-term birth
Constriction rings	Diabetes

blood flow patterns can identify in some cases an infant with poor cardiac output and therefore reduced cerebral blood flow. Often, however, it is only by being aware that a condition predisposing to cerebral asphyxia in labour is present that it can be anticipated and these are contrasted with causes of traumatic injury in Table 10.1. The baby who is at greater risk can often, but not always, be identified during labour by characteristic abnormal patterns of heart rate on the fetal cardiotocograph recording (p. 35).

It is not always possible to predict from the baby's condition immediately after birth – e.g. as shown by the Apgar score – whether signs of cerebral injury will follow. Most infants with low scores at birth will show no permanent abnormal cerebral sequelae, whilst some who seem in good condition initially develop signs of brain damage.

Clinical features of cerebral injury

By clinical signs alone it is often difficult to localize a cerebral lesion or distinguish between cerebral injury from trauma and that from asphyxia, because the baby behaves in the same way in both situations at different stages. Many infants who have suffered from prenatal or intrapartum asphyxia will have poor cardiorespiratory function after birth and this can reduce cerebral blood flow further and cause additional brain injury. Apnoea, or depressed respiration, and systemic hypotension may be the only initial signs of cerebral damage.

Birth asphyxia sufficient to cause permanent brain damage is often followed by a clinical picture of a cerebral nature described as hypoxic-ischaemic encephalopathy. Those babies who suffer milder insults have a more favourable outcome but unfortunately the clinical signs of encephalopathy do not always reflect the severity of the underlying biochemical insult to the brain.

Mild hypoxic-ischaemic encephalopathy

In most cases when the asphyxial insult to the baby has been mild, following a period of a few hours in which the baby is quiet and apparently well, the picture of cerebral irritation emerges. In this state the baby will lie quietly most of the time but is easily disturbed into excessive jittery muscular activity. There may also be a shrill high-pitched persistent cry which is recognizably different from the normal cry of a hungry baby. Often there is abnormal wakefulness, the eyes remaining constantly open with an anxious or frowning expression. Rapid eye and tongue movements may occur and short myoclonic twitching movements are sometimes seen. Head retraction and hyperextension of the limbs are less common features. Occasionally rhythmical alternating extension and flexion of the limbs may occur, resembling bicycling or boxing movements. These movements should be readily distinguishable from fits, being persistent for long periods, whereas fitting movements are less complicated and usually brief. Where there is doubt, an electroencephalogram (EEG) recording may help.

Severe hypoxic-ischaemic encephalopathy

After more profound asphyxia, the baby has a diminished level of consciousness and respiration may be periodic from birth. Seizures may occur and these may be clonic, myoclonic or tonic (p. 149). There is profound hypotonia (described below) and immobility which may last from a few hours to several days and results from brain stem dysfunction. The infant is unresponsive to handling and most reflex responses are lost. He is unable to suck well enough to feed adequately.

Over the next 24 hours, a period of cerebral

irritation occurs with extensor hypertonia associated with rising intracranial pressure from cerebral oedema. The head is retracted, the trunk and limbs tend to extend, and reflex responses are brisk. The asymmetrical tonic neck response (p. 66) is consistently obtainable and may be initiated through spontaneous movements of the body. Although this exaggerated extension posture may be the prelude to later development of permanent cerebral palsy, it is also occasionally seen as a purely temporary phenomenon in low birth weight babies. Its presence makes feeding difficult and, because the baby arches away from his mother, development of the normal emotional attachment between them may be impaired. Subsequently there is a slow return to a more normal pattern of behaviour unless the cerebral injury has resulted in permanent damage.

A tense or bulging fontanelle is common and reflects raised intracranial pressure. Cerebral ultrasound examination or CT or MRI scanning should distinguish whether the increased pressure results from intracranial bleeding or cerebral oedema. Papilloedema is rarely seen. An inability to suck, low body temperature, vomiting, abnormal crying and cyanotic attacks are additional features of more severe cerebral dysfunction and may accompany any form of brain injury whether hypoxic-ischaemic or traumatic. A lumbar puncture seldom clarifies the diagnosis and should be avoided unless there is a suspicion of meningitis.

Investigation in cerebral injury

An increasing number of techniques can now be applied to the investigation of cerebral conditions. In cerebral injury from trauma or hypoxic-ischaemic encephalopathy, these can give useful information for the management of the infant but they have only limited value in predicting the outcome.

Ultrasound

Ultrasound scanning through the open anterior fontanelle can identify haemorrhagic lesions in the periventricular white matter and intraven-

tricular haemorrhage, which occur mainly in the pre-term infant with respiratory distress syndrome (Figs 9.7 and 9.8, p. 137). It can also reveal localized and generalized areas of ischaemic damage. It is a particularly valuable investigation since it can be carried out in the infant's cot or incubator, involves no radiation, does not require the baby to be sedated or anaesthetized, and frequently provides important information necessary for correct treatment and for assessing the prognosis.

CT scanning

Computerized tomography (CT) scanning which, like MRI scanning, involves much greater disturbance to the infant can show more accurately the distribution of hypoxic-ischaemic changes in the brain parenchyma (Fig. 10.1), the more diffuse lesions being associated with a higher incidence of permanent residual brain damage. It can visualize the subdural space which is often difficult to locate with ultrasound.

MRI scanning

Magnetic resonance imaging (MRI) can, in addi-

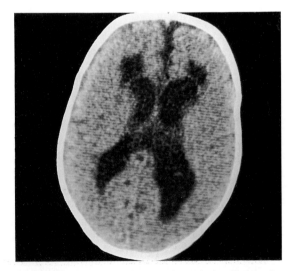

Figure 10.1 Cerebral oedema and ventricular dilatation in hypoxic-ischaemic encephalopathy demonstrated by CT scan.

tion, reveal recent infarcts in the brain and is superior to other techniques in examination of the spinal cord.

Electroencephalography

The electroencephalogram (EEG) pattern has limited value but may be able to confirm that certain abnormal movements are fits. A normal EEG pattern is usually an indication of a favourable prognosis for the baby, although in severe cerebral injury a pattern of low voltage activity with bursts of high voltage sharp waves, known as burst suppression (Fig. 10.2), indicates a poor prognosis with residual brain damage. The more rapidly any abnormalities on the EEG resolve, however, the better the prospects for full recovery of the infant.

Intracranial pressure monitoring

Intracranial pressure monitoring by measuring at the anterior fontanelle can identify at an early stage those infants developing raised intracranial pressure and can monitor its changes during treatment, but the technique is not commonly available.

Cerebral blood flow

Cerebral blood flow measurements using Doppler ultrasound techniques can give some indication of the adequacy of perfusion of the brain but the usefulness of this test remains uncertain at present.

Management

Mild hypoxic-ischaemic encephalopathy

The most important aspect of management is prevention. Careful monitoring of the fetus during labour, particularly where fetal growth retardation has been confirmed during the antenatal period, will identify most, but not all, asphyxiated infants and expedite their delivery, by caesarean section if necessary.

Since it is difficult to tell initially how severe the results of a cerebral injury will be, all infants with cerebral symptoms should be nursed in quiet surroundings in an incubator to maintain body temperature and to facilitate observation. The baby should be handled only as much as is needed for essential observations, feeding and changing the nappy, although the importance of encouraging practical parental involvement within the limits of safety must not be ignored.

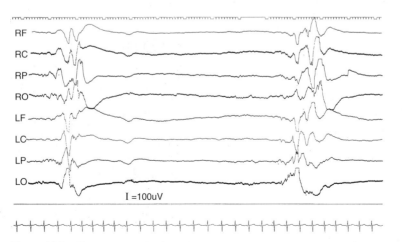

Figure 10.2 'Burst suppression' pattern on an EEG in severe hypoxic-ischaemic encephalopathy. An indication of a poor prognosis for later cerebral function. (Reproduced with the kind permission of Dr Christian Wulff.)

The blood glucose level should be maintained by small frequent feeds, if necessary by nasogastric tube. Sedation may be needed if the baby is distressed and so long as vomiting does not preclude oral administration, chloral hydrate may be given in a dose of 40–80 mg in a term infant repeated at up to 6-hourly intervals while restlessness persists. Transcutaneous oxygen monitoring is useful to ensure normal oxygen levels since both too much and too little oxygen can cause additional damage.

Severe hypoxic-ischaemic encephalopathy

The management of severe hypoxic-ischaemic encephalopathy is outlined in Box 10.1. Since cardiorespiratory function is likely to be compromised and hypoxia with CO_2 retention tends to raise intracranial pressure, blood gas analysis is essential to assess the need for assisted ventilation. The blood pressure should be monitored closely and hypotension treated by increasing the blood volume with transfusions of human albumin solution. The blood glucose values should be kept in the range 4–5.5 mmol/L (75–100 mg/dl) since both hypoglycaemia and hyperglycaemia can accentuate existing brain injury.

If seizures occur, they should be treated with intravenous phenobarbitone followed by daily oral maintenance doses (p. 150), since persistent fits can reduce cerebral blood perfusion and exhaust brain glucose even in the presence of normal blood glucose levels. (See also page 150 for a fuller discussion of the treatment of neonatal fits.)

Box 10.1 Management of severe hypoxic-ischaemic encephalopathy

- Avoid unnecessary disturbance
- Prevent hypoxia and hyperoxia
- Prevent hypercapnia
- Maintain normal blood pressure
- Maintain normal blood glucose level
- Control seizures
- Restrict fluids
- Monitor fluid and electrolyte balance

Fluid intake should be restricted to minimal maintenance levels with close monitoring of the electrolytes and osmolality of both blood and urine. This prevents fluid overload and electrolyte imbalance, both of which can easily occur.

There is little evidence to validate the effectiveness of steroids or hyperosmolar solutions to reduce intracranial pressure, although their occasional use in severe cerebral oedema may be justified.

Chronic subdural haematoma is a rare later sequel developing over several months which may cause vomiting, failure to thrive, fits and enlargement of the head. It can be treated by repeated subdural taps if strict attention is paid to aseptic technique.

Prognosis of cerebral injury

Infants who have shown signs of what is thought to be traumatic cerebral injury and who survive the neonatal period only exceptionally have permanent damage. Follow-up studies have shown the incidence of neurological disability to be approximately 1 in 10 severely affected babies treated with the intensive management described above. Such disabilities range from a specific learning difficulty with clumsiness of movement and poor attention span to more serious forms of cerebral palsy, epilepsy or mental retardation. The great majority of more mildly affected babies fully recover without sequelae.

Cerebral injury from prolonged asphyxia, as opposed to trauma, is much more likely to result in permanent ill-effects, particularly if the baby's growth in utero was impaired or if the baby was of low birth weight. It is difficult to tell from the features in the newborn period which babies will fail to make a full recovery, although the occurrence of certain features on imaging investigations are associated with a worse outlook. These include evidence of cerebral infarction, periventricular leucomalacia, haemorrhagic necrosis or cyst formation, most of which result in cerebral palsy, developmental delay or epilepsy. The occurrence of repeated fits in the first few days, continued failure to suck and the persistence of other neurological signs of cerebral injury for more than about 4 days are also features of bad prognostic significance. Failure to establish normal respiration within 30 minutes of birth despite adequate artificial ventilation makes full recovery extremely unlikely; however, the absence of such features gives no guarantee of a good prognosis and only prolonged follow-up will show the full extent of any neurological deficit. Research using magnetic resonance spectroscopy has shown some of the biochemical changes which occur in the brain cells as a result of asphyxia, and studies are underway to assess whether keeping the infant mildly hypothermic or using drugs such as magnesium sulphate or allopurinol can protect the brain and reduce the risks of long-term damage.

Physiotherapy

After the acute stage of cerebral injury is over, the baby may have persistence of abnormal tone and motor responses which can be indicators of an emerging neurological deficit. Although the eventual degree of handicap is not known at this time, a paediatric physiotherapist with understanding of neurological development can begin to advise the parents on ways of positioning the baby during sleep and handling while awake to make possible a more normal sequence of development and modify the progression of the neurological signs. Not only can this improve the outlook for the child, but it also increases the parental confidence in handling him and gives the opportunity to identify and treat at an early stage any deviations from normal development.

NEONATAL FITS

It is important to recognize fits in the neonatal period since, in contrast to fits in older children, they are frequently a pointer to an underlying condition and their treatment may materially affect the infant's prognosis. Seizures may themselves cause injury to the neonatal brain and may continue unrecognized for some time. Occasionally they result from an inherited metabolic disease which, if diagnosed early, may affect the family's decision on having further children.

Fits in the first few weeks of life have a different pattern from the common seizures of later infancy and childhood. Instead of the generalized 'grand mal' type of convulsive fit, the most usual pattern is one of jerking or twitching of a focal nature, often rapidly shifting from one part of the body to another. Sometimes these movements change site so rapidly that they appear almost to be generalized, whilst at other times a truly repetitive twitching of one extremity or side of the face is all that is seen. Tonic seizures of a more general distribution, with hyperextension of the trunk, neck and limbs, are another variation. More difficult to recognize as fits are momentary changes of respiratory pattern (perhaps apnoeic attacks), flickering of the eyelids, tonic deviation of the eyes to one side, drooling or lipsmacking. Focal fits do not, as in later life, necessarily signify a localized brain lesion, but may even be seen when the cerebral involvement is clearly a diffuse one in metabolic disorders such as hypoglycaemia or hypocalcaemia. Sometimes the diagnosis of fits can only be established for certain by a continuous EEG recording.

The causes of neonatal fits can broadly be classified as follows:

- Common causes
  - hypoxic-ischaemic encephalopathy
  - intracranial haemorrhage or oedema from birth trauma
  - infection, particularly meningitis
  - metabolic disturbances, including hypoglycaemia, hypocalcaemia and hyponatraemia
- Less common causes
  - structural abnormalities such as hydrocephalus or an arteriovenous malformation
  - withdrawal of drugs, e.g. heroin, barbiturates, alcohol
  - inborn errors of metabolism, e.g. phenylketonuria and pyridoxine dependency
  - benign familial neonatal seizures
  - toxicity from local anaesthetics or theophylline.

Fits at this stage of life must always be regarded as potentially serious and every effort made to find a reason for them. In many cases the baby will already have a condition in which fits are not unexpected. If this is not the case and the baby seems healthy between the fits, benign familial seizures, hypocalcaemia or an arteriovenous malformation should be considered. However, if the baby is sick, he needs urgent investigation to exclude meningitis or metabolic disorders. The investigations will include estimation of blood glucose, calcium and urea, a lumbar puncture and a skull X-ray with a standard EEG or a continuous EEG recording. An ultrasound scan performed through the anterior fontanelle may show haemorrhage, dilatation of the ventricles or a space-occupying lesion. Occasionally a CT scan will be required, particularly if a lesion on the surface of the cortex is possible, and MRI scanning if a cerebral infarct is suspected. Urinary amino acid chromatography or gas chromatography on the urine for organic acids should be performed to exclude rare metabolic disorders if no diagnosis is made. Phenylketonuria should be excluded by the routine screening test for the condition (p. 67).

Diagnosis and management of fits

Because fits are potentially so serious, an intravenous infusion should be set up to give the appropriate drugs and an urgent search made for an underlying cause. If the blood glucose is below 2.5 mmol/L, hypoglycaemia should be assumed and the term baby given 5–10 ml/kg of 10% glucose (0.5–1.0 g/kg) intravenously immediately, followed by an infusion of 10% dextrose to maintain a blood glucose level of 5–10 mmol/L (75–100 mg/dl). A response to this regimen suggests that a low blood glucose is the cause, but other conditions should be sought if no improvement is obtained.

Hypocalcaemia is confirmed if the serum calcium level is below 1.7 mmol/L. In most cases this condition occurs towards the end of the first week of life and is associated with a high phosphate load in the milk. Most modified cow's milk formulas now have low levels of phosphate so that the condition is becoming increasingly

uncommon. If the hypocalcaemic infant is hypertonic and irritable with increased tendon reflexes (the condition known as hypocalcaemic tetany), oral calcium gluconate 200 mg/kg per day or 50% magnesium sulphate 0.1–0.2 ml/kg intramuscularly will raise the calcium level, but if fits occur, 10% calcium gluconate 0.2 ml/kg should be given intravenously over 10 minutes under ECG monitoring. Babies suffering from hypocalcaemia in the newborn period have been found to suffer from dental enamel hypoplasia in the milk teeth. It seems probable that maternal vitamin D deficiency in late pregnancy may also play a part in its causation.

Occasionally a baby may have many fits without apparent cause and be surprisingly well inbetween. If there is a family history of neonatal fits of similar type, it is likely that the infant has the syndrome of benign familial neonatal fits. The fits subside spontaneously and there is a normal neurological outcome in the majority of cases.

Anticonvulsant drug treatment

In the absence of an easily treated metabolic cause, anticonvulsant drugs form the mainstay of treatment. Continuous fitting is relatively uncommon and drugs are not often needed to terminate a fit, but if necessary paraldehyde 0.1 ml/kg rectally or intravenously is usually effective. Diazepam 0.5 mg/kg intravenously can also be used but may cause apnoea and accentuate jaundice by releasing the bilirubin from its binding sites on albumin. It should therefore be used with caution.

For longer-term control of fits, phenobarbitone remains the drug of choice. An intramuscular loading dose of 20 mg/kg is given to achieve a therapeutic blood level of approximately 20 mg/ml quickly and this can be maintained with daily oral doses of 3–4 mg/kg. The rate of excretion of phenobarbitone is slow but very variable and blood level monitoring is desirable to avoid sedation from overdosage.

Phenytoin 8 mg/kg given by slow intravenous injection followed by 5 mg/kg per day orally for maintenance is often effective if phenobarbitone is not. Sodium valproate is a less effective anti-convulsant in the newborn period than it is at other ages but may occasionally be used. Anti-convulsant treatment is usually given for only 2–3 months after control of neonatal seizures, since recurrence of the fits is unusual after this time.

If no response is obtained from anticonvulsants, a therapeutic trial of pyridoxine 50 mg daily will reduce fitting in the rare infant with pyridoxine dependency.

Pertussis immunization following neurological Illness

Although it was believed that there was a small risk of neurological damage from the pertussis fraction of the diphtheria / pertussis / tetanus vaccine used for routine immunization of infants, its dangers were greatly exaggerated. Nevertheless it is wise to defer the pertussis fraction until later in infancy for those infants who have had fits or severe hypoxic-ischaemic encephalopathy, until it is clear that the infant has no continuing neurological disorder. There are no other perinatal contraindications to its use and for all other infants it should be recommended.

Prognosis of neonatal fits

The outcome in later childhood for those babies who have suffered from fits in the first week depends more on the prognosis of the underlying cause than on the fits themselves, although the greater the number of fits, the more likely it is that there will be continuing neurological damage. When fits are due to transient hypocalcaemia, normal development is the rule. When caused by intracranial haemorrhage or oedema, the outlook is also good in 90% of cases, but there is a high incidence of subsequent neurological handicap when fits result from cerebral anoxia, hypoglycaemia or meningitis, particularly when this is associated with other neurological signs such as apathy, hypotonia, apnoea and poor feeding. When an associated structural abnormality of the brain is identified, or when a bleed, periventricular densities or cyst formation is found within the cerebral cortex, the likelihood of abnormal development is strong.

HYPOTONIA – THE FLOPPY INFANT

Muscular hypotonia is a feature of many conditions in the newborn infant. The pre-term infant of less than 34 weeks of gestation is always hypotonic and its extent is used in the estimation of gestational age (p. 106). It is a prominent feature in Down's syndrome and often helps to confirm the diagnosis when it is suspected from a dysmorphic facies (p. 220). Cerebral injury from trauma or asphyxia (p. 145), hypoglycaemia (p. 97), hyponatraemia (p. 51) and any infection, especially with septicaemia or meningitis, are also causes, although in many cases other manifestations of these conditions are present. Certain drugs such as diazepam and opiate analgesics can also cross the placenta and cause sedation or hypotonia.

Localized hypotonia

Cervical spinal cord trauma may result in sparing of facial movement when there is severe loss of movement and tone below the injury. In a baby with a myelomeningocele affecting the lumbar spine, the legs are floppy from incomplete innervation whereas the arms are normal.

Generalized hypotonia

More rarely, low muscle tone or weakness of the muscles is found in an otherwise well infant which results from one of a group of neuromuscular diseases which are either present at birth or develop during the first weeks of life. The differentiation of these conditions is difficult. The family history, cytogenetic studies and DNA analysis can be helpful in diagnosing some cases since many are genetically inherited, but often extensive investigation, including biochemical testing, electromyography and muscle biopsy, is needed.

A degenerative process involving the anterior horn cells in the spinal cord is the cause of the muscular weakness in a group of conditions included under the term Werdnig–Hoffmann disease or progressive infantile spinal muscular atrophy. The condition is recessively inherited and, although weakness and hypotonia become noticeable only after the first few weeks or months, they can be present at birth. Progressive weakness of all muscle groups, particularly the trunk and respiratory muscles, leads to death in the first year in all but a few exceptional cases.

Another group includes the familial myopathies and muscular dystrophies. In these, the rate of progression of the weakness is very variable, but ultimately most have a relentless downhill course with slowly increasing paralysis. For certain types of myopathy, there are diagnostic blood tests. For example, with Duchenne muscular dystrophy a raised blood creatine phosphokinase level in the first few days of life can be diagnostic. The disease can even be predicted with some certainty antenatally using DNA analysis (p. 20).

Hypotonia in a male infant with cryptorchidism suggests the possibility of the Prader–Willi syndrome (Fig. 10.3) with its later obesity and mild mental retardation. The diagnosis is confirmed by finding a characteristic abnormality on chromosome 15 in cytogenetic studies (Plate 15).

Myasthenia gravis is extremely rare except in the transient form which occurs when the mother has the condition (p. 26), and in myotonic dystrophy one of the parents may show some signs of the condition such as a characteristic facies or difficulty in relaxing a clenched hand.

In many 'floppy infants', no specific diagnosis is found despite complete investigation and the baby's muscle power and tone improve gradually. This group probably comprises a mixture of different conditions but the term 'benign congenital hypotonia' has been used to describe it.

SPINAL INJURY

Injury involving the spinal cord or its nerve roots is probably not as uncommon as is generally supposed. Dislocation in the upper cervical spine may follow hyperextension of the neck during a difficult delivery. The clinical picture is variable and not easy to recognize, but extreme floppiness and immobility together with respiratory difficulty are usually prominent and occasionally may progress to spastic quadriplegia, although if the brain itself is unaffected the child will not usually have learning difficulties.

EYE INJURIES

Subconjunctival haemorrhage, showing itself either as a bright red ring around the cornea or as a flare spreading more widely outwards, is common. It resolves within a few weeks without treatment or complications. Reassurance is all that is needed. More rarely, orbital haemorrhage may result in proptosis of the eye, but spontaneous reabsorption of the haemorrhage almost always occurs without any residual damage. Forceps injury to the cornea may very occasionally produce permanent corneal opacities, and haemorrhage into the anterior chamber may cause a secondary glaucoma.

HEARING

The inner ear can be damaged by trauma or asphyxia at birth, infection by the rubella virus in pregnancy, or aminoglycoside antibiotics such as gentamicin (p. 168). There also appears to be an increase in sensori-neural deafness in some ethnic minority groups in the UK. Hearing can now be tested with some accuracy in the newborn

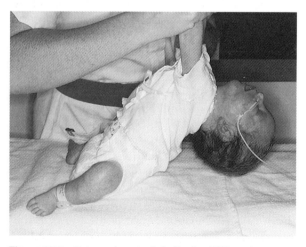

Figure 10.3 Extreme hypotonia in Prader–Willi syndrome.

period using oto-acoustic responses or by performing auditory brain stem-evoked response tests. Severe deafness from birth is followed in many cases by very poor speech development. The early provision of hearing aids and speech training may improve the acquisition of speech and it is recommended that babies in the following categories should be considered for neonatal hearing testing:

- a family history of early sensori-neural deafness
- moderate or severe hypoxic-ischaemic encephalopathy
- babies with parenchymal brain damage on ultrasound scans
- babies given aminoglycoside antibiotics
- those with evidence of intrauterine infections
- chromosomal anomalies
- congenital malformations of the head and neck, including cleft lip and palate
- consanguineous parents.

NERVE INJURIES

Brachial plexus injuries

Injury to the cervical nerve roots may cause paralysis of the arm which varies in extent and distribution depending on which nerves are involved. Erb's palsy, the commonest abnormality, is due to contusion, or more rarely rupture, of the upper nerves of the brachial plexus from downward traction of the arm or shoulder during, for instance, a delivery complicated by shoulder dystocia, producing paralysis of the muscles supplied by the fifth and sixth cervical nerves – the abductors of the shoulder, the flexors of the elbow and the supinator. Thus the resulting characteristic posture is a relatively immobile arm held extended down the side and pronated (Fig. 10.4). Loss of movement in the arm can be shown by demonstrating that only the unaffected arm moves when performing the Moro reflex (p. 66). It is very occasionally accompanied by phrenic nerve palsy, causing paralysis of the diaphragm on the same side.

Less commonly, the eighth cervical and first thoracic nerves are injured by upward traction on the arm. The resultant paralysis (Klumpke's

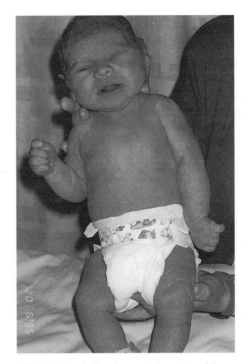

Figure 10.4   Extended and pronated posture of the arm in Erb's palsy.

palsy) involves mainly the intrinsic muscles of the hand and the flexors of the wrist and fingers. Sensory loss may be present but is not easily demonstrable with certainty. Rarely, complete paralysis of the whole arm may occur from more extensive plexus injury.

Injury is sometimes caused to the radial or posterior interosseous nerves due to traction or local pressure. Wrist drop is the presenting feature and recovery is the rule.

Differential diagnosis

The only difficulty lies in distinguishing these brachial plexus injuries from pseudoparalysis due to a painful lesion in the arm itself such as a subperiosteal haemorrhage, osteomyelitis or even a fracture. The arm is held limply and no movement can be demonstrated, but it is usually possible to elicit tenderness on pressure and swelling or bruising may be present as an additional sign.

Prognosis and treatment

Fortunately all but a few of these nerve injuries are due to contusion and complete division is rare. Movement generally begins to return gradually within a month, continues for up to 18 months and eventually around 80% get a reasonable recovery of hand and arm function. Encouraging movement of the arm and preventing contractures by means of physiotherapy are important, but nerve grafting using microsurgical techniques and later release of soft tissue contractures can improve the outlook when there is little evidence of recovery in the first 3 months.

Facial nerve palsy

Facial nerve palsy is sometimes caused by trauma to the facial nerve by forceps, although more often it occurs after normal delivery and is thought to be due to abnormal pressure on the nerve from the maternal sacrum. Unilateral facial weakness becomes obvious as the baby cries, the eye on the affected side failing to close and the mouth being pulled across to the opposite side (Fig. 10.5). There is no interference with feeding and recovery is usually complete within a few weeks. When bilateral, there is just a remarkable lack of facial expression when crying, but this is rarely due to pressure and other causes such as nuclear agenesis (Moebius syndrome) have to be considered.

FRACTURES OF THE LONG BONES

The bones most often broken during delivery are the clavicle, humerus and femur. The fractured clavicle, if not noticed at delivery, is often missed for it causes little swelling and practically no interference with arm movements. Fractures of the other bones are usually recognized by the sound or feel of the break at the time and later confirmed by the immobility of the limb with perhaps bruising or swelling. Occasionally crepitus is the only sign.

When a fracture is suspected, ultrasound examination is often better than X-rays in diagnosing neonatal fractures in the early stages. There is no

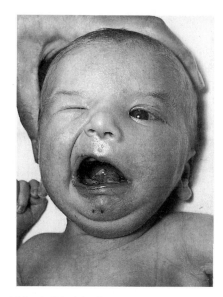

Figure 10.5 Left facial palsy.

more remarkable example of the infant's potential for natural repair than the way in which union occurs with eventual return to normal contour of the bone in spite of severe displacement. Accurate reduction of the fracture is not of great importance. Immobilization need not be complete and in the case of the fractured humerus, bandaging the arm to the side suffices. For the femur, bandaging the leg to a light lateral splint extending upwards beyond the pelvis is sometimes advocated, but union with normal final alignment almost always results even if no immobilization is used.

DISLOCATION OF JOINTS

Congenital dislocations of the knee result in an alarming reversed angulation of the leg at the knee. It is usually only necessary to reposition the leg progressively by serial splintage, and eventually a stable knee and good function are obtained. Occasionally other joints such as the elbow can be dislocated during delivery, but conservative treatment usually restores the joint to normal.

OTHER INJURIES

Rupture of the liver or spleen with intra-abdominal haemorrhage is a rare complication of a difficult delivery but should not be forgotten when there is increasing pallor, restlessness and tachypnoea.

Bruising of the external genitalia is not uncom-mon after breech delivery. Occasionally there is a large haematoma which causes temporary difficulty with passing urine, but this always subsides spontaneously within a few days.

FURTHER READING

David T J (ed) 1994 Recent advances in paediatrics 13. Birth asphyxia. Churchill Livingstone, Edinburgh, ch 2

Dubowitz V 1992 The muscular dystrophies. Postgraduate Medical Journal 68: 500–506

Eken P, Toet M C, Groenendaal F, de Vries L S 1995 Predictive value of early neuroimaging, pulsed Doppler and neurophysiology in full term infants with hypoxic-ischaemic encephalopathy. Archives of Disease in Childhood 73: F75–F80

Freeman N V, Burge D M 1994. Surgery of the newborn. Churchill Livingstone, Edinburgh

Levene M, Liford R (eds) 1995 Fetal and neonatal neurology and neurosurgery. Churchill Livingstone, Edinburgh

Martin E, Barkovich A J 1995 Magnetic resonance imaging in perinatal asphyxia. Archives of Disease in Childhood 72: F62–F70

Roberton N R C (ed) 1992 Textbook of neonatology. Churchill Livingstone, Edinburgh

Rutherford M A, Pennock J M 1994 Cranial ultrasound and magnetic resonance imaging in hypoxic-ischaemic encephalopathy: a comparison with outcome. Developmental Medicine and Child Neurology 36: 813–825

Sinclair J, Bracken M 1992 Effective care of the newborn infant. Oxford University Press, Oxford

Temple C M, Dennis J et al 1995 Neonatal seizures: long term outcome and cognitive development among normal survivors. Developmental Medicine and Child Neurology 37: 109–118

11

Infections

MECHANISMS OF PROTECTION FROM INFECTION

The full-term newborn baby is more vulnerable to attack from bacteria, viruses and fungi than the older infant because her defence mechanisms are immature and some organisms which are non-pathogenic in the older child can cause serious infection in the neonatal period. In the preterm infant these defences are even less mature so that serious consequences of infection are more likely. Male babies are more susceptible to infection than females. Some protection, however, is afforded through the following immune responses.

Immunoglobulins (antibodies)

Until about 3–4 months of age the baby has only a limited capacity to produce antibodies in response to infection. Some passive immunity is gained by transfer of some immunoglobulin G (IgG) antibodies from the mother in the last weeks of pregnancy but the infant has no IgM or IgA antibodies since neither is able to cross the placenta. This gives the infant protection from viral diseases such as measles, mumps, chickenpox and rubella for 4–6 months as long as the mother has immunity following exposure to these infections. However, antibodies against such bacteria as *Escherichia coli*, group B streptococci, *Haemophilus influenzae* and *Streptococcus pneumoniae* are not usually transferred, which may partly explain why these organisms in particular are more likely to infect the newborn baby.

Complement

Complement is a group of substances which damage the cell membranes of invading organisms and enable their further destruction by phagocytes. These are present in reduced amounts at birth.

Cellular immune systems

Lymphocytes

Lymphocytes which produce immunoglobulins are immature at birth and those which recognize invading organisms or have cytotoxic activity have only limited function in the term infant.

Polymorphonuclear leucocytes

Polymorphonuclear leucocytes, which accumulate at the site of infection under the influence of the complement system and phagocytose or kill bacteria, migrate less well in the neonatal period, but their killing capacity is mature once the baby approaches term. With overwhelming infections, the bone marrow becomes unable to keep up an adequate production of white cells and neutropenia may result, causing a reduction in the infant's capacity to eradicate bacteria.

Colostrum

Colostrum from breast feeding affords some protection against infection by providing the infant with substances such as IgA, lysozymes, lactoferrin and lymphocytes. Later on, breast milk reduces the proliferation of organisms in the gut since the acidity produced by the breakdown of the excess lactose in the large bowel favours the growth of harmless lactobacilli and inhibits the more pathogenic E. coli organisms.

SOURCES AND ROUTES OF INFECTION

Before birth, infection may take place either across the placenta or by ascending the birth canal. Amongst infections acquired principally by the transplacental route are rubella, cytomegalovirus, toxoplasmosis, syphilis, tuberculosis and HIV infection. Those organisms which reach the fetus via the birth canal, especially after prolonged rupture of the membranes, include the group B streptococcus, E. coli, Pseudomonas aeruginosa, Listeria monocytogenes and Mycoplasma hominis. More often, members of this latter group infect the baby during delivery – as do the gonococcus, hepatitis B virus, Candida albicans (Monilia), echovirus, Coxsackie virus and Chlamydia trachomatis.

Within the first few days of life, the baby becomes colonized by bacteria which are usually harmless but which can occasionally cause disease, and the pattern of pathogenic organisms changes over the years. The skin and umbilicus are colonized by staphylococci, the lower gut by E. coli and the upper respiratory tract by streptococci. Spread from one baby to another is a constant risk. For instance, a mild staphylococcal 'sticky eye' which is trivial in itself can be a source of much more serious infection like staphylococcal pneumonia or osteomyelitis in other infants at a later stage. Staphylococcal, streptococcal and E. coli infections often originate from care givers carrying the organisms and much less frequently from the mother.

Some mechanical apparatus is easily contaminated and it is essential to ensure the adequate sterilization of incubators, ventilators, suction apparatus, breast milk pumps and weighing scales after use. Some organisms like P. aeruginosa, on the other hand, tend to live in moist places like wash basins and their traps and have even been found in some 'disinfectant' fluids and soaps.

Clinical factors predisposing to infection are pre-term birth, low birth weight, hypothermia, prolonged rupture of the membranes and the presence of certain congenital malformations, particularly superficial lesions such as meningomyelocele, and abnormalities of the urinary tract.

Organisms causing neonatal infection

Although in the past Staph. aureus was the commonest cause of serious neonatal infections, more recently in the UK *E. coli* and group B β-haemolytic streptococi have been the most commonly isolated organisms in cases of septicaemia, pneumonia and meningitis. *E. coli* is a universal bowel organism and between 5 and 20% of mothers carry the group B streptococcus in the birth canal; this may be acquired by the infant during vaginal delivery, but treatment of the mother with penicillin before and during labour reduces the risk of infection in the baby. Only rarely, however, does either organism cause serious illness. *Staph. epidermidis* (coagulase-negative staphylococcus) is increasingly recognized to cause serious infection in pre-term infants, but in the majority of healthy term infants it is a harmless commensal organism.

Although it has been traditional to take swabs for bacterial culture from several sites on each infant admitted to a special care baby unit, they rarely identify either the baby who will develop a serious infection or the pathogen if she becomes ill. However, the swabs may identify an increasing rate of colonization by potentially pathogenic bacteria or show when it is necessary to take additional precautions to prevent cross-infection within the unit. Although there has been an increase in some virus infections in the newborn, e.g. herpes simplex encephalitis and echovirus 11 infection, most outbreaks have been small and confined to one unit, although each has had its fatalities.

MINOR INFECTIONS

Infections of skin and subcutaneous tissues

Isolated superficial pustules caused by staphylococcal infection are common, occurring singly or in crops. They are most troublesome in moist areas like the groins or axillae, although they can arise anywhere. Sometimes the lesion is just a small blister with no surrounding erythema, and although usually trivial in itself and rarely the primary cause of a disseminated staphylococcal infection, it is a source of cross-infection to others, so it should never be passed over casually. The little yellowish-white spots on an erythe-

matous or urticarial base which characterize urticaria neonatorum (p. 57) are sometimes mistakenly diagnosed as pustules.

Paronychia

Reddening of the skin in the nail fold area is also common and may proceed to pus formation, usually involving more than one finger at a time.

Bullous impetigo

Bullous impetigo (pemphigus neonatorum) is now rarely seen. Large vesicles arise containing thin pus, rupturing and leaving raw areas which may form scabs. Ritter's disease, or the scalded skin syndrome, is a more serious variety of the same infection in which the lesions rapidly coalesce and large areas of exfoliation of skin result, resembling a scald. Both conditions are caused by staphylococci.

Periumbilical infection

Infection of the periumbilical skin bears a special risk of spread via the umbilical vein, giving rise to thrombophlebitis and possibly leading to suppuration in the liver itself with severe jaundice. Some cases of portal hypertension with oesophageal varices arising in later childhood have been attributed to this cause.

Treatment of skin sepsis

Culture of material from any skin lesion should always be attempted because information about the type of organism and its sensitivity to antibiotics is of value in minimizing its spread. For minor lesions, local application of an antiseptic powder is sufficient. Systemic antibiotic treatment is not usually necessary and in general should be avoided since the overenthusiastic use of antibiotics encourages the development of resistant organisms such as methicillin-resistant *Staph. aureus* (MRSA) which is increasing in prevalence in hospitals in the UK and elsewhere. When they are needed, flucloxacillin is a good first choice since the majority of skin infections are caused by staphylococci which are almost all sensitive to it.

Acute mastitis

This infection usually occurs in an engorged neonatal breast and is usually caused by *Staph. aureus*. It appears as an inflamed red swelling under the nipple and the infant is usually febrile. Occasionally it may develop into an abscess which requires surgical incision and drainage, but if it is treated early with antibiotics the infection will usually resolve. Flucloxacillin is the drug of choice, given orally if the infection is minor, but systemically if the baby is ill.

Eye infections

Sticky eye

A sticky eye in the first one or two days of life is often due only to chemical irritation and clears spontaneously. The only treatment necessary is to wipe away the secretions with cooled boiled water when they accumulate. After this age it is likely to be infective in origin.

Conjunctivitis

Conjunctivitis with a purulent discharge from the eye is relatively common. Staphylococci, *E. coli* or streptococci are frequently grown in culture but it is difficult to be sure that they are the true cause. After taking swabs for culture, treatment should be started immediately with chloramphenicol 1.0% eye ointment applied at least four times a day and should be continued for 5 days or until it has resolved.

More persistent infection not responding to routine treatment may be caused by *Chlamydia trachomatis*, but the organism is difficult to culture in the laboratory (Plate 16). The conjunctiva tends to be more 'fleshy' in appearance and is associated with swelling of the eyelids. Treatment with tetracycline eye ointment 4- to 6-hourly is usually effective combined with oral erythromycin in more severe cases. Topical

chloramphenicol suppresses infection with this organism but does not cure it.

Dacrocystitis

Dacrocystitis is occasionally seen as a complication of conjunctivitis, with a reddened swelling over the region of the lacrimal sac at the root of the nose. Pressure over the sac produces a little purulent discharge from the lacrimal duct in the lower eyelid and this can be gently carried out three or four times daily as a therapeutic measure, combined with local instillation of chloramphenicol ointment and systemic flucloxacillin.

Ophthalmia neonatorum

Ophthalmia neonatorum due to gonococcal infection is uncommon where treatment of sexually transmitted diseases is readily available but is a common cause of blindness worldwide. Prevention can be achieved by giving an infant born to an infected mother a single intramuscular dose of penicillin 50 mg/kg at birth. Maternal gonorrhoea is often asymptomatic, but in the infant the effect is dramatic. It is a serious acute infection beginning as a purulent conjunctivitis but liable to involve deeper structures of the eye, causing irreparable damage if left untreated. The diagnosis can usually be made quickly from a direct Gram stain on a smear of pus, but culture to determine antibiotic sensitivity is essential since penicillin resistance is becoming common throughout the world.

Treatment. The eye should be irrigated with chloramphenicol eye drops as frequently as is needed to reduce the profuse production of pus. In addition, benzylpenicillin 50 mg/kg should be given intramuscularly 12-hourly for at least 7 days to clear the infection, although cefotaxime intravenously should be given if the organism is penicillin-resistant.

Respiratory tract infections

'Snuffles'

An excess of nasal secretion which partially

blocks the nasal airway is common in the first few weeks of life. It is sometimes present at birth when it may be a clear mucoid discharge or, much less commonly, a mucopurulent one. Although included amongst the infections, it is likely that many of these cases are not infective. Respiratory syncytial virus is occasionally the cause of relatively mild upper respiratory tract infection in the newborn, in contrast to the more familiar acute bronchiolitis seen in older infants.

Although congenital syphilis is rare where antenatal screening and treatment are available, it is a cause of purulent or blood-stained nasal discharge often associated with other features of congenital syphilis (p. 173).

No treatment for the common variety of 'snuffles' is usually necessary, but interference with feeding due to nasal obstruction justifies the sparing use of 0.25% ephedrine nasal drops in normal saline given before feeds. Otitis media is often missed in the newborn period because it is not suspected or because the ear drum sometimes cannot so easily be seen. It gives rise to irritability and failure to feed and thrive. Needle aspiration of the middle ear is the only means of proving the diagnosis but this is obviously too painful and hazardous a procedure to use in most circumstances and is unnecessary. *Staphylococcus aureus* and streptococci are the commonest infecting bacteria and nearly all cases respond well to a combination of oral ampicillin and flucloxacillin.

Infections of the alimentary tract

Thrush

Thrush or moniliasis, which is caused by the fungus *C. albicans*, most commonly affects the mouth but may also involve the oesophagus and gastrointestinal tract, resulting in diarrhoea and vomiting. It is a common cause of rashes in the nappy area at this age, as described on page 102 (Plate 17). The source of monilial infection is usually the vagina of the mother, but the organism is commonly found on the skin, including that of the breast. Oral thrush shows itself as numerous small white plaques (resembling curds of milk) on the tongue and inside the mouth which are difficult to dislodge. The resulting soreness sometimes causes refusal of feeds. Nystatin suspension, 1 ml (100 000 units), given by a dropper directly into the mouth after each feed for 7–10 days is usually an effective treatment, but it may have to be repeated. Other effective topical preparations include miconazole and clotrimazole.

SERIOUS ACUTE INFECTION

The incidence of serious acute infections in the newborn period is about 3 per 1000 live births in the UK and they include meningitis, pneumonia and urinary tract infection, often with septicaemia. Making a specific diagnosis may be difficult because clinical signs pointing to the site of the infection are often absent.

Immaturity of the immune responses allows the infection to become rapidly disseminated in the body and thus more damaging. For this reason it is important to recognize the clinical signs which should raise the suspicion of an infection and, after investigating thoroughly to locate the infection and isolate the organisms responsible, to begin antibiotic treatment immediately (p. 167).

Clinical signs of infection

The warning signs of sepsis include:

- pyrexia or hypothermia
- reluctance to feed
- lethargy
- vomiting
- failure to gain weight
- an anxious look
- pallor of the skin
- irritability
- apnoea
- jaundice
- abdominal distension
- sudden collapse.

Other signs are more specific to the site of the infection – for instance respiratory distress (tachypnoea, costal recession and grunting) in pneumonia.

A white cell count in the blood may be helpful in diagnosis at an early stage, since either a depressed or a raised neutrophil count strongly suggests infection. Additionally, acute phase reactants such as C-reactive protein may be found in the blood but they often add little to the early diagnosis of infection.

Rarely transitory fever can be associated with dehydration alone but it is not seen in infants fed right from the time of birth. The body temperature may reach 39–40°C (103° or 104°F) and it occurs typically on the third or fourth day. It is associated with crying and restlessness, but not with the general signs of infection, and is relieved within 24 hours by giving extra water.

Investigation in suspected infection

In any infant showing the clinical signs of more than a trivial local infection, it is mandatory to carry out the following investigations to confirm the diagnosis and find the causative organism:

- full blood count
- blood culture
- urine culture – either a clean-catch or suprapubic sample
- swabs from the throat, nose, ear and any evidently infected site
- lumbar puncture and CSF culture
- chest X-ray.

In addition to these, the blood electrolytes and blood gases may be measured if the infant is particularly ill. A raised level of C-reactive protein in the blood may give an early indication of infection.

Septicaemia

Infection may originate before, during or after birth and the commonest organism identified in the first 2 days of life is the group B haemolytic streptococcus. Other organisms often responsible are *E. coli*, *P. aeruginosa* and *Listeria monocytogenes*. Viruses of various types are less commonly isolated. In very pre-term babies, *Staph. epidermidis* and strains of *Streptococcus viridans* are becoming recognized more frequently as pathogens (Ch. 9).

A blood culture must be taken from a peripheral vein after skin sterilization because the use of the femoral and umbilical veins for the purpose is liable to give false-positive results from contamination.

The disseminated intravascular coagulation syndrome may complicate the clinical picture and usually presents as circulatory failure and haemorrhage from one or more sites (p. 179).

Treatment

Intravenous antibiotic treatment should start before the diagnosis is confirmed with either a combination of penicillin or ampicillin and gentamicin, or alternatively with a broad-spectrum second or third generation cephalosporin such as cefuroxime or cefotaxime. A positive blood culture enables any necessary change in treatment to be made according to the sensitivity of the organism found and the antibiotics should be continued for 14 days. If the baby is gravely ill, an infusion of immunoglobulin at the outset may improve the prognosis.

Close attention should also be paid to other aspects of treatment such as maintenance of body temperature, fluid and electrolyte balance, blood glucose values and nutrition.

Meningitis

Fortunately this infection is rare, affecting only 1 in 3000 newborn infants. Most neonatal meningitis is due to infection by group B streptococci, *E. coli* or occasionally *L. monocytogenes*. *Pseudomonas aeruginosa* and other Gram-negative enteric organisms may cause it in pre-term infants undergoing intensive care, but bacteria such as *H. influenzae* which so commonly cause meningitis in older infants or children are rarely implicated. Occasional outbreaks of enteroviral meningitis are recorded, caused by such viruses as echovirus II or Coxsackie B.

Infection of the meninges usually follows a stage of septicaemia, and it is vital to examine the cerebrospinal fluid (CSF) in all babies in whom generalized infection is suspected, since in the early stages of the illness there are no signs to localize the infection to the meninges. The usual clinical features include listlessness, a reluctance to feed, vomiting, pallor and temperature instability, and only later does fullness of the anterior fontanelle become detectable. Fits may occur occasionally but neck rigidity is often completely absent until the late stages of the disease.

Diagnosis should be made as early as possible by lumbar puncture, which is a relatively simple procedure and not hazardous if done correctly. Early diagnosis, and thus more effective treatment, of one case justifies the investigation of many which turn out to be negative.

Technique of lumbar puncture

The infant should be held gently but firmly by the assistant in either a sitting or lying position so as to flex the spine and enlarge the interspinous spaces (Fig. 11.1). Strict asepsis must be maintained throughout to prevent the introduction of organisms to the CSF. After sterilization of the skin with spirit and iodine, a suitable small lumbar puncture needle with a stilette is inserted into a space between the vertebral spines approximately on a level with the upper border of the iliac crests. After the initial puncture of the skin, the operator waits until the infant remains still and then gently and slowly inserts the needle at a

right angle to the surface, not deviating to either side of the midline. A definite click is felt as the dura is punctured in many cases, but it is advisable to advance the needle very slowly until spinal fluid flows. If inserted too far, it invariably causes bleeding and it can then be difficult to confirm the high white cell count or see the infecting organisms on Gram staining.

The normal neonatal CSF often contains up to 20 white cells/mm^3, 1.5 g/L of protein and a glucose level of 2.7–4.4 mmol/L. Although usually the white cell count and protein levels are higher and the glucose value lower than these in meningitis, the overlap is large and they are not often helpful in making the diagnosis. A Gram stain of a smear of the fluid will often demonstrate bacteria and guide the choice of antibiotic, but it is essential to culture the CSF to identify the organism and confirm its antibiotic sensitivities. A specific latex agglutination test can be used to confirm group B haemolytic streptococcal infection.

Treatment

All the general measures to investigate and treat septicaemia must be instituted and suitable antibacterial therapy started immediately. The chosen antibiotics must pass freely into the CSF

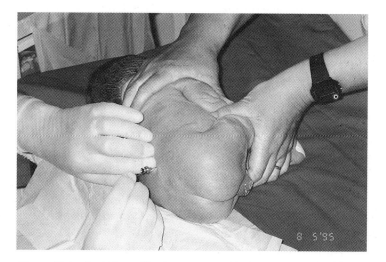

Figure 11.1 Technique of lumbar puncture showing the position in which the baby should be held.

and be given intravenously in maximal doses to give adequate bactericidal concentrations to cover the most likely organisms. Amoxycillin or ampicillin, to which *Listeria monocytogenes* is normally sensitive, together with cefotaxime or ceftriaxone is a commonly recommended combination which penetrates well into the CSF and will be effective against most group B streptococci and *E. coli*. Gentamicin penetrates poorly into the CSF and is no more effective when instilled directly into it either by lumbar puncture or directly into the cerebral ventricles. It is not routinely recommended, therefore, for the treatment of meningitis, although it is commonly used in combination with a cephalosporin. Amikacin may also be used with cefotaxime or ceftriaxone. Ceftazidime may be used if the infecting organism is *P. aeruginosa*.

Chloramphenicol is occasionally used because it is so well concentrated in the CSF when given systemically, although it is probably not adequate for the treatment of *E. coli* or other Gram-negative organisms. It can cause the 'grey baby syndrome' (p. 167) if given in excessive dosage, and blood levels of the drug must be measured if this is to be avoided.

Whatever antibiotic is chosen initially, it is essential to confirm that the causal bacteria are sensitive to it, and monitoring of both blood and, if possible, CSF levels of the drug used is advised in view of the risk of toxicity at this age (p. 167).

The duration of treatment depends upon the cause and severity of the meningitis but, in general, systemic treatment should continue for 10–14 days after CSF culture becomes negative. There is some evidence that the administration of steroids to babies with meningitis may reduce the incidence of deafness in survivors.

Outlook

The overall mortality rate for neonatal meningitis treated in the UK is around 25%, deaths often being related to a delay in diagnosis. Of those that recover, approximately 30–50% have permanent neurological handicaps, including deafness and blindness, since complications like hydrocephalus, subdural effusion and ventriculitis are common, but the development of new antibiotics has certainly improved the prognosis in recent years.

Congenital pneumonia

This is generally part of an acute septicaemic illness acquired prenatally, especially when the membranes have been ruptured for more than 24 hours before the onset of labour. It is most commonly due to the group B haemolytic streptococcus and may be rapidly fatal if not treated immediately. Respiratory distress is often the chief presenting sign but all the features of septicaemia may be present.

Prevention is possible only if the organism has been grown from a maternal vaginal swab, in which case the prophylactic administration of penicillin to the mother during labour and to the baby immediately after birth is effective in reducing the risk of serious infection.

Pneumonia of later onset is due to aspiration of infected material or droplet infection, and Gram-negative bacilli are the most usual organisms involved. *Staphylococcus aureus* may also cause pneumonia but is much less common.

Clinical features

The clinical features are those of acute infection with the signs of respiratory distress. Local signs are generally confined to fine râles on auscultation. A chest X-ray is essential for differentiating infection from the many other causes of respiratory distress. In staphylococcal pneumonia, a lung abscess or the formation of a tension cyst, with or without pneumothorax, may complicate the picture.

Treatment

The baby is best nursed lying prone or on the side but should be gently moved at intervals to prevent local accumulation of secretions. The head end of the cot or incubator platform should be tipped upwards. Humidified oxygen given in adequate concentration to maintain a normal Po_2 or oxygen saturation is essential, together with intravenous antibiotics. If the infant is only mildly ill, she may be given small frequent bottle feeds although it is often better to conserve her energy by passing a nasogastric tube to administer fluids and nutrients.

Urinary tract infections

Urinary infection, usually caused by *E. coli* but less often by other Gram-negative organisms, may remain undiagnosed in the newborn baby unless the possibility is borne in mind, since its clinical features are so non-specific. The evidence shows that progressive kidney damage leading ultimately to chronic renal failure often begins in the neonatal period, due to vesicoureteric reflux of infected urine or to severe pyelonephritis associated with septicaemia.

Symptoms and signs

Symptoms and signs are non-specific and consist of reluctance to feed, drowsiness, vomiting, failure to thrive and sometimes jaundice. Pyrexia may or may not be present.

Diagnosis

Infection will be missed unless urine is cultured in all babies with such clinical features. The diagnostic difficulty lies in collecting an uncontaminated specimen. It is often possible, with patience, to obtain a 'clean catch' midstream specimen after cleansing the external genitalia with sterile water, and sometimes a baby can be induced to empty the bladder by holding her erect over a container and tapping the lower abdomen with the finger about once per second. Collection in an adhesive polythene bag appliance frequently results in contaminated urine, making the results of the investigation hard to interpret. As an approximate guide, for a 'clean catch' specimen, 50×10^6 pus cells/L of uncentrifuged urine in the female and 25×10^6/L in the male suggest infection, and a pure bacterial growth of more than 10^8 organisms/L confirms the diagnosis.

Suprapubic aspiration of the bladder, using a

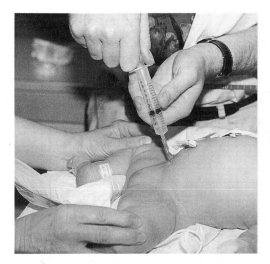

Figure 11.2 Technique of suprapubic aspiration of urine. The needle is inserted half way between the pubic bone and the umbilicus to a depth of 2 cm.

5 ml syringe and no. 1 needle inserted perpendicularly to the skin about 2 cm deep and midway between the top of the symphysis pubis and the umbilicus (Fig. 11.2), is relatively quick and safe provided that it is done with full aseptic precautions and a single needle insertion. The bladder at this age is more an abdominal than a pelvic organ, so the procedure is often successful if attempted about 30 minutes after a feed, but ultrasound imaging of the bladder can improve the success rate of the procedure. Any growth of organisms in urine obtained by this method is indicative of infection.

Treatment

This should be started before results of the urine culture are obtained if the baby is obviously ill. Intravenous cefotaxime is probably the most effective antibiotic to use at the present time. Alternatively, gentamicin or netilmicin may be given intravenously, but their blood levels must be carefully monitored and the size and frequency of the doses adjusted accordingly, especially if renal function is impaired. If sensitivity tests allow, amoxycillin, trimethoprim or co-trimoxazole may be used after the first week of life and continued for 10–14 days. Subsequent urine

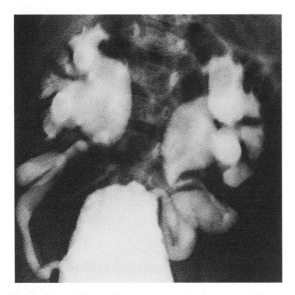

Figure 11.3 Micturating cystogram showing gross reflux and dilatation of the pelves of the kidneys and the ureters in a baby with a urinary tract infection. (By kind permission of Dr Jo Fairhurst.)

checks are essential, with careful follow-up of progress in the first year.

Imaging of the renal tracts after completion of treatment is essential since there is a relatively high incidence of congenital anomalies or vesicoureteric reflux. An isotope scan can demonstrate evidence of scarring in the renal parenchyma and may show the relative function of the two kidneys; an ultrasound scan can demonstrate any obstructive lesion or malformation; and a micturating cystogram will identify any reflux (Fig. 11.3). If such problems are identified, the baby should be referred for a paediatric surgical assessment.

Acute gastroenteritis

Infective diarrhoea and vomiting are fortunately uncommon in the newborn. Colostrum and breast milk confer some degree of protection against this infection so it is less common in breast-fed than in formula-fed babies. Outbreaks do occur from time to time in maternity or newborn baby units, and the condition is most commonly due to infection with a rotavirus.

Occasionally bacteria such as *Salmonella*, *Shigella* or campylobacter are identified in the stools. The disease can be rapidly fatal at this age, especially when it affects either low birth weight infants or those with a severe congenital malformation.

The newborn baby rapidly becomes ill from dehydration and electrolyte imbalance when diarrhoea and vomiting are profuse. The signs of dehydration are an inelastic skin, sunken eyes and fontanelle, dryness of the mouth and oliguria. Later, if left untreated, there is tachycardia, hypotension and a greyish pallor from circulatory impairment.

Treatment

Isolation from other babies is essential since the organisms are highly contagious. In addition to the clinical evaluation of the infant, estimation of blood electrolytes and urea is necessary to assess the effect of the fluid losses and to monitor the infant's progress. Replacement of excess losses of fluid and electrolytes is central to successful treatment. An initial rapid intravenous infusion of 20 ml/kg of albumin solution to improve the blood pressure and restore the circulating volume is needed for the more severely dehydrated infant, but in most cases a slower correction with 0.9% saline is sufficient. Once the initial replacement is complete, intravenous fluid volumes should be calculated to provide the normal daily fluid requirements plus the estimated deficit and additional losses from diarrhoea and vomiting, restoring the baby's fluid balance over 48 hours. Regular measurements of blood electrolytes and urea will guide the choice of fluids and indicate in particular whether additional sodium or potassium replacement is required. Breast feeding should be continued unless the baby is vomiting, although cow's milk formula should not be given during treatment. Antibiotics are needed only when an accompanying septicaemia is suspected.

Acute osteomyelitis and septic arthritis

Although it is an uncommon occurrence, staphylococcal infection in bone or a joint occasionally follows some apparently minor superficial sepsis after a latent period of 2 or 3 weeks. Other organisms such as group B haemolytic streptococci and *H. influenzae* may also cause a similar infection. In the case of a long bone of the arm or leg, attention may be drawn to the condition simply by the fact that the limb is not used (pseudoparalysis), but there is often local swelling and redness of skin. The general constitutional disturbance is surprisingly slight, although fever is almost always present. Appropriate systemic antibiotic treatment (usually flucloxacillin) is continued for several weeks, and provided that resistant organisms are not encountered, surgical intervention is seldom needed.

USE OF ANTIBIOTICS IN THE NEWBORN PERIOD
General principles

Widespread indiscriminate use of antibiotics, especially those with a broad spectrum of activity, is to be strongly deprecated for there is evidence that usually harmless organisms can become pathogenic when the normal bacterial flora of the baby is disturbed and increasing numbers of antibiotic-resistant organisms will emerge. Prophylactic antibiotic treatment should be used only exceptionally. On the other hand, since the outcome of serious infections at this age is so much better if early treatment is given, the non-specific clinical features of suspected infection do justify the use of appropriate antibiotics before a specific bacterial diagnosis has been reached.

The choice of antibiotic

When the bacterial diagnosis is certain on clinical grounds, a single appropriate antibiotic can sometimes be used from the start. Benzyl penicillin is the drug of choice for the group B streptococci. Gentamicin or netilmicin will cover both staphylococci and most Gram-negative organisms, and the newer cephalosporin antibi-

otics are also effective against these bacteria, although they are less effective against group B streptococci and are ineffective against *L. monocytogenes*. If listeriosis is suspected, it should be treated with ampicillin. Anaerobic infections with *Bacteroides* require treatment with metronidazole. When the causative organism has been isolated and its antibiotic sensitivity established, the treatment can be modified accordingly.

Treatment of suspected sepsis

For a *relatively mild infection* in which an organism has not yet been identified, a combination of ampicillin and flucloxacillin is commonly used initially.

For the *more seriously ill infant* with probable septicaemia, a combination of penicillin or ampicillin with gentamicin or netilmicin, or alternatively a cephalosporin such as cefotaxime or cefuroxime, should be given intravenously until the specific causative organism is isolated. The policy of which antibiotic is to be used in these circumstances must, however, depend upon which bacteria are prevalent at that time and their likely sensitivities.

Certain antibiotics have special disadvantages if used for the neonate but are mentioned here since they may be needed for particular infections. Chloramphenicol can cause hypotension from cardiovascular failure with muscular hypotonia and a pallid cyanosis, a situation known as the grey baby syndrome, if used in high dosage. It is more likely to occur in the pre-term infant. Although a highly effective antibiotic, chloramphenicol should therefore be used only exceptionally in the newborn period in reduced dosage, and the blood levels should be measured to avoid these toxic effects. Tetracycline is deposited in the growing bones and teeth and causes yellowness of the first dentition with some increased susceptibility to caries, but it is rarely needed. Sulphonamides, including co-trimoxazole, can precipitate kernicterus by displacing bilirubin from the albumin to which it is normally bound, making it available to cross from blood to brain. Co-trimoxazole is, however, the drug of choice for the rare *Pneumocystis carinii* pneumonia.

Dosage

The pathways of metabolism and excretion of many antibiotics are immature in the newborn baby. Blood levels of all antibiotics, therefore, tend to be higher and are sustained for longer in the first few days of life on a given dose, particularly if the baby is born prematurely. It is essential to measure the blood levels of gentamicin and netilmicin and to adjust the dose accordingly to avoid accumulation in the blood, since high concentrations of these may cause nerve deafness and renal failure (Table 11.1).

Table 11.1 gives the single doses of a selected group of antibiotics. For mature infants (37–42 weeks' gestation), the dose is given 12-hourly for the first 48 hours, 8-hourly between the third and 14th day, and 6-hourly thereafter. For preterm infants (less than 37 weeks) the dose is given 12-hourly for the first week, 8-hourly for the second, third and fourth weeks, and 6-hourly thereafter. Absorption from the gut of antibiotic preparations given orally is uncertain and irregular during the first week of life and so intravenous or intramuscular administration is preferable for the more seriously ill baby.

Table 11.1 Antibiotics commonly used in the newborn baby

Antibiotic	Single dose per kg body weight	Route of administration	Number of doses per day*	Comments
Amikacin	7.5 mg/kg	iv	2	
Ampicillin or amoxycillin	30–50 mg/kg	iv/im/oral	2–3	
Azlocillin	100 mg/kg	iv	2	Dose should be halved in pre-term infants
Benzylpenicillin	15–30 mg/kg	iv/im	2–3	Dose may be increased to 50 mg/kg in severe infections
Cefotaxime	50 mg/kg	iv/im	2–3	
Ceftazidime	30 mg/kg	iv/im	2–3	
Cefuroxime	30 mg/kg	iv/im	2–3	
Chloramphenicol	12.5 mg/kg	iv/oral	2	Dose may be doubled after 2 weeks of age; blood levels should be monitored
Cloxacillin or Flucloxacillin	25–40 mg/kg	iv/im iv/oral	4	Dose may be increased up to 100 mg/kg in severe infections
Erythromycin	12.5 mg/kg	Oral/iv	4	iv by slow infusion
Gentamicin	3.0 mg/kg	iv/im	2–3	Monitor blood levels; keep peak level 8–10 mg/L and trough level < 2 mg/L
Isoniazid	5 mg/kg	Oral	1	Pyridoxine supplement required
Metronidazole	7.5 mg/kg	iv/oral	3	Infuse over 1 hour
Netilmicin	3.0 mg/kg	iv/im	2–3	Monitor blood levels; keep peak level 8–10 mg/L and trough level < 2 mg/L
Tobramycin	2.0 mg/kg	iv	2–3	Monitor blood levels as for gentamicin
Vancomycin	10–15 mg/kg	iv	2–3	Infuse over 60 minutes
Antifungal agents				
Amphotericin	0.25–1.0 mg/kg	iv	1	Infuse over 6 hours; use higher dose in severe infections
Flucytosine	50 mg/kg	Oral/iv	4	Infuse over 30 min
Miconazole	10 mg/kg	iv	2	Infuse over 1 hour
Nystatin	100 000 U	Oral	4	Give after feeds
Antiviral agents				
Acyclovir	10 mg/kg	iv	3	Infuse over 1 hour

* The lower dose frequency should be used in the first 7 days in term infants and for 10–14 days in pre-term infants; iv, intravenous; im, intramuscular. For further details consult the current British National Formulary or the Neonatal Vade Mecum.

VIRAL AND PROTOZOAL INFECTIONS

Antenatal infection

Transmission of bacterial infections across the placenta to the fetus is a remarkably rare event but any infection which produces severe illness in the mother may affect fetal growth by interference with its nutrition. Certain microorganisms, however, are able to pass the placental barrier, infect the fetus and interfere with its growth, differentiation or development. Toxoplasmosis, rubella, cytomegalovirus, herpes simplex virus and syphilis are the best known examples, and their effect on the fetus can be devastating. Human immunodeficiency virus (HIV) may infect the fetus. It does not cause malformation of the infant, but has long-lasting effects by means of damage to the immune system after birth. Exceptionally, transplacental infection occurs from Coxsackie and varicella viruses, whilst the bacteria causing tuberculosis and listeriosis have been known to spread to the fetus in this way also. Hepatitis B probably does not cross the placenta but commonly affects the infant during labour.

Congenital rubella

When contracted in early pregnancy, rubella virus can cross the placenta and cause serious damage to the developing fetus. In the first 12 weeks, there is a 90% chance of fetal infection which may cause malformation of the eyes (microphthalmia, retinopathy and cataracts), the brain (microcephaly and mental retardation) and the heart (especially between the fifth and eighth weeks), and sensori-neural deafness. Infection in the third month causes the deafness alone in up to 30% of cases, the risk diminishing during the fourth month. In addition, maternal infection at any stage up to 20 weeks may result in non-specific signs at birth such as hepatosplenomegaly, jaundice, thrombocytopenia and growth retardation. X-rays of the long bones may show changes characteristic of rubella osteitis. There appears to be no significant risk if the fetus is exposed after this time. Because of such high rates of damage in the early weeks, termination of pregnancy is often considered if maternal infection can be proved by rising antibody levels.

Confirmation of the infection in the neonate may be made by virus culture from the stools or CSF or by demonstrating IgM antibodies to the virus or a persisting titre of IgG antibody over the first few months of life. Infection in the nervous system is accompanied by a high protein level and an increase in mononuclear cells in the CSF. Despite the presence of antibody, these infants continue to excrete the active virus for many months after birth and may therefore spread the infection, which can be dangerous to women in early pregnancy. Appropriate isolation precautions must therefore be taken.

No treatment is available for the infection, but if the woman has anti-rubella antibodies before pregnancy, infection of the fetus is prevented. In the UK, the long-standing rubella immunization programme and the national campaign in 1994 to immunize all schoolchildren against rubella have almost eradicated the risk of fetal infection in the offspring of these children. However, a small number of adult women are still found to be susceptible to the infection at routine screening at their first antenatal visit and they should be offered immunization immediately after the birth of the baby. This is particularly important for Asian women who arrived in the UK as young adults and missed the school immunization programme. It is for this reason that the incidence of congenital rubella is doubled in this ethnic group.

Congenital cytomegalovirus infection

Cytomegalovirus (CMV) infection in the fetus can result in spontaneous abortion, serious multisystem disease or mental retardation and it is estimated that undetected CMV infection of the brain may be responsible for serious intellectual impairment in approximately 400 children in Britain each year. About 1% of susceptible women acquire the infection during pregnancy and in 40% of cases it affects the fetus no matter at what stage of pregnancy it occurs. Over half of women of child-bearing age have already been exposed to the virus, as shown by the presence of circulating antibodies, but reactivation of the virus during pregnancy can still involve the baby. Only about 10% of infected infants show clinical evidence of the disease at birth, but many of these infants go on to have serious long-term neurological problems A minority of asymptomatic infants may also develop nerve deafness or other neurological deficits, although about 90% will develop quite normally.

The affected infant may be stillborn or, if alive, of low birth weight. The full clinical picture is one of widespread involvement of many systems of the body with early jaundice, purpura, haemolytic anaemia, hepatosplenomegaly, pneumonia with cough and respiratory distress, or, less commonly, fits, rigidity, microcephaly, choroidoretinitis and osteitis. Longer-term complications include hepatitis, leading to cirrhosis of the liver, and progressive neurological disorders with mental retardation and cerebral palsy.

The diagnosis is confirmed by isolation of the virus from cultures of the urine and a throat swab together with identification of CMV antibodies in the mother and child. In symptomatic infants the CSF protein level is raised and mononuclear cells are found in the fluid. The antiviral agent gancyclovir is occasionally used if the baby is seriously affected, although subsequent brain damage is often not prevented by this treatment and the baby may continue to excrete the virus for some years. Prevention is not yet possible.

Congenital toxoplasmosis

Toxoplasmosis is caused by the protozoon *Toxoplasma gondii* which behaves in a similar way to the cytomegalovirus. Symptomatic infection is very common in childhood and early adult life, and by the age of 20 years about a quarter of the population has acquired the antibody. Primary maternal infection occurs during two pregnancies in every 1000, but it is only in less than half of these that the organism passes across the placenta to the infant. Infection in the first trimester is accompanied by a high risk of fetal damage, fetal death and abortion but later infection has fewer complications. Although only 10% of babies infected before birth have clinical signs of it in the newborn period, it is these infants who will develop the later problems, the asymptomatic infants probably having no lasting effects.

The incidence of the disease in pregnancy may be partially reduced by recommending the avoidance of undercooked meat and contact with cats, which are the alternative host for the organism. If a maternal acute infection is confirmed, treatment with spiramycin throughout the pregnancy reduces the incidence of congenital disease. If fetal toxoplasmosis is diagnosed in pregnancy, the mother should be treated with spiramycin, although its efficacy in treating the fetus remains uncertain.

Although congenital toxoplasmosis may present as a fulminating type of illness, with anaemia, purpura due to thrombocytopenia, jaundice and enlargement of liver and spleen, the more usual presentation is a widespread involvement of the central nervous system. In this form of the infection, fits and the signs of cerebral irritation are followed by the development of hydrocephalus and choroidoretinitis which leads ultimately to blindness. Intracranial calcification is a later characteristic radiological finding. The diagnosis is confirmed if the organism itself and the antibody to it are found in the CSF, but in the absence of CNS disease, the diagnosis relies on finding antibody in the serum of the mother and baby. An affected newborn baby should be treated with alternating courses of spiramycin and a combination of sulphadiazine, pyrimethamine and folic acid for the whole of the first year to reduce the risk of choroidoretinitis.

Other virus infections

Coxsackie B virus may occasionally be responsible for severe illness in the neonatal period, sometimes as an epidemic outbreak in a hospital unit. It is usually manifested as acute myocarditis or meningoencephalitis and no specific treatment is available.

Echoviruses, usually of type 11, have been increasingly recognized as a cause of neonatal illness. Infection arises mainly from the mother during delivery but may also be postnatal from others who come into contact with the baby. Outbreaks have been reported in maternity or special care neonatal units.

The clinical features vary from mild disturbance of general health to a fulminating septicaemia-like illness. Almost any system may be involved but outbreaks of gastroenteritis are perhaps most usual.

Viral cultures are essential for prevention of the spread of the infection in an outbreak, but they only help with treatment to the extent that antibiotics may be omitted. Fortunately the great majority of echovirus infections are mild and the infant successfully uses her own defence mechanisms to achieve full recovery. Normal human immunoglobulin contains antibody to this virus, which may be of some value in treatment in the early stages of the illness.

Varicella. Maternal infection in the first few weeks of pregnancy may cause fetal varicella syndrome which results in eye, limb and brain defects. Infection around the time of delivery can pass to the infant either before or just after birth. The chickenpox which results may be more severe than that seen in older children and has a high mortality. For these babies, treatment with intravenous acyclovir together with a dose of zoster immune globulin should be given.

CHRONIC INFECTIONS
Tuberculosis

Neonatal tuberculosis is rare although there is a higher risk in some ethnic Asian families where pulmonary tuberculosis is more common. It occurs more frequently in many developing countries, particularly those with a high incidence of HIV infection. It can be acquired from the mother before or after birth and the symptoms are non-specific refusal of feeds, loss of weight, vomiting, a slight pyrexia, and enlargement of the liver and spleen. Death may occur from miliary tuberculosis within a month if it is not treated. The tuberculin test is of no value in diagnosis at this age since the infant is unable to react to it. The chest X-ray of an infected infant is

likely to show miliary shadowing in the lungs. Treatment with rifampicin and isoniazid is likely to be fully successful if started in good time and continued for 6 months to a year. Protection against neonatal tuberculosis is discussed on page 28.

EFFECTS OF MATERNAL SEXUALLY TRANSMITTED DISEASES
HIV infection

Although still an uncommon infection during pregnancy in the UK, except in some drug abusers, HIV infection is extremely common in many developing countries, particularly in Africa. It is wise to consider the possibility of infection in recent arrivals and displaced people from such countries.

The acquired immune deficiency syndrome (AIDS) is a fatal disease caused by the human immunodeficiency virus (HIV). Pregnancy appears to reactivate the virus, and in approximately 25% of asymptomatic carriers, the baby will be infected either across the placenta or through contact with infected blood at delivery, but this falls to around 8% if the mother has been treated with AZT during the pregnancy. The rate of fetal infection is higher in women with symptomatic disease and in those who are vitamin A deficient or who suffer from other sexually transmitted diseases. There does not appear to be any increase in the incidence of pre-term labour or stillbirth. Infection of the baby is more likely if she is growth-retarded or pre-term, or if there has been prolonged rupture of the membranes or a prolonged second stage of labour.

The diagnosis of true HIV infection in the infant is difficult since maternal antibody readily transfers across the placenta and may persist in the baby's blood for many months. It may in some cases be possible to culture the virus or identify antigen in the baby's blood, but it is often only by the emergence of the characteristic clinical picture in the baby that infection is confirmed. Although the affected infant will be well in the neonatal period, the characteristic repeated serious infections with opportunistic

Table 11.2   Immunization schedule for HIV-infected infants

Vaccine	Age for immunization
Diphtheria, tetanus and pertussis	2, 3 and 4 months
Polio – inactivated i.m. vaccine*	2, 3 and 4 months
Influenza vaccine	At 6 months
Haemophilus influenzae type B (Hib)	2, 3 and 4 months
Mumps, measles, rubella (MMR)	At 15 months
Pneumococcal vaccine	At 2 years

*Oral (live) polio vaccine should not be administered.

organisms, such as cytomegalovirus and *Pneumocystis carinii*, will begin to appear, leading commonly to the baby's death within the first 2 years of life.

Currently no specific treatment exists other than that of the infections as they occur, but each potentially infected infant should receive all the vaccines in Table 11.2. Live vaccines must not be given in view of the infant's diminished immunity. The risk of contracting *P. carinii* infection can be reduced by continuous treatment with co-trimoxazole orally once the baby's immune status is shown to be compromised.

Management

During labour in an HIV-positive woman, it is essential to avoid the use of fetal scalp electrodes or taking fetal blood samples, to prevent the direct inoculation of the virus into the bloodstream of the infant. It is not yet certain whether delivery by caesarean section protects the infant from infection although some studies suggest that it may do so.

Since the mother and baby are both potentially infected there is a risk of transmission of the virus to those caring for the infant, but only from contact with infected blood. It is wise for care givers to wear protective gloves whenever contact with the infant's blood is likely, e.g. when taking venous or heel prick blood samples, and to wash the hands thoroughly after the procedure. Contact with other body fluids is safe since they are most unlikely to contain the virus. Isolation of the infant is not necessary although the mother should be made aware of the importance of washing her hands before and after handling the infant.

Postnatal infection through ingestion of infected maternal lymphocytes in breast milk can occur, but the risk of this is considerably smaller than intrapartum transmission of the virus. It is wise to advise HIV-positive mothers not to breast feed their infants when safe bottle feeding can be provided as an alternative, although the small risk of transmission of infection through breast milk must be balanced against the known benefits of breast feeding and other medical and social hazards which may affect the infant.

Prevention of neonatal HIV infection can only be achieved by measures designed to limit spread of the infection to HIV-negative women. Screening by HIV testing at antenatal clinics remains a sensitive ethical issue and is not yet widely practised. All these facts must be carefully explained to the parents when counselling them about the risks to the infant in further pregnancies.

Social aspects of HIV infection

HIV-infected mothers have a higher incidence of other sexually transmitted diseases and in the UK are more likely to be drug abusers. Both situations may have an independent effect on the health of the baby (pp. 160 and 14). Social deprivation is also common and may result in adverse emotional consequences for the child (p. 14). Serious maternal ill-health from progression to AIDS may occur during the child's infancy and some mothers may die from it. As a result of these circumstances, up to 20% of children will not be living with their natural parents by 1 year of age and many will need the support of the social services. However, early follow-up studies show that the health and development are not adversely affected in the majority of uninfected infants.

Hepatitis B infection

Hepatitis B infection or carriage is widespread throughout the world but is particularly common in many developing countries, occurring in up to 10% of the population in some parts of the Far East. It is also more common amongst women who have many sexual partners or who are intravenous drug abusers. Although it may cause acute hepatitis in the mother, it more commonly results in asymptomatic chronic carriage of the virus in apparently healthy people. It can be transmitted to the baby through blood and body secretions during birth, or later, by infected mothers. The risk of infection is particularly high if the mother carries the hepatitis B e antigen (HBeAg) or the HB s antigen (HBsAg). If the baby contracts the infection, she may rarely develop fulminant, and often fatal, hepatitis, but otherwise the asymptomatic chronic carrier state develops in the large majority of infants. Immunization of the infant of a known carrier within 12 hours of birth with hepatitis B vaccine together with 200 IU of hepatitis B immunoglobulin intramuscularly reduces the risk of infection to under 5%. Without immunization, about 70% of infants born to infected mothers will become carriers with the risk of developing chronic active hepatitis or cirrhosis of the liver in later childhood. The colostrum and milk of HB e antigen-positive mothers is always infected and their babies should not breast feed until they are fully protected by the immunization schedule.

Since the baby's blood may be infectious, the same precautions should be taken to protect the carers of the infant as were described for HIV infection.

Herpes simplex

Neonatal herpes simplex infection is uncommon, although its incidence seems to be increasing. There is an increased risk of pre-term birth, and, very occasionally, intrauterine infection results in microcephaly, choroidoretinitis and microphthalmia. More usually, the infection is acquired from direct contact with infected areas on the maternal genitalia and it occurs much more commonly in the offspring of mothers with recently acquired infection.

In the infant, the disease may either be localized as an eye, skin or mucous membrane infection or spread in a generalized and often fatal form. Jaundice, hepatosplenomegaly, meningoencephalitis and sometimes haemorrhage as a result of the syndrome of disseminated intravascular coagulation (p. 179) are all features of the more serious form of the disease. Diagnosis is achieved by culture of the virus from any available area such as a vesicle on the skin, but to be successful treatment must be given as soon as the possibility of infection is identified, often from birth, and certainly before the disease becomes widely disseminated. Apart from general supportive measures, specific treatment of the baby with intravenous acyclovir can reduce the severity of the disease and hasten the eradication of the virus, but many survivors of the encephalitic form of the disease will remain brain-damaged.

When the maternal genital herpes infection is diagnosed antenatally, caesarean section is justifiable to prevent exposure of the infant to the virus, although it is probably only necessary if there are active vesicles on the vulva at the time of delivery. It is not yet clear whether antenatal administration of antiviral agents is beneficial for the baby, but it is not necessary to use it prophylactically in asymptomatic babies after birth.

Congenital syphilis

Syphilis, which is caused by infection with the spirochaete *Treponema pallidum*, though common in many other parts of the world is fortunately now rare in Britain and results in only about 10–15 cases each year of congenital infection. Stillbirth occurs in about one-third of cases and an affected liveborn child in about half of cases. The more recently the mother has acquired the disease, the more likely the baby is to be affected.

Routine antenatal blood tests for maternal syphilis have resulted in almost complete elimination of the congenital form in the UK, but as it is a rarity, the clinical picture tends to be forgotten and an occasional case still goes unrecognized. The infection involves the placenta and is not acquired by the fetus before the fourth month of pregnancy, which means that, when a positive serological test is found, treatment of the mother's disease should be given before then.

The clinical features are sometimes present at birth, but more often they appear between the

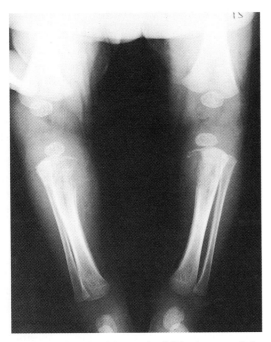

Figure 11.4 Osteitis of the proximal tibiae in congenital syphilis.

second and sixth weeks. The classical signs of the condition include the following: purulent rhinitis with a profuse and sometimes bloody discharge; various skin eruptions (generally maculopapular with a copper tinge fading to brown); splenic enlargement which is almost invariable; jaundice with enlargement of the liver due at first to fatty infiltration and later to pericellular cirrhosis. Anaemia is a usual finding and bone involvement shows radiologically as a thickened dense epiphyseal line at the end of the long bones with a zone of rarefaction proximal to it (Fig. 11.4). The finding of specific IgM antibody is now the most useful diagnostic test. The Venereal Disease Research Laboratories (VDRL) test on serum may be falsely negative or positive at birth and during the first few weeks. False-positive reactions occur often in those whose mother's reaction is positive, so in the absence of other clinical signs the test should be repeated at 3 months before regarding it as a reason to start treatment. The CSF should be examined once the diagnosis is made because involvement of the CNS influences the duration of the treatment. Penicillin G 15 mg/kg body weight twice daily by intramuscular injection for a minimum of 10 days is the treatment of choice.

MALARIA

This infestation should be considered in any febrile baby whose mother, during pregnancy, visited a country where malaria occurs. Pregnant women seem more susceptible to infection with malarial parasites in countries where it is common. *Plasmodium falciparum* may infect the placenta, reducing its function and causing intrauterine growth retardation in the fetus. It can also cause premature labour. The organism only rarely crosses the placenta to the fetus, but if it does the baby is usually well at birth but develops a fever, jaundice, anaemia and splenomegaly within 10–20 days. Infection is confirmed by finding the parasite by microscopic examination of a blood smear, and treatment with chloroquine 10 mg/kg by mouth at once, repeated 6 hours later and followed the next day with two doses of 5 mg/kg, should overcome the initial illness. A blood transfusion may be needed if the anaemia is severe.

FURTHER READING

Beath S V, Boxall E H, Watson R M, Tarlow M J, Kelly D A 1992 Fulminant hepatitis in infants born to anti-HBe hepatitis carrier mothers. British Medical journal 304: 1169–1170

Boue A (ed) 1995 Fetal medicine – prenatal diagnosis and management. Oxford University Press, Oxford

British National Formulary (current edition). British Medical Association and Royal Pharmaceutical Society of Great Britain, London

Department of Health 1996 Immunisation against infectious disease. HMSO, London

Fleming P, Speidel B, Marlow N, Dunn P 1991 A neonatal vade mecum. Edward Arnold, London

Greenough A, Osborne J, Sutherland S 1992 Congenital perinatal and neonatal infections. Churchill Livingstone, Edinburgh

Isaacs D (ed) 1996 Seminars in neonatology – fetal and neonatal infections. W B Saunders, London de Louvois J 1994 Acute bacterial meningitis in the newborn. Journal of Antimicrobial Chemotherapy 34: 61–73

Levene M, Liford R (eds) 1995 Fetal and neonatal neurology and neurosurgery. Churchill Livingstone, Edinburgh

Levin M, Heyderman R 1991 Bacterial meningitis. In: David T J (ed) Recent advances in paediatrics 9. Churchill Livingstone, Edinburgh, ch 1

Logan G S, Peckham C 1991 Congenital infections. Hospital update July 1991: 586–591

McIntosh D, Isaacs D 1992 Herpes simplex virus infection in pregnancy. Archives of Disease in Childhood, Fetal and Neonatal Edition 67: 1137–1138

Mok J Y Q 1992 Management of HIV infection. In: David T J (ed) Recent advances in paediatrics 10. Churchill Livingstone, Edinburgh, ch 1

Roberts R, Dinsmore W 1992 Sexually transmitted diseases in pregnancy. British Journal of Hospital Medicine 47: 674–679

Seidman D S Stevenson D K, Arvin A M 1996 Varicella vaccine in pregnancy. British Medical Journal 313: 701–702

Sherwen L N 1995 Human immunodeficiency virus infection in the perinatal period: a review of the literature concerning women and neonates. Journal of Perinatology 15: 54–66

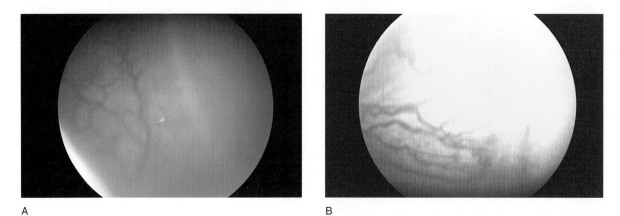

A   B

Plate 12 Fundal photographs in retinopathy of prematurity. A: Mild disease – an avascular (pale) peripheral retina with a visible ridge. B: Active progressive disease showing engorgement of the posterior pole vessels. (By kind permission of Mr David Clark.)

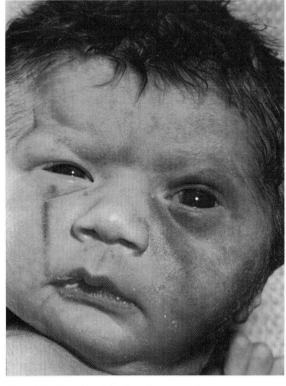

Plate 13 Facial bruising from forceps delivery.

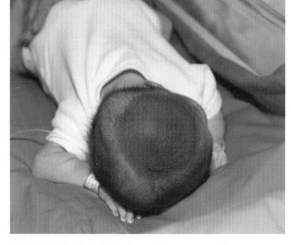

Plate 14 Scalp bruising from a Ventouse suction cup.

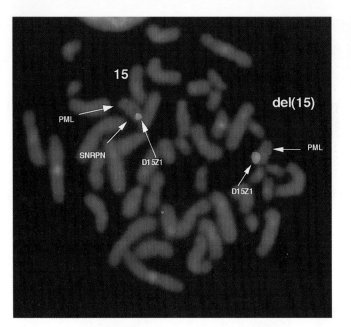

Plate 15 Fluorescence in situ hybridization (FISH) demonstrates the deleted gene SNRPN in Prader–Willi syndrome. The red signal from a probe for the SNRPN gene is present on the normal chromosome (15) and absent from the deleted chromosome (del(15)). (By kind permission of MS Christine Joyce.)

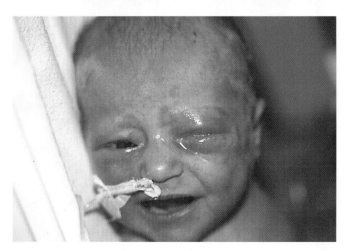

Plate 16 Chlamydial conjunctivitis.

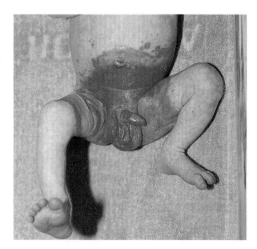

Plate 17 Monilial nappy rash.

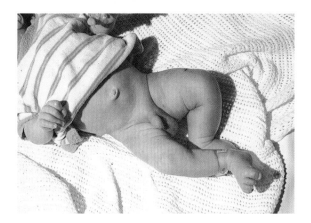

Plate 18 Large haematoma in the left thigh caused by femoral venepuncture in a baby with haemophilia.

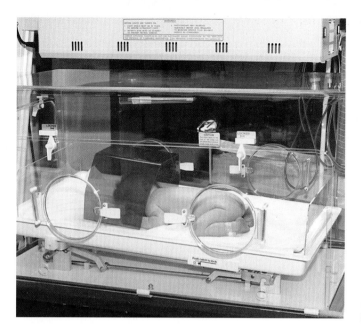

Plate 19   Phototherapy in an incubator showing a yellow hood to protect the eyes from glare.

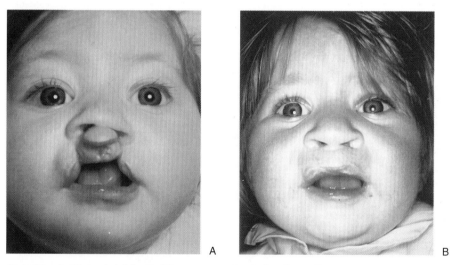

A   B

Plate 20   A: Bilateral cleft lip. B: After surgery at 3 months of age. (By kind permission of Mr R McDowall.)

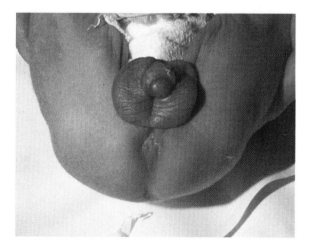

Plate 21   Anal atresia (note also the bifid scrotum).

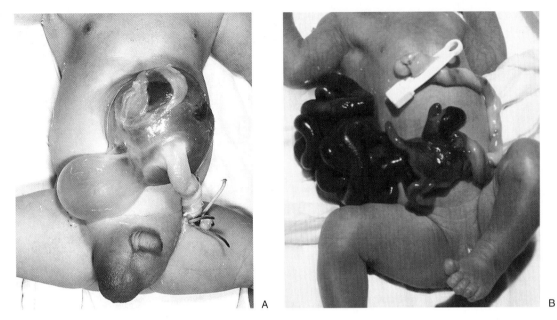

Plate 22   A: Exomphalos. B: Gastroschisis.

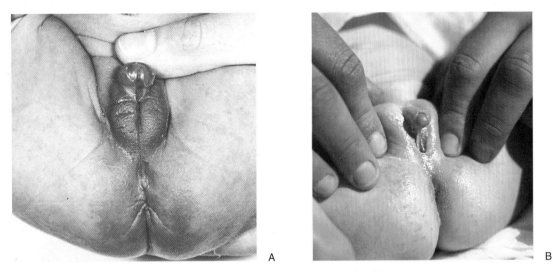

Plate 23   Ambiguous genitalia. A: An infant with congenital adrenal hyperplasia. B: A baby with androgen insensitivity syndrome.

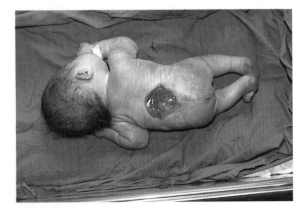

Plate 24   Spina bifida with meningomyelocele.

12

Haematological problems and jaundice

POLYCYTHAEMIA AND ANAEMIA AT BIRTH

The fetus produces large numbers of red cells containing fetal haemoglobin to enable them to obtain sufficient oxygen for the fetus direct from the maternal red cells across the placental membrane. As a result, the haemoglobin concentration of the newborn infant is high, ranging from 15–20 g/dl. Certain antenatal factors, such as intrauterine growth retardation from placental insufficiency and maternal diabetes, increase the red cell production still further. Haemoconcentration occurs in all babies in the first few hours of life, resulting in a small additional rise, and occasionally in these circumstances the blood becomes excessively viscous and the circulation sluggish. Whilst this polycythaemia usually causes no obvious trouble, at a packed cell volume (PCV) of over 65% the viscosity rises steeply and may give rise to respiratory difficulty or cerebral symptoms within the first few days of life. If the PCV is greater than 70%, cerebral blood flow may be compromised and the blood should be diluted by removing some and replacing it with the same volume of plasma.

A mild degree of anaemia may result from clamping the umbilical cord before the baby has received the full quota of placental blood through the umbilical vein. Holding the baby above the level of the placenta after birth, for instance by delivering the baby up onto the mother's abdomen, does not prevent this placental transfusion of blood. During the first 6–8 weeks of life, the haemoglobin level slowly falls, since the bone marrow does not initially replace the expired red cells. The iron in these cells is stored and used in haemoglobin synthesis as the red cell production restarts at 8–10 weeks of age. At the lowest point, the haemoglobin concentration may fall as far as 9 g/dl, or lower in the pre-term infant, and iron supplements do not prevent the fall. As long as there are no symptoms from this 'physiological anaemia', it requires no investigation or treatment. If, on the other hand, the infant becomes tired, breathless or slow to feed, it may be sufficient to check that the reticulocyte count (immature red cells in the blood which indicate that the bone marrow is actively producing red cells) is elevated and follow the rise in haemoglobin level at weekly intervals, although it is occasionally necessary to give a small top-up transfusion of blood.

HAEMORRHAGIC DISORDERS

Bleeding

Fetal haemorrhage

Blood loss from the baby may occur before, during or after birth. The antenatal loss of blood from fetal to maternal circulation is a recognized occurrence although it is rarely diagnosed. It may occur spontaneously across the placental membrane or be a complication of amniocentesis or fetal blood sampling. It can be confirmed, if suspected, by finding red cells containing fetal haemoglobin in the mother's blood (p. 184). Transfer of blood from one twin to another is commonly diagnosable at birth as it can result in substantially different haemoglobin concentrations in the two infants. Occasionally this may result in heart failure in the baby receiving the extra blood in utero, but it is more usual for one twin to require a top-up transfusion because of a significant anaemia.

Bleeding into the liquor or birth canal during delivery from rupture of vessels on the fetal side of the placental circulation or from the umbilical cord may cause a serious enough loss to require an emergency blood transfusion to restore the blood volume and haemoglobin level. It is more likely to occur if there is placenta praevia or a velamentous insertion of the cord, and the bleeding can be difficult to distinguish from maternal blood. Since the fetal blood volume is only 80 ml/kg of body weight, the loss of as little as 50 ml of blood can rapidly put a newborn baby into hypovolaemic shock, which causes pallor, tachycardia and tachypnoea. Unless blood loss is thought of as a possible cause of these symptoms, they can easily be misinterpreted as asphyxia and the vital blood volume replacement omitted. Transfusion of a minimum of 20 ml/kg body weight should be given immediately the condition is identified, further volumes being given if needed to raise the haemoglobin above 12 g/dl.

Haemorrhage due to birth trauma in the cranial cavity or intraabdominally is described in Chapter 10 in the section on 'birth injury'.

Haemorrhage in the newborn baby

Haemorrhage after birth may occur from many sites. The umbilical cord stump may bleed but this is usually prevented by proper cord clamping. Enough blood may accumulate in a cephalhaematoma to cause loss of blood volume. Haematemesis and melaena most commonly result either from maternal blood being swallowed during delivery or from blood-contaminated milk being ingested during breast feeding. The maternal origin of the blood can be confirmed by identifying exclusively adult haemoglobin in the vomit or stool. Pulmonary haemorrhage and intraventricular bleeding are almost always complications of severe hyaline membrane disease in pre-term infants. Vaginal bleeding, which results from hormonal changes after birth, is common, benign and resolves rapidly without treatment.

These conditions usually cause relatively limited blood loss and treatment is confined to that of the underlying cause, although if it is thought that the blood loss is significant, the haemoglobin level, platelet count and clotting studies should be checked and blood cross-matched against the mother's blood in case a transfusion is needed. All infants who have had a bleed should be given intramuscular vitamin K to prevent or reverse haemorrhagic disease of the newborn.

Haemorrhagic disease of the newborn

Vitamin K is required for the production of blood clotting factors II, VII, IX and X by the liver. It is derived from food and is also synthesized in the gut by intestinal bacteria. If deficient, the baby may bleed spontaneously from one or more sites. This condition, known as haemorrhagic disease of the newborn, most commonly occurs between the third and sixth days of life in fully breast-fed infants as breast milk contains little of the vitamin.

Most commonly, bleeding occurs from the gastrointestinal tract, either as haematemesis or melaena. Less often it presents as an intracranial haemorrhage, haematuria or umbilical stump bleeding. Haemorrhagic disease should be considered likely if the prothrombin time, which measures the vitamin K-dependent blood clotting factors, and partial thromboplastin time are prolonged and the platelets normal, but it must be remembered that the normal prothrombin time in the newborn is only some 20–50% of the adult value.

Once haemorrhage has occurred, the treatment depends on its severity. In the milder cases with little or no general disturbance or evidence of circulatory impairment, it may be sufficient to give 1 mg of vitamin K intramuscularly. The baby is kept warm and observed carefully with half-hourly pulse charting. Increasing pallor with tachycardia above 160/minute and a falling blood pressure or a repetition of the bleeding are definite indications for more specific treatment. Fresh frozen plasma contains the deficient clotting factors and rapid intravenous infusion of about 20 ml/kg body weight is sufficient both to stop bleeding and to restore the blood volume. This may have to be followed by a transfusion of fresh blood if the loss has been great enough to cause symptomatic anaemia.

Prevention

Prevention of this form of haemorrhagic disease (Box 12.1) is almost assured by the routine administration of 1 mg of vitamin K to all new-

---

Box 12.1 Prevention of haemorrhagic disease of the newborn – recommendations of the College of Paediatrics and Child Health

- All newborn infants should receive vitamin K
- Intramuscular vitamin K ensures adequate prophylaxis in normal term infants
- One dose of vitamin K orally is adequate prophylaxis for the majority of normal term infants; further doses should be considered for breast-fed infants.
- Infants with jaundice suggestive of cholestasis and infants with unexplained bleeding should receive further vitamin K, preferably parenterally

---

born infants either intramuscularly or orally on the first day of life (p. 33), a procedure which is widely practised in maternity units. If liver function is impaired, for example when the baby is pre-term or has neonatal liver disease, it is less effective and must be given intramuscularly to ensure adequate utilization.

A recent epidemiological study suggested that the incidence of leukaemia was increased in infants given vitamin K intramuscularly, but further studies have not confirmed the association. To ensure that the proven benefits of vitamin K were not forgotten, the British Paediatric Association recommendations (Box 12.1) on vitamin K administration were issued while further studies were carried out.

Disseminated intravascular coagulation

A more severe haemorrhagic state may arise when the circulating clotting factors and platelets are consumed in a widespread process of clotting in small blood vessels. This uncommon condition, known as disseminated intravascular coagulation (DIC), usually occurs as a complication of septicaemia. The bleeding which results from the consequent lack of clotting factors may occur from any site and the falling platelet count may cause purpura to appear in the skin. The diagnosis is made by finding red cell fragmentation on microscopy of blood smears and an increase in fibrin degradation products (FDP) in the blood.

Treatment is directed primarily towards the

underlying condition. The use of heparin by intravenous infusion to prevent further intravascular clotting is of little value in the newborn period. Fresh frozen plasma may help by replacing depleted clotting factors and exchange transfusion may occasionally be needed.

Hereditary clotting factor deficiencies

Disorders such as haemophilia (factor VIII deficiency) and Christmas disease (factor IX deficiency) rarely cause prolonged bleeding in the neonatal period, but when there is a family history, extra care should be taken to observe sites of potential haemorrhage such as the umbilical cord stump and the site of heel pricks. These problems may be reduced if the haemophilia has been identified in early pregnancy by DNA analysis on samples of fetal blood.

Venepunctures in the femoral vein and neck vessels should be avoided on any baby in whom a clotting abnormality is suspected (Plate 18). In all other venepunctures and heel pricks, local pressure should be applied after removal of the needle to prevent bruising. Intramuscular injections should not be given until a clotting factor deficiency has been excluded by the appropriate tests.

Purpura and bruising

Bruising into the skin most commonly occurs during delivery, particularly during breech presentation when the buttocks and genitalia may be affected. In very pre-term infants it may result from deficient clotting factors and an excess capillary fragility, both related to the baby's immaturity. Petechiae from capillary leakage are often seen in term infants due to congestion – as in 'traumatic cyanosis' (p. 57) – asphyxia or a deficiency of platelets.

Thrombocytopenia may be a consequence of any severe infection, including the antenatal infections described on page 169. It is also found in disseminated intravascular coagulation. Platelet deficiency also occurs in about 50% of infants whose mothers suffer from thrombocytopenic purpura, due to transmission of maternal platelet antibodies across the placenta. The purpura and bleeding may be severe enough to require fresh platelet transfusion, although they are usually mild and transient. Corticosteroid treatment is ineffective but infusion of immunoglobulin may raise the platelet count in some cases. Very occasionally, thrombocytopenia is found to be due to incompatibility of the platelets between the mother and baby, in a way that is quite similar to that of rhesus haemolytic disease of the newborn. It may be the presenting feature of congenital leukaemia and is also seen in cases of congenital hypoplastic anaemia.

HAEMOGLOBINOPATHIES

Although thalassaemia and sickle cell disease cause few problems in the neonatal period, they are included here since both are inherited as recessive disorders which makes early diagnosis desirable, particularly for genetic counselling of the parents (p. 194).

In thalassaemia, defective haemoglobin synthesis causes a severe anaemia requiring repeated blood transfusions if the sufferer is to survive. It occurs mainly in peoples from the Mediterranean countries and those from the Indian subcontinent. Prenatal diagnosis by DNA analysis of chorionic villus samples and termination of affected pregnancies have almost eliminated thalassaemia in Cypriots in Britain, but so far this approach has been less acceptable to the UK Pakistani population.

Sickle cell disease results in crises of haemolytic anaemia throughout childhood and primarily occurs in those originating from black African countries.

Both these conditions can be identified by haemoglobin electrophoresis from the 'Guthrie' blood spot, and screening for both conditions is now routine in certain parts of the USA where people from many ethnic groups live (p. 68).

JAUNDICE

Although jaundice occurs in many babies in the first week of life, it has many causes and is a potentially serious condition which may threaten life or impair normal development. When it exceeds the accepted normal limits, therefore, the cause must be urgently sought and appropriate treatment given.

A reminder of how bilirubin is formed and metabolized should assist in the understanding of the causes of jaundice in newborn infants and how it may best be investigated. Bilirubin, the yellow pigment which shows in the skin as jaundice, is formed by the normal breakdown of haemoglobin after the red cells die, and is fat-soluble. It is conjugated with glucuronic acid by an enzyme in the liver and is thus rendered water-soluble so that it may be excreted in the bile into the gut.

The liver enzyme glucuronyl transferase, which is necessary for this process, becomes effective slowly after birth and so it takes several days for conjugation to become sufficiently active to cope with the amount of bilirubin produced by the normal turnover of haemoglobin. The consequent rise of unconjugated bilirubin concentration in the blood and its deposition in the skin and other tissues may be sufficient to cause visible jaundice. This occurs in about one-third of healthy term infants and is called 'physiological' jaundice. Table 12.1 gives a brief representation of bilirubin metabolism and shows the origins of several of the causes of neonatal jaundice.

More severe jaundice associated with raised levels of unconjugated bilirubin follows an unusually rapid breakdown (haemolysis) of red cells, which is most often the result of incompatibility between the blood groups of the mother and baby. As the bilirubin in this type of jaundice is fat-soluble, the kidneys cannot excrete it and the urine is not bile-stained, but it does contain an excess of urobilinogen derived from the breakdown of bilirubin in the gut. If there is obstruction to the outlet pathways for bile in the liver or bile ducts, the resultant jaundice is due to an accumulation of bilirubin which has been normally conjugated by the liver. Being water-soluble, this form of bilirubin is excreted in the urine which is thus dark in colour.

When jaundice occurs because of impairment of liver cell function, as in hepatitis, there is usu-

Table 12.1 Bilirubin metabolism and the origins of neonatal jaundice

Metabolism of bilirubin	Pathological mechanisms affecting bilirubin breakdown
Haemoglobin breakdown ↓	Excess breakdown of red cells, e.g. rhesus haemolytic disease, ABO incompatibility, G6PD deficiency,* congenital spherocytosis
Porphyrins ↓	
Unconjugated bilirubin ↓	
Conjugation by liver enzymes ↓	Diminished activity of enzymes, e.g. physiological jaundice, prematurity, urinary infection, breast milk jaundice, hypothyroidism
Conjugated bilirubin ↓	Many causes of neonatal hepatitis prevent excretion of conjugated bilirubin
Passes through bile duct ↓ Excreted in stools	Obstruction to the flow of bile, e.g. biliary atresia, choledocal cyst

*Glucose-6-phospate dehydrogenase

ally some intrahepatic obstruction to the flow of bile as well as liver enzyme failure, so the excess bilirubin is partly unconjugated but mainly conjugated and will therefore be excreted in the urine because it is water-soluble. Jaundice associated with dark yellow or brown urine is never normal and investigation must be undertaken to find its cause (p. 189).

Conversion of unconjugated bilirubin deposited in the skin to a water-soluble product that can be excreted also takes place through the action of daylight or its equivalent. This disposal mechanism is made use of in phototherapy (p. 187).

Patterns of jaundice

Jaundice is a common physiological event occurring in around one in three full-term infants during the first week of life. Nevertheless, the possibility of a pathological process should always be considered because of both the risk to the infant from the jaundice itself and the importance of identifying the cause and instituting treatment. The level of bilirubin is notoriously difficult to gauge clinically, especially in dark-skinned babies, and should always be measured in the blood where there is any clinical suspicion either that the level is high or that the infant has a serious underlying cause for it. Any jaundice with a serum bilirubin level over 200 μmol/L should be investigated to identify the underlying cause.

Jaundice may appear with one of a number of characteristic patterns (Fig. 12.1). If it occurs within the first 24 hours and the bilirubin level rises at a rate of more than 10 μmol/L (0.5 mg/dl) per hour, the likely cause is a serious haemolytic process (p. 183). When it rises more slowly over 3–4 days and then falls towards normal, it is likely to be physiological and due to immaturity of the hepatic bilirubin conjugation enzymes. The level of bilirubin can be increased by, for example, an excessive load of haemoglobin from a large cephalhaematoma, polycythaemia, dehydration, calorie deprivation or even sepsis. Prolongation of moderately high levels of bilirubin beyond the 10th day of life may be associated with prematurity, urinary infection, hypothyroidism or most commonly breast feeding (p. 188). Very rarely, galactosaemia may be a cause. Later-rising jaundice is often associated with the accumulation of conjugated bilirubin due either to obstruction of the bile ducts or to hepatitis (p. 190).

Investigation in neonatal jaundice

It is important to establish at the outset whether the baby's bilirubin is conjugated or unconjugated, since the investigations required are very different. If unconjugated, investigation should seek to exclude a blood group incompatibility between mother and baby, sepsis, red cell enzyme abnormalities and serious metabolic disease such as galactosaemia. If it is conjugated, liver function tests, blood clotting studies (to exclude a deficiency of vitamin K-dependent factors produced by the liver) and specific tests to identify the cause of obstruction to bile flow should be performed (p. 190).

KERNICTERUS AND BILIRUBIN ENCEPHALOPATHY

When unconjugated bilirubin in the plasma rises above a threshold value it is deposited in the body tissues. The brain is particularly vulnerable since it contains so much fat, and damage from excessive bile pigment there is known as kernicterus, which causes the clinical picture of bilirubin encephalopathy. The infant becomes lethargic, refusing to suck, and may show muscular twitching, eye rolling, rigidity with arching of the back and finally respiratory failure. In the absence of treatment, two-thirds of these babies would die at this stage, whilst the remainder would be handicapped in later life by the choreoathetoid form of cerebral palsy, mental handicap or nerve deafness. The point at which hyperbilirubinaemia becomes a danger to the developing brain is not determined by a critical blood level but is influenced by many other factors. Albumin in the blood binds a proportion of the circulating bilirubin, rendering it innocuous, so kernicterus occurs more readily when the albumin level is low. Partly for this reason the brain is vulnerable at lower bilirubin levels in pre-term infants. The danger is increased by any substance which competes with bilirubin for binding sites with albumin; the vitamin K analogue Synkavit caused much damage in this way in the past and is no longer used, but certain sulphonamides and the benzoate preservative in diazepam injection solution, for instance, have a similar action. A period of asphyxia, acidosis, hypoglycaemia or hypothermia may add significantly to the risk of kernicterus.

At what point is there a serious risk of brain damage?

Taking all these factors into account it is only possible to give general guidance about the bilirubin level at which brain damage is likely to occur. In the term baby a level of 425 μmol/L (25 mg/dl) or more of unconjugated bilirubin

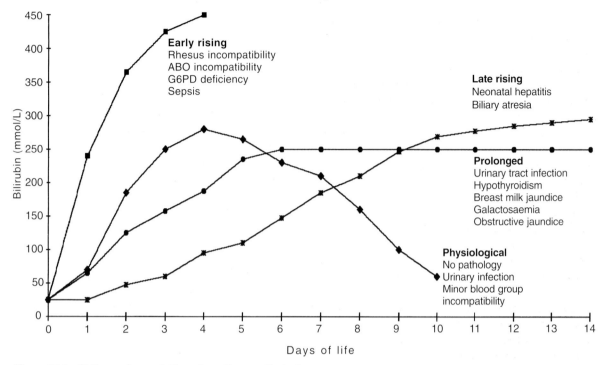

Figure 12.1 Patterns of neonatal jaundice with some illustrative causes.

may be regarded as dangerous. When less than 36 weeks of gestation, or when there has been a period of asphyxia, the blood level must be kept below 300 μmol/L (18 mg/dl) and in the very low birth weight or very pre-term infant it should be kept below 250 μmol/L (15 mg/dl).

JAUNDICE WITH UNCONJUGATED BILIRUBIN

Haemolytic disease of the newborn

Icterus gravis neonatorum was first described by Morgagni in 1761 but has only been attributed to blood group abnormalities between the fetus and mother since the 1940s. In its simplified form there are two main types of disease. In one, the mother, who is rhesus (Rh)-negative, forms Rh antibodies in response to a transfer of red cells from a Rh-positive fetus across the placenta in pregnancy or, more usually, during the birth

of the child. In a subsequent pregnancy, this maternal antibody is in turn passed back across the placenta and, if the developing child is Rh-positive, causes haemolytic disease by destroying fetal red cells. If haemolytic disease were to occur in every case of an Rh-negative mother bearing an Rh-positive child, it would affect about one pregnancy in 10. Fortunately, the development of antibodies is liable to occur in only 10% of such cases – approximately 1 in 100 pregnancies – and the administration of anti-D to mothers (p. 184) after delivery has made the condition a relative rarity.

In the other type, known as ABO incompatibility, the anti-A or anti-B haemolysins which are present in the blood of the group O mother are transferred to the developing group A or B infant, and in a very small proportion of cases, this results in haemolytic disease and jaundice. The incidence of significant disease in the baby is about 1 in 200 births and many of these are only mildly affected. There are also incompatibilities involving other rarer blood groups which occasionally cause similar trouble.

The nomenclature of the blood groups and their subdivisions is complicated, but some appreciation of the way in which rhesus antigens are inherited is necessary for practical purposes, so it is described here in simplified form.

All cells in the body, except the ova and sperm, carry a double set of rhesus genes and the more common ones are given the letters C, c, D, d, E, e. A group of three (containing one of each letter) is inherited from each parent so that individuals may be designated, for example, as CDe/cDE. The most important one in connection with this disease is the D antigen and any person whose group contains any D antigen is known for practical purposes as Rh-positive. Someone without any D (e.g. cdE/Cde) is Rh-negative. A person who has D in both components of the pair (e.g. cDe/CDe) is homozygous positive. Such a father is bound to endow his offspring with a D antigen (i.e. his offspring will all be Rh-positive), while a heterozygous father with only one D antigen has only a 50% chance of doing so. The proportion of people who are Rh-negative varies greatly between races. For example, the incidence is around 15% in ethnic white peoples, but is only 1–2% in black West Africans. Thus the risk of rhesus haemolytic disease will vary considerably from one ethnic group to another.

Haemolytic disease due to rhesus incompatibility

The disease may take one of three main forms:

- hydrops fetalis in which the infant is often stillborn with gross oedema, ascites and anaemia
- jaundice arising during the first few hours after birth associated with a variable degree of progressive haemolytic anaemia; the jaundice is not obviously present at birth because until then the excess of bilirubin has been excreted through the placenta by the mother
- gradual onset of anaemia during the course of

the first few weeks with no more than slight jaundice.

Other cases may show variations of these patterns – for instance, the liveborn infant with oedema, anaemia and a rapid onset of severe jaundice within an hour of birth. In severe instances, the liver and spleen are enlarged, and there may be petechial haemorrhages and, if left untreated, cardiac failure from the anaemia. The blood picture shows a high proportion of primitive red cells, and hence the name 'erythroblastosis fetalis' which is sometimes used to describe this condition.

The main threats to the life of an affected baby, if not stillborn, are either a rapidly progressive anaemia or cerebral damage from hyperbilirubinaemia. The depth of jaundice reached depends on the rate of red cell destruction and the rate of bilirubin excretion. The latter varies with the efficiency of liver enzyme function which may be impaired by this disease. Preterm infants have even less efficient bilirubin conjugation mechanisms so the shorter the gestation period the more likely is severe jaundice to occur (p. 187).

Prevention

The use of anti-D immunoglobulin has now become a well established and almost completely effective method of prevention except where maternal Rh antibodies are already present. Using the Kleihauer technique of acid elution on blood preparations, it is possible to show immediately after the birth of the first baby whether or not red cells of the fetus have passed across into the maternal circulation and, if so, the size of the 'transfusion'. It is this which causes the initial sensitization and production of maternal Rh antibodies, but if the mother and child are ABO-incompatible (mother O, infant A or B) the leaking cells are destroyed in the maternal circulation and no sensitization ensues. In a similar way, giving the mother anti-D globulin intramuscularly within 48 hours after delivery of the baby destroys the 'transfused' fetal Rh-positive red cells; 100 μg of the immunoglobulin is generally used but the dose depends on the size of the fetomaternal transfusion.

Antenatal prediction

Blood grouping is done at the first antenatal visit and all Rh-negative women should then be tested for Rh antibodies. If antibodies are not present, the test should be repeated at 28, 32 and 36 weeks, but, if found, the quantity of antibody should be re-estimated at more frequent intervals. In some cases, amniocentesis between the 30th and 36th weeks of pregnancy adds greatly to the accuracy of prediction and helps to assess the severity of the disease; the degree of staining of the liquor with bile pigment and the actual quantity of the antibody are estimated.

Predictions based on maternal antibody level alone are not sufficiently accurate, but if combined with previous history, the exclusion of ascites and heart failure by ultrasound of the fetus, the results of amniocentesis and the knowledge of the gestational age of the baby, the obstetrician and paediatrician together can judge better whether the risk to the baby is higher from early delivery, with the combined risks of prematurity and rhesus haemolytic disease, or from giving the baby an intrauterine blood transfusion to prevent the death of the fetus in utero. In general, intrauterine transfusion is preferable before 30 weeks of gestation, whilst premature delivery is the lesser hazard after that point.

Management at birth

Since the presence of maternal antibodies does not always imply an affected baby, the first objective is to establish the diagnosis and decide as early as possible whether exchange transfusion is required. For this purpose, specimens of cord blood are taken for haemoglobin estimation, blood grouping (for both ABO and rhesus groups), the Coombs' or anti-human globulin test, and for estimation of the serum bilirubin level. Such samples should be taken in all cases where there is any suspicion of Rh incompatibility. In most centres it is advocated for all Rh-negative mothers regardless of whether antibodies

were found antenatally. A positive Coombs' test on the cord blood means an affected infant; a negative one means that no sensitization of the infant's red cells has taken place and that he will not develop the disease. Many babies with a positive Coombs' test are, however, so mildly affected that little more than a slight anaemia or mild jaundice develops and exchange transfusion is not required.

The treatment of rhesus haemolytic disease depends on the severity of the condition. It is aimed at restoring a normal haemoglobin concentration and preventing the rise of bilirubin to a dangerous level. An immediate guide to the severity can be obtained by examining the cord blood. If its haemoglobin level is below 10 g/dl or if the bilirubin concentration is above 85 µmol/L (5 mg/dl), the disease is severe and immediate exchange transfusion is indicated. Otherwise the rate of rise in the level of bilirubin is monitored at intervals of not more than 8 hours, and an exchange transfusion is carried out if it exceeds 10 µmol/L (0.5 mg/dl) per hour.

These guidelines for treatment may have to be modified in favour of earlier exchange transfusion in a pre-term baby of less than 36 weeks' gestation or where a previous infant has been severely affected. In exceptional circumstances, where there is a severe anaemia resulting in oedema and ascites at birth, resuscitation and urgent replacement of 20 ml of the baby's blood with a smaller volume of packed group O Rh-negative red cells will be needed. This must be followed by administration of a diuretic such as frusemide before proceeding with a limited exchange transfusion.

In less severely affected infants, the rate of rise of bilirubin can be reduced by giving phenobarbitone to the mother for 2 weeks before the birth of the baby to stimulate the baby's liver enzymes into action. Continuous phototherapy from birth may also reduce the need for an exchange transfusion in some infants. The rise in serum bilirubin gradually slows as the liver becomes able to metabolize and excrete it, and eventually the jaundice disappears. However, the haemolysis continues as long as there is some rhesus antibody in the baby's circulation and this may result in a further fall of haemoglobin for which a top-up transfusion of blood is required.

The introduction of anti-D globulin injections has resulted in a substantial fall in the incidence of Rh haemolytic disease and thus experience in the management of the severely affected infant is becoming limited. Treatment of mothers with very high antibody levels now often involves complicated early intrauterine fetal blood transfusion and elective pre-term delivery. These mothers are often treated and delivered at special centres with adequate expertise to provide the necessary complex intensive neonatal care after the birth.

Prognosis

With careful management, over 95% of infants born alive can be expected to survive, the deaths being those with severe hydrops fetalis and those of very low birth weight. About 40% of affected babies require no treatment. Later disability from kernicterus is now a rarity although minor degrees of deafness have been found in prospective studies.

Exchange transfusion

The aim of exchange transfusion is to reduce the level of circulating bilirubin, to restore the blood volume and the haemoglobin concentration to normal, and to remove as much as possible of the circulating maternal Rh antibody from the baby's blood in order to reduce the risk of further haemolysis.

The techniques for performing exchange transfusions vary, but they are normally carried out using catheters inserted into the umbilical artery and vein, continuously running the cross-matched blood into the venous catheter while slowly removing an equivalent amount from the arterial line. This is continued until about 200 ml/kg body weight of blood has been exchanged and will take between 1.5 and 2 hours to complete. Monitoring of the ECG, heart rate and body temperature must be carried out throughout the procedure. Although in many cases one exchange is sufficient, in more severely affected infants further exchanges may be required.

Haemolytic disease due to ABO incompatibility

Diagnosis and management

Unlike rhesus haemolytic disease, ABO haemolytic disease is as likely in the first born child as it is after subsequent pregnancies. Prediction during pregnancy is much less precise than in Rh incompatibility and the severity does not relate to the level of antibody in the maternal serum. The Coombs' test on the baby's blood is usually negative and the cord bilirubin and haemoglobin levels do not have predictive value. The essential diagnostic observation is the development of clinically obvious jaundice within the first 24 hours – a situation which always requires laboratory investigation. Anaemia is rarely marked and is less of a feature than the rapidly rising level of bilirubin. Although exchange transfusion may be necessary when the jaundice is early and severe, in most cases of ABO haemolytic disease, phototherapy effectively prevents a rise in bilirubin to dangerous levels (p. 187).

Inherited causes of haemolytic disease

Glucose-6-phosphate dehydrogenase deficiency

Deficiency of glucose-6-phosphate dehydrogenase, an enzyme which protects the haemoglobin molecules from oxidation, is inherited as an X-linked recessive disorder. It affects males severely and the carrier females less so. It occurs substantially more commonly in certain ethnic groups, notably those from the Mediterranean area, the Middle and Far East and some parts of Africa where it is the commonest reason for exchange transfusion. The red cells of affected babies are highly susceptible to haemolysis when challenged by certain drugs such as antimalarials, sulphonamide-containing antibiotics, aspirin and paracetamol, or when the baby has an infection. Under these conditions, and sometimes without apparent provocaton, neonatal haemolytic jaundice may occur. It should be remembered that certain drugs are excreted in the mother's milk and even these small quantities may cause haemolysis in the predisposed child. It is treated by phototherapy or exchange transfusion according to criteria similar to those described for rhesus haemolytic disease.

Hereditary spherocytosis

In this condition the red cells are spherical, in contrast to the usual biconcave disc shape, and are unusually susceptible to destruction by haemolysis. Anaemia with mild jaundice is often present in the newborn period but severe hyperbilirubinaemia is exceptional. It is usually inherited as an autosomal dominant condition, so the family history may give warning of the condition.

JAUNDICE IN PRE-TERM INFANTS

This is simply an exaggerated form of the jaundice commonly seen in term infants. It is due to a greater functional inadequacy of the liver enzyme system which normally conjugates bilirubin with glucuronic acid and enables it to be excreted. Arising on the second or third day, the jaundice reaches a peak between 5 and 7 days and, on the whole, the shorter the gestation period, the greater the hyperbilirubinaemia and the later its peak. There is evidence that in some immature infants, the passage of bilirubin to the brain causing kernicterus occurs at a relatively low blood level (p. 183).

Clinical estimation of the depth of jaundice by simple observation of skin colour is notoriously inaccurate, particularly in pre-term infants, because it depends on the type of lighting, reflection from surrounding objects and the state of the baby's skin capillary blood flow. This is even more so when there is dark racial pigmentation. Serial laboratory estimations of serum bilirubin at intervals of 12–24 hours are therefore necessary.

Treatment

Exchange transfusion is now rarely needed but phototherapy is often helpful in keeping the serum bilirubin concentration below danger levels. However, the photodegradation of retinoids as well as the bilirubin may, rarely, leave the infant deficient in vitamin A (p. 117).

PHOTOTHERAPY

Exposing the skin to blue light of wavelength 400–500 nm and in an intensity of 4–10 microwatts/cm^2 converts the bilirubin in the superficial capillaries to harmless water-soluble metabolites which are then excreted in the urine and bowel. Although it is not as effective as exchange transfusion in removing bilirubin rapidly from the blood, this treatment can often prevent the bilirubin from reaching dangerous levels.

Exposing the baby's skin to sunlight effectively reduces the bilirubin level but is impractical for treatment in the UK. Most phototherapy treatment equipment uses either banks of fluorescent tubes which emit light of the correct wavelength or diffused light from a halogen bulb source. To receive effective treatment, the baby should be nursed naked in a suitably warm environment, such as an incubator, with some protection for the eyes to reduce the discomfort from the intense glare, although there is little evidence that it does any permanent harm (Plate 19). The most recent systems use a matrix of fibre-optic strands bonded to a flexible backing sheet which is applied directly to the skin under the baby's clothing. A cold light source illuminates the light filaments on the sheet through a connecting fibre-optic cable (Fig. 12.2). Thus the baby can be cared for in almost a normal way while the treatment is given and does not become overheated.

To judge whether a baby requires treatment, many maternity departments use charts on which the measured bilirubin levels are plotted against the baby's age at the time the sample was taken. Action lines drawn on the charts indicate the bilirubin level at which phototherapy should be given, although the lines should be interpreted in the light of the underlying cause of the jaundice, whether the baby is well or sick, and the level of maturity – the more premature the

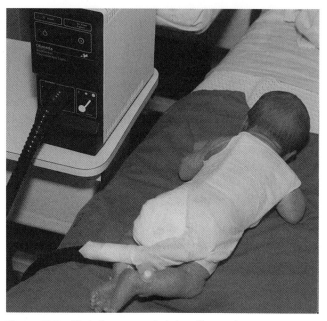

Figure 12.2 Phototherapy applied via a fibre-optic system.

baby, the lower the level at which treatment should be started (Fig. 12.3). Treatment usually continues for 2 or 3 days, with serial estimations of serum bilirubin once or twice a day to monitor its progess, and it is more effective in preventing a rise in serum bilirubin to a high level than in causing a significant fall once it has risen. Additional fluids are not normally needed during phototherapy, as long as the infant is taking the correct amounts of feed.

Although no serious sequelae have been shown to follow this form of therapy, fretfulness, fluid loss from overheating, looseness of the stools and vomiting have all been reported. Clearly the need for phototherapy must take into account the age of the baby, for the chances of a natural fall in the serum bilirubin after the fifth day are high.

OTHER CAUSES OF JAUNDICE

Common causes

Breast milk jaundice

Jaundice with serum bilirubin above 200 μmol/L

and continuing for more than 10 days is frequently associated with breast feeding. So long as the baby is well and the other causes of prolonged jaundice have been excluded, the diagnosis of breast milk jaundice can be made with confidence even though there is no specific test for the condition. Withdrawal of breast feeding temporarily with substitution of artificial milk results in a fall of bilirubin level but is rarely needed as a test since the slow decline in bilirubin value over the next week or two confirms the diagnosis. Although it may be that some factor in breast milk affects the conjugation and excretion of bilirubin, it may also result from interference with bilirubin metabolism in the gut which allows reabsorption of unconjugated bilirubin back into the circulation. Only rarely should discontinuation of breast feeding be recommended since the jaundice rarely reaches a level requiring treatment and within 6–8 weeks it normally resolves.

Jaundice due to sepsis

Apart from thrombophlebitis ascending from

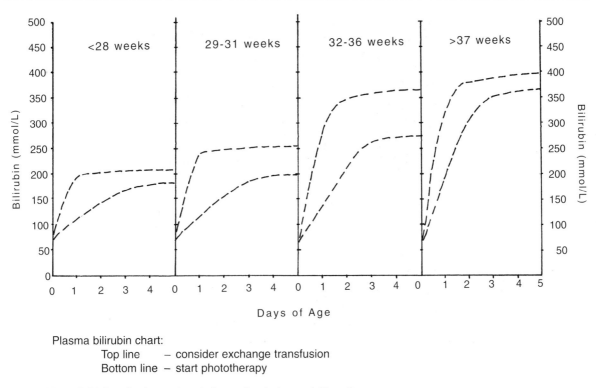

Plasma bilirubin chart:
　　Top line　　　– consider exchange transfusion
　　Bottom line – start phototherapy

Figure 12.3　Guidelines for the treatment of unconjugated neonatal jaundice.

umbilical sepsis into the portal vein, which is extremely rare, jaundice may be a feature of any septicaemic illness in the first week of life. Unexplained jaundice, especially if associated with reluctance to feed, drowsiness or vomiting, should therefore always raise the suspicion of infection, particularly in the urinary tract (p. 165).

Rarer causes

Congenital hypothyroidism

Congenital hypothyroidism should not be forgotten as a possible cause of abnormally prolonged jaundice, although the thyroid-stimulating hormone (TSH) screening test carried out on the seventh day of life should now identify these babies at an early stage. The clinical signs are described on page 222.

Congenital galactosaemia

This rare error of metabolism is described on page 223 but is mentioned here since persistent jaundice is one of the early signs and because, if the condition can be detected in the first few weeks of life, the treatment is rewarding and can minimize the mental retardation, permanent liver damage or death which may result from late diagnosis.

Congenital infection

Congenital infection by the rubella virus, cytomegalovirus, toxoplasmosis and syphilis may all present with jaundice as a prominent clinical feature. Initially of haemolytic type, the jaundice later has obstructive features and has to be differentiated from the many causes of neonatal hepatitis.

OBSTRUCTIVE JAUNDICE

Jaundice may result from obstruction to the flow of bile either within the liver or from blocked extrahepatic bile ducts. In this situation bilirubin passes to the liver where it is conjugated normally within the cells into its metabolites. Because they cannot pass through the bile ducts to the bowel, they are reabsorbed into the blood. These water-soluble pigments circulate to the kidneys where they are excreted, colouring the urine a dark yellowish-brown. The stools remain pale, as little or no bile flows into the gastrointestinal tract. Since the conjugated bilirubin is not fat-soluble, it cannot cross the blood–brain barrier so there is no risk of kernicterus.

This uncommon clinical picture of a baby with persistent jaundice, conjugated hyperbilirubinaemia, pale stools and dark urine can result from both congenital atresia of the bile ducts and the many causes of neonatal hepatitis and requires urgent investigation. The initial tests required in such a baby are given in Box 12.2, but extensive additional specific investigation is usually needed to reach a complete diagnosis. The most common conditions identified are biliary atresia and idiopathic neonatal hepatitis. In the UK, alpha-1 antitrypsin deficiency is a relatively common cause, although it is rarely seen in Australia and South Africa where, respectively, cytomegalovirus infection and syphilis are more frequent causes.

Congenital biliary atresia

Biliary atresia is a rare condition which may affect either the small intrahepatic ducts or the common bile duct or both. It is not a simple congenital malformation and may occur with meta-bolic causes of neonatal hepatitis such as alpha-1 antitrypsin deficiency, and it appears to progress in the first few weeks of life. Jaundice may arise from birth or may be delayed until 2–3 weeks of age and the conjugated bilirubin level often fluctuates. The jaundice has a greenish tinge and the spleen may be enlarged. Liver function tests are not often helpful in diagnosis although the transaminases are usually mildly elevated and the prothrombin time may be elevated.

A progressive dilatation of the bile duct from partial or complete localized obstruction at the ampulla of Vater may cause a palpable choledochal cyst which can be confirmed by ultrasound imaging.

Early surgery may relieve the obstruction provided the intrahepatic ducts are patent, and a portoenterostomy is usually recommended. In this operation, known as the Kasai procedure, a loop of small bowel is opened and anastamosed directly onto the surface of the liver to allow bile to drain straight into the gut lumen. If this is carried out before 8 weeks of age, the jaundice clears in nearly all infants, who then have about a 65% chance of long survival. Surgery is much less effective beyond this age and it is for this reason that the investigation of obstructive jaundice should be carried out urgently. If the operation is not successful, the only treatment which can prevent early death from cirrhosis is liver transplantation.

Neonatal hepatitis

Neonatal hepatitis is twice as common as biliary atresia and may be difficult to differentiate from it. The cause is not always established, but in the UK about 20% of cases are associated with recessively inherited alpha-1 antitrypsin deficiency, in which case cirrhosis of the liver is likely to follow and siblings have a high risk of being affected. The condition is diagnosed by protease-inhibitor (Pi) typing which can also detect carriers and enable genetic evaluation of the risk of recurrence of the disease in other family members. Various intrauterine infections including hepatitis A and C, rubella, cytomegalovirus, toxoplasmosis, Coxsackie and herpes simplex viruses

---

Box 12.2 Initial investigation in conjugated hyperbilirubinaemia

- Standard liver function tests
- Prothrombin time
- Bacterial culture of blood and urine
- Viral culture of urine
- Reducing substances in urine
- Alpha-1 antitrypsin level and Pi type
- Serum and urine amino acids
- Hepatitis A, B and C antigens
- Serum thyroxine and TSH levels
- Ultrasound examination of the liver and bile ducts

make up a further 10%, and maternal carriers of hepatitis B antigen can transmit the viral infection to the baby during labour (p. 172). Cystic fibrosis and a large number of very rare recessively inherited metabolic disorders, including galactosaemia and fructosaemia, can cause a similar clinical picture. In many cases, however, no cause is identified.

The course of the illness is very variable and in many cases the baby is not apparently unwell. Jaundice gradually appears over the first few weeks and there may sometimes be a low-grade pyrexia or reluctance to feed. When none of the serious causes mentioned above are identifiable, the chances of complete recovery are good. Among the rest, a few affected babies die in the early stages and about half of those who seem to be recovering develop later cirrhosis of the liver in addition to the other consequences of the underlying cause.

Diagnosis

Differentiation of biliary atresia and neonatal hepatitis is never easy and usually requires specialized experience. Moderately raised transaminases, high serum alpha fetoprotein and low alpha-1 antitrypsin levels, though favouring hepatitis, may be found in either condition. Ultrasound examination of the liver may reveal a choledochal cyst, but rarely helps otherwise since the intrahepatic ducts are usually not dilated in biliary atresia. Metabolic and infective causes should be investigated. It is usually possible to distinguish the two disorders with a combination of isotope excretion scans and histological examination of a liver biopsy, although occasionally laparotomy is needed to exclude extrahepatic biliary atresia. There is some evidence, however, that surgery may worsen the outlook for some babies who prove to have neonatal hepatitis.

FURTHER READING

Brown L P, Arnold L, Allison D, Klein M E, Jacobsen B 1993 Incidence and pattern of jaundice in healthy breast fed infants during the first month of life. Nursing Research 42(2): 106–110

Freeman N V, Burge D M 1994 Surgery of the newborn. Churchill Livingstone, Edinburgh

Hamosh M 1990 Breast milk jaundice. Journal of Paediatric Gastroenterology and Nutrition 11: 145–149

Hughes R G, Craig J I, Murphy W G, Greer I A 1994. Causes and consequences of Rhesus (D) haemolytic disease of the newborn: a study of a Scottish population, 1985–1990. British Journal of Obstetrics and Gynaecology 101(4): 297–300

McNinch A, Tripp J 1991 Haemorrhagic disease of the newborn in the British Isles: a two year prospective study. British Medical Journal 303: 1105–1109

Mowat A 1994 Liver disorders in childhood. Butterworth Heinemann, Oxford

Roberton N R C (ed) 1992 Textbook of neonatology. Churchill Livingstone, Edinburgh

13

Congenital malformations and genetic disorders

The identification of a physical malformation or a metabolic or genetic disorder in a baby before or after birth is very distressing for the parents and wider family, since such a defect may have an effect on the baby's health or threaten her life or developmental progress in the future. In many cases, remedial measures can result in near normality, while in others intervention only corrects a physical feature while leaving the child permanently handicapped or requiring prolonged medical or surgical attention and special educational and social provision. Whilst in most cases there is little debate about the appropriateness of medical or surgical intervention, in a small minority of situations the parents and paediatricians may have different views which may be difficult to resolve. When the problem is genetically inherited, it is possible in an increasing number of cases to identify the abnormal gene both in the baby and in other family members in order to identify sufferers and carriers, often

193

before the disease becomes evident. In these cases the parents may have a greater choice about whether to have the tests performed or not, a decision which is often very difficult to make. It is therefore important both to know something of the anomalies themselves and the social, emotional and psychological consequences which result from them.

INCIDENCE

Estimates of the total incidence of congenital abnormalities vary widely depending upon what is regarded as serious enough to include and up to what age the infants surveyed are followed. Many defects, e.g. those of the urinary tract, may not become apparent until middle or late childhood. On average, however, a congenital abnormality of significance occurs about once in every 30 live and stillbirths; in 25% of these babies there is more than one defect. Minor abnormalities occur in about another 3% of total births.

AETIOLOGY

Although much has been learnt about the experimental production of congenital malformations in animals, disappointingly little is known about their causation for human application, with a few notable exceptions.

Genetic inheritance

Although many congenital anomalies have some genetic basis, a distinct pattern of inheritance is uncommon in structural abnormalities but is more often found in the rarer inborn errors of metabolic or biochemical function. The three main modes of transmission of inherited disorders are dominant, recessive and X-linked inheritance.

In the dominant pattern of inheritance, offspring of one affected parent have a 1 in 2 risk of showing the same disorder, e.g. in achondroplasia. In recessively inherited conditions, such as cystic fibrosis, phenylketonuria or the mucopolysaccharidoses, both apparently normal parents are carriers of the abnormal gene and each of their offspring has a 1 in 4 chance of having the condition. The occurrence of such conditions is greater when the two parents are blood relatives and may therefore share a recessive gene. The increased incidence of malformations in Asian families in Britain has been attributed to the high rate of cousin marriages in some of these ethnic groups and to child-bearing at an older age. In X-linked inheritance, e.g. haemophilia, an abnormality is seen only in the male children of a mother who is carrying the gene without being affected herself. More often there is a mixed aetiology with heredity playing a less well-defined role, e.g. in cleft palate, pyloric stenosis, congenital heart disease and many others.

The study of the chromosomes in the nucleus of cells can identify a limited number of major anomalies and has helped the geneticist to understand their pattern of inheritance, but the vast majority of congenital malformations show no detectable chromosome abnormality by the present methods of examination. These include conventional light microscopy, banding of the chromosomes with Giemsa staining and examination after culturing the chromosomes in special media, chromosome 'painting' and other more specialized techniques. The identification of 'fragile X chromosomes' (p. 221) in some children with unexplained mental retardation is an example of the application of newer cytogenetic methods. The development of DNA technology means that we are no longer limited to looking at whole chromosomes but can identify the specific chromosome on which the abnormal gene responsible for a disorder is located and the precise position of the gene on the chromosome. In a rapidly increasing number of disorders (Table 13.1), the condition can be diagnosed by identifying the abnormal gene itself. These techniques are particularly valuable in confirming that the baby has a genetically determined condition, even though its underlying biochemical abnormality is not known.

In some conditions there is a substantial difference in the occurrence rate of abnormalities in different racial groups. For instance, sickle cell disease is confined to those originating from Black Africa; thalassaemia is seen mainly in those of Mediterranean or Far Eastern origin; and glucose-6-phosphate dehydrogenase deficiency is com-

Table 13.1 Some conditions diagnosed by DNA analysis (A) and FISH (B)

A: DNA analysis

Diagnosis	Mode of inheritance	Diagnostic findings
Cystic fibrosis	Autosomal recessive	Mutation of CFTR gene on chromosome 7 identified in 50–90% of cases
Werdnig–Hoffmann disease	Autosomal recessive	SMN and NAIP gene deletions found on chromosome 5 in over 95% of cases
Congentital adrenal hyperplasia	Autosomal recessive	Mutations of 21 hydroxlase gene on chromosome 6 in most cases
Myotonic dystrophy	Autosomal dominant	Trinucleotide repeat mutations of specific gene on chromosome 19 in almost all cases
X-linked hydrocephalus	X-linked	Mutation in L1CAM gene identified in most familial cases
Wiedemann–Beckwith syndrome		Visible deletion on chromosome 11 in 5%; uniparental disomy for 11p15 markers in 20%

B: Fluorescent in situ hybridization (FISH)

Condition	Diagnostic findings
Prader–Willi syndrome	Deletions on short arm of 15 chromosome in 5%; maternal uniparental disomy for chromosome 15 in the rest
Williams syndrome	Deletion of elastin gene on chromosome 7 in 95% of cases
Velocardiofacial syndrome	Gene deletion on short arm of chromosome 22 in 90% of cases

moner in many tropical and subtropical countries (p. 186).

Social class differences also occur, neural tube defects being more common where the father has an unskilled occupation whereas congenital dislocation of the hip is more prevalent in managerial and professional families.

Malnutrition may play some part; folic acid deficiency is a major factor in the origin of neural tube defects since there is a 75% reduction of recurrence of the condition if folic acid supplements are taken before conception and while the fetus is differentiating (p. 21). Maternal ageing is known to be a factor in the production of at least one major abnormality – Down's syndrome – and probably in all trisomic chromosomal anomalies. Birth order is of significance in anencephaly, spina bifida and congenital dislocation of the hip, which are all more common in first pregnancies.

The majority of malformations, however, are likely to be caused by factors adversely affecting the fetus in the early stages of its development.

Infections

The best known of these is rubella with its effects on ears, eyes, heart and brain. These and the abnormalities caused by antenatal infection with toxoplasmosis and cytomegalovirus are described in Chapter 11. Some viral infections, including Coxsackie A and B and echoviruses, may also cause anomalies but associations with other viruses are less certain.

Drugs

The thalidomide incident in the 1960s had the beneficial side-effect of promoting caution in the use of all drugs in early pregnancy. Many other substances have been suspected but few are proven to be the sole cause of malformation. It seems likely that some drugs contribute to the production of a defect only in conjunction with other factors such as nutritional deficiency, hypoxia or a genetic predisposition. The excess of babies with cleft palate and congenital heart disease born to mothers taking sodium valproate or carbamazepine is a possible example of this. The effect of harmful drugs varies according to which organs are undergoing differentiation at the time of exposure. Other toxic pollutants such as sulphur dioxide, carbon monoxide, solvents, lead and dioxins are all suspected of contributing to congenital malformations but are not linked to any particular ones. Cigarette smoking affects the growth of the fetus and may predispose an infant to the adverse effects of other factors. Alcohol ingestion undoubtedly causes a dysmorphic syndrome in some infants (p. 13).

Irradiation is undoubtedly a potential danger to fetal development, but proven ill effects have only occurred after very heavy exposure, or following preconceptional irradiation of parental gonads.

Other factors

The incidence of malformations is doubled when the mother suffers from diabetes mellitus in pregnancy (p. 25), and in multiple births the risk is also increased, but this may affect only one fetus. Some defects such as those seen in cocaine-addicted mothers may result from vascular accidents and others from episodes of hypoxia at sensitive periods during fetal life.

PREVENTION

Careful and comprehensive history-taking from the pregnant mother at the first antenatal visit to identify familial inherited disorders is of the utmost importance, but opportunities for prevention are still often missed at this stage.

Identification of carriers of inherited disorders

Although the pattern of inheritance of many diseases is known, the accurate identification of carriers of X-linked and recessive conditions has until recently been possible in only a minority of cases. For instance, carriers of the phenylketonuria gene can be identified reasonably accurately by measuring the ratio of phenylalanine to tyrosine in the blood, but haemophilia carriers can be identified by estimation of factor VIII activity with no more than a moderate degree of certainty. Recently, methods of identifying the site of individual genes on the chromosomes have been developed. DNA material is examined by complex genetic engineering techniques and, as a result, geneticists are now able to demon-

strate accurately in an increasing number of conditions which family members are carrying the abnormal gene (Table 2.4). It is not necessary to know the underlying biochemical abnormality for accurate gene analysis and these techniques can predict the onset of certain genetic diseases which occur later in life.

Genetic counselling for families in which an inherited abnormality has occurred is of great value and expert counselling clinics are growing in numbers. Antenatal diagnosis of certain developmental disorders with the help of either blood testing of the mother or fetal ultrasound and amniocentesis, including gene analysis, to identify some genetic disorders has become increasingly available and is discussed on page 19.

Publicity aimed at decreasing the proportion of women who reach antenatal clinics too late in pregnancy, and education about the importance of adequate nutrition before conception and during the early months of pregnancy might lead to some reduction in the incidence of genetic diseases.

Immunization against infections to which the fetus is susceptible is at present only practicable in the case of rubella and to be effective and safe this has to be done before conception.

Prenatal identification of congenital malformations

Clinical findings which point to an increased chance of malformation in the current pregnancy and help in predicting the possibility include polyhydramnios, oligohydramnios and intrauterine growth retardation, all of which justify a careful ultrasound examination of the fetus. A newborn infant with a single umbilical artery is also at increased risk of renal tract anomalies.

Deformities

Deformities, as distinct from true developmental malformations, can undoubtedly be caused by abnormal mechanical stresses or pressures upon the developing fetus; examples of these are talipes deformities of the feet and congenital scoliosis, although in both there may also be a hereditary predisposing factor. Amniotic bands can cause amputations of digits or even whole limbs.

Lethal anomalies

A small proportion of malformations can result in the death of the baby before or shortly after birth, although timely treatment can save life in many cases. In some cases where a lethal anomaly such as renal agenesis or anencephaly has been identified by ultrasound examination in early pregnancy, a termination may be recommended. Around 20% of lethal malformations are identified at postmortem examination of stillborn babies and about 50% cause death within the first month. In the remainder, death occurs during later infancy or childhood. The great majority affect the heart, central nervous system, gut and urinary systems, but many are associated with chromosomal abnormalities or are only one of several malformations in the same infant. Mortality rates from congenital malformations vary markedly between racial groups, the risk in the offspring of Asian-born mothers being more than twice as high as UK-born mothers. By contrast, the rate is low in Afro-Caribbean mothers. Examples of these most serious defects are given in Table 13.2.

Table 13.2 Examples of lethal congenital malformations

Central nervous system	Anencephaly
	Spina bifida
	—with hydrocephalus
	—encephalocoele
	Spinal muscular atrophy
Cardiovascular system	Hypoplastic left heart syndrome
	Transposition of the great arteries
	Pulmonary atresia
	Cardiomyopathy
Gastrointestinal tract	Diaphragmatic hernia
	Exomphalos
	Gastroschisis
	Intestinal atresias
Urinary tract	Renal agenesis
	Dysplastic or cystic kidneys
Chromosomal disorders	Trisomy 18
	Trisomy 13
Multiple abnormalities	Recognizable 'syndromes'
Metabolic disorders	MCAD deficiency

THE CLASSIFICATION OF CONGENITAL ANOMALIES

Sometimes a congenital abnormality will have been identified before birth by ultrasound examination, e.g. hydrocephalus, spina bifida, hydronephrosis, severe congenital heart disease and many others (p. 18). Most are either obvious at birth or are identified in the first few days or weeks, e.g. gut atresias, but some are only revealed by a deliberate search (congenital dislocation of hips, phenylketonuria).

In the following descriptions stress is laid mainly upon those malformations in which early recognition is important so that appropriate management or advice can be given; most of the rarer anomalies are omitted unless some specific form of early treatment is essential.

ALIMENTARY TRACT

Cleft lip and cleft palate

This type of deformity occurs between 1 in 300 and 1 in 600 births. The lip is involved in 60% of these, the remainder involving the palate alone. Both genetic inheritance and environmental factors are involved in its causation. If either parent has the condition, the occurrence in their offspring is up to 1 in 20, but even with a family history, 1 in 25 siblings of an index case will be affected. For an isolated midline cleft palate, which is a genetically distinct condition comprising about a quarter of the total, the risk is about half this figure. Around 10% of clefts are associated with other congenital malformations, particularly trisomies and other chromosome anomalies. Maternal anticonvulsants taken in pregnancy increase the risk and small 'epidemics' of cleft lip and palate have been reported in association with outbreaks of Coxsackie B4 virus infections.

The cleft lip may be single (Plate 5) or double (Plate 20A), and if double, the central portion (globular process) between the clefts may protrude forward.

Management

Although the parents are often shocked by their

baby's appearance, the main problem for the child in the neonatal period is difficulty with feeding. The method of feeding depends upon the extent of the deformity. In many cases of cleft lip alone, or small clefts of the soft palate, breast feeding is possible and should be recommended. For those infants who, from choice or because breast feeding is unsuccessful, are to be bottle fed, feeding can often be managed remarkably well using an ordinary bottle and a big soft teat, with an enlarged hole in it if necessary, even when the cleft is quite severe. Specially designed flanged teats are available to try and close the gap during suction, but they are seldom helpful; however, in some cases a fitted solid palatal prosthesis may help. If this fails, spoon or cup feeding is always possible and should be practised at some time before operation in order that mother and child will be accustomed to it when it is used temporarily after repair of the lip. Great parental anxiety is natural at first and a full explanation of the management and the likely outcome of operation, including showing the parents photographs of the final result in other children (Plates 20A and B), is time well spent.

Respiratory difficulty occurs only in a rare group, known as the Pierre Robin syndrome, in which a midline cleft of the soft palate is associated with micrognathia (short mandible); the tongue tends to protrude upwards and backwards through the cleft, obstructing the respiratory passages. Life may even be endangered from the resulting cyanotic attacks, but they may almost always be prevented by nursing the infant in the prone position, which sometimes requires a special arrangement for supporting the head face downward whilst keeping the airway clear.

Surgical treatment

Most plastic surgeons like to operate on the lip when the baby is about 3 months old, although occasionally it is done within a few days of birth. The palate is commonly left until 6–9 months.

Middle ear infections are common even after closure of the defect and frequently grommets will be inserted in the tympanic membranes to prevent hearing loss associated with chronic serous otitis media. Orthodontic care is required to ensure a good cosmetic appearance of the teeth and speech therapy will frequently be required later to improve speech, although the end result is nowadays generally excellent.

Oesophageal atresia

In this anomaly, the upper part of the oesophagus is present only to the level of the second to fourth thoracic vertebrae (about one-third of its length), where it ends blindly. In 90% of cases, there is also a fistula between the trachea and the lower section of the oesophagus which leads to the stomach. In about 8% there is a blind oesophagus without a tracheo-oesophageal fistula, and the remainder consists of other variations. The anomaly occurs about once in 3000 live births.

Diagnosis

A large amount of amniotic fluid is normally swallowed by the infant each day, but this is impossible when the oesophagus is blocked and polyhydramnios results. About 1 in 30 cases of polyhydramnios is associated with upper intestinal obstruction or diaphragmatic hernia. It should therefore be routine practice to pass a nasogastric tube to exclude oesophageal atresia soon after delivery in all cases of polyhydramnios. The abnormality should also be suspected in any newborn infant who accumulates excessive saliva and mucus secretions in the mouth and pharynx, particularly when this secretion is frothy and the baby has periodic attacks of choking with obstruction to breathing and perhaps cyanosis.

It is clearly vitally important to make the diagnosis before the first feed is given, for this will lead only to immediate choking and aspiration of feed into the lungs. Every midwife must be alert to these early signs and, having suspected the condition, should, without delay, attempt to pass a firm polythene nasogastric tube through the mouth and down the oesophagus. If atresia is present, the tube is held up by an obstruction

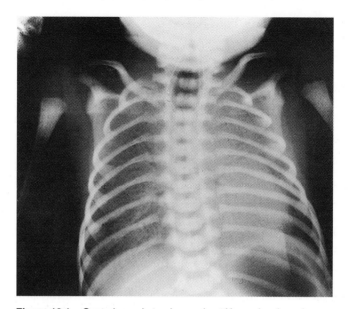

Figure 13.1 Oesophageal atresia – a chest X-ray showing a large bore nasogastric tube coiled in the upper oesophagus. (By kind permission of Dr Jo Fairhurst.)

when 7–10 cm have been passed, although if the tube is not fairly rigid it may curl up in the oesophageal pouch (Fig. 13.1). However, the absence of acid in the fluid aspirated from the tube should suggest that the oesophagus is blocked. Instillation of a radio-opaque medium is contraindicated since the inevitable aspiration into the lungs adds to the problem already present. Gas in the intestine on X-ray indicates the presence of a tracheo-oesophageal fistula as well as atresia (Fig. 13.1), but absence of gas does not exclude it.

Management

The accumulated secretions in mouth, pharynx and blind oesophagus must be aspirated frequently and a search made for other congenital malformations. Prompt transfer of the infant to the care of an experienced paediatric surgical team for operative repair is essential. In most cases the surgeon mobilizes the two ends of the oesophagus and makes an immediate anastomosis by a thoracic approach. A temporary gastrostomy will allow enteral feeding if more extensive

surgery is required later, but it is essential to fashion an oesophagostomy which opens to the outside at the root of the neck to allow the infant to retain the art of sucking and swallowing until the oesophagus is finally joined to the stomach. The main risk to the infant is from pneumonia following aspiration of the oesophageal contents into the lungs, from any accompanying anomalies or from prematurity.

Congenital oesophageal hiatus hernia

Congenital oesophageal hiatus hernia, in which there is upward protrusion of the cardiac portion of the stomach through the oesophageal hiatus in the diaphragm, usually remains undiagnosed until later infancy and may in fact sometimes be intermittent with a sliding hernia. There is free reflux of gastric contents up the oesophagus due to interference with the valvular mechanism at the cardia and ulceration is liable to occur at the junction of oesophageal and gastric mucosa, followed occasionally by stricture formation. The condition is not an uncommon one but it seems probable that some cases remain undiagnosed, for they may become symptomless soon after mixed feeding begins at about 4 or 5 months.

Vomiting is usually noted from birth but it is not always profuse or consistent; later the vomit characteristically contains small amounts of blood due to oesophagitis, and very occasionally anaemia from persistent occult bleeding is the presenting feature. Confirmation of the diagnosis can only be made by X-ray screening during a barium feed, which demonstrates the pouch of stomach above the diaphragm. The reflux of gastric contents into the oesophagus is not in itself enough to make the diagnosis, because it may occur to some extent in many normal infants. Medical treatment, consisting of the use of thickened feeds and maintaining the semi-upright position throughout the day and night for several months, successfully tides over most cases until they become symptomless towards the end of the first year. Persistent oesophagitis, which may be suspected when there is continued altered blood in the vomit and confirmed by oesophagoscopy, may necessitate surgery.

Congenital hypertrophic pyloric stenosis

In this condition the muscle at the pylorus of the stomach hypertrophies over the first few weeks of life causing an increasing obstruction to the passage of milk feeds. It is doubtful whether this relatively common disorder should be classed as congenital or as a malformation, even though it presents so early in life. Heredity plays a part in its causation, for the normal incidence of about 2/1000 births is much increased where either the parent or a previous child has suffered from it, and it is five times as common in boys as in girls. The risk of occurrence of the condition in the children of women who have had pyloric stenosis is 1 in 5 for sons and 1 in 15 for daughters. In the case of an affected father, the risks are 1 in 20 for sons and 1 in 40 for daughters.

Clinical features

Whether or not there is some pyloric hypertro-

phy present at birth, the obstruction rarely begins until after the second week. Vomiting, which is the major presenting feature, sometimes starts in the first week but more often it is delayed until the third to fifth weeks or even occasionally as long as 2 months. It starts as small possets but gradually becomes projectile and occurs immediately after feeding, the vomit usually containing no bile; weight is lost, but unless dehydration or electrolyte disturbances become severe enough to cause apathy the infant will continue to take the feeds hungrily. Stools may become infrequent and small.

Visible gastric peristalsis in the left upper quadrant of the abdomen after a feed is characteristic but not diagnostic and only palpation of the thickened pylorus during a feed, which requires patience and some experience, is conclusive evidence. Occasionally an ultrasound examination or barium meal (Fig. 13.2) will confirm the diagnosis in a case where the tumour cannot be felt.

Surgical treatment by means of Ramstedt's pyloromyotomy, in which the hypertrophied muscle is split along its length to widen the pyloric canal, relieves the problem rapidly and

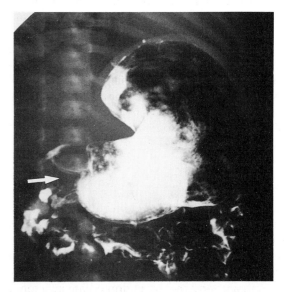

Figure 13.2 Barium meal in congenital hypertrophic pyloric stenosis showing the pyloric canal (arrowed) narrowed to a fine line by the hypertrophied surrounding muscle.

effectively. It is never a surgical emergency and significant fluid and electrolyte imbalance should be rectified intravenously before the operation.

Duodenal atresia

This is another condition in which surgery is required within the first day or two of life. The site of obstruction is usually, but not always, at a point in the third part of the duodenum below the opening of the common bile duct. Maternal polyhydramnios is a warning sign and the infant frequently has evidence of intrauterine growth retardation. There is a substantially increased incidence in babies with Down's syndrome. If a congenital abnormality scan has been carried out in the early stages of pregnancy, this anomaly is identifiable since the stomach and duodenum are shown distended with fluid in contrast to the rest of the gut which is empty.

After birth, the condition presents as repeated vomiting of bile starting within the first 2 or 3 days of life without noticeable distension of the abdomen. Meconium may be passed normally at first. The yellowish staining of vomit due to pigment in swallowed colostrum is to be distinguished clearly from the greener colour of bile. Also, it must be remembered that, on the rare occasions where the atresia is above the bile duct opening, no bile will be present in the vomit. Straight X-ray of the abdomen in the erect posture is diagnostic, the double gas shadows of the dilated stomach and duodenum only being visible, usually with fluid levels. The operation of duodenojejunostomy usually relieves the condition.

Duodenal stenosis

This is more difficult to diagnose. Vomiting is usually present from birth and is often bile-stained. Since the obstruction is only a partial one, meconium and normal 'changing' stools are passed.

Straight X-ray of the abdomen is not likely to be conclusive; screening after a small feed containing contrast medium may safely be used for diagnosis if there is no evidence of lower intestinal obstruction from straight X-ray films.

Neonatal intestinal obstruction below the duodenum

Obstruction below the duodenum gives rise to a recognizable clinical picture, for which there are several different causes. The onset of vomiting of bile-stained or brownish coloured material and an increasingly distended abdomen over which there may sometimes be visible peristalsis within the first few days of life are the characteristic features, and a straight X-ray of the abdomen in the erect posture will confirm the diagnosis by showing the characteristic dilated loops of bowel and fluid levels in the gut.

Differential diagnosis of the site and cause of the obstruction can often be made from the clinical signs and X-ray appearance, and the principal types are described here with their main characteristic features.

Atresia of the jejunum or ileum

Abdominal distension is early in onset and erect straight X-ray shows the large gas shadows of dilated small intestine – usually with fluid levels but with no gas in the colon (Fig. 13.3). Occasionally the X-ray appearance of slight general dilatation of the gut with occasional fluid levels may be caused simply by swallowing a lot of air, but in atresia of the small gut the distended loops of intestine terminate abruptly at the point of obstruction. Early operation is usually successful, but it is often necessary to resect a portion of the very dilated gut before anastomosis.

Meconium ileus

Meconium ileus is not strictly a congenital malformation but is included here because the clinical presentation is again one of small gut obstruction. It is an early complication of cystic fibrosis which is itself a congenital condition affecting the mucus-secreting glands throughout the body. Because of a deficiency of pancreatic

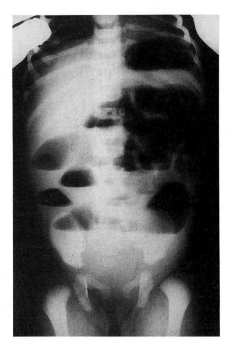

Figure 13.3 Multiple fluid levels in an erect abdominal X-ray in ileal atresia.

enzymes, the contents of the small intestine become hardened and obstruct the lumen. The diagnosis may be suspected before operation on three possible grounds: a family history of cystic fibrosis in siblings, the abnormally solid nature of the meconium together with a positive meconium protein (BM meconium) test, and a characteristic finely mottled appearance of the small intestine on X-ray due to small bubbles of gas trapped in the meconium-filled lumen. Operation to remove the obstructing meconium is not always straightforward and irrigation may be necessary via a temporary ileostomy.

Cystic fibrosis

Cystic fibrosis only rarely presents in the first few days as meconium ileus but the diagnosis should be sought at an early stage whenever a family history in siblings is known. A case can be made for the routine screening of all newborn babies for the condition by blood testing for raised levels of immunoreactive trypsin and this is now performed in certain parts of Britain and the USA and is widely used in Australia. The diagnosis can only be confirmed, however, by the finding of raised sodium content of the sweat – a test which is difficult to perform accurately in the first week or two of life. The identification of one of the several known gene mutations associated with the condition may in time improve the early diagnosis of this disorder (pp. 20 and 195).

Meconium peritonitis

This may be a complication of meconium ileus or necrotizing enterocolitis, or may be due to congenital defects in the intestinal wall. X-ray of the abdomen shows gas in the peritoneal cavity and sometimes calcification outside the bowel. Exploratory laparotomy is essential to detect the site of the perforation and to repair it.

Malrotation of the midgut

Malrotation of the midgut, though often remaining undetected and symptomless until later childhood, may also cause obstruction in the neonatal period. There may be either duodenal obstruction from compression by the abnormal mesentery or a volvulus involving the ileum and jejunum.

Meckel's diverticulum

Meckel's diverticulum is usually asymptomatic but may cause intestinal obstruction after the first 2 days of life. There is nothing diagnostic about the clinical features except the timing of onset which is generally after the first 2 days of life.

Hirschsprung's disease

Hirschsprung's disease may show itself in the neonatal period as abdominal distension with gas and severe retention of faeces amounting sometimes to obstruction. It is almost entirely a disease of males, with an incidence of 1 in 5000 births and, like duodenal atresia, is relatively more common in children with Down's syndrome. The hold-up in the passage of faeces through the lower part of the colon is caused by a length of large gut which lacks parasympathetic ganglion cells (the 'aganglionic segment') and fails to pass on the peristaltic wave. This segment may be a short one extending from the rectum into the last few inches of sigmoid colon, or less commonly it may extend upwards for a variable distance in the colon. Persistent dilatation of the normal gut behind it results in the so-called megacolon.

Usually no meconium is passed at all in the first few days, but sometimes there are infrequent loose offensive stools thereafter. The outstanding feature of Hirschsprung's disease is in the abdominal distension from retained gas. On rectal examination, it is possible sometimes to produce a temporary dilatation of the aganglionic segment with relief of symptoms by a rush of gas and faeces. A barium enema may reveal the characteristic narrowed segment of colon but a rectal biopsy showing the absence of ganglion cells is necessary for diagnosis; however, even these can be difficult to interpret.

The use of repeated saline washouts may help to postpone surgery during the neonatal period. If a laparotomy is required to exclude other causes for the obstruction, it is usual to fashion a colostomy and take a biopsy of the rectal mucosa for histological diagnosis. The colostomy may have to remain for several weeks or months before the operation of rectosigmoidectomy is performed, consisting of resection of the aganglionic segment and most of the rectum followed by anastomosis of the proximal colon to the remaining rectal stump. In subsequent pregnancies, there is a risk of about 1 in 5 for any male child developing the same condition.

Meconium plug

Temporary obstruction from the presence of a meconium plug (not in association with meconium ileus) is relatively common. The plug occupies the lower colon and rectum, and its leading end consists of white mucoid jelly which may sometimes be removed by gentle rectal examination. Occasionally a small repeated saline washout may be necessary to do so.

Necrotizing enterocolitis

This serious disorder, the presenting signs of which are often those of intestinal obstruction, occurs largely in pre-term babies and has therefore been included in Chapter 9.

Incarcerated inguinal hernia

Incarcerated inguinal hernia is another occasional cause of obstruction, usually occurring in the pre-term male baby (p. 121).

Milk curd obstruction

Obstruction from hardened milk curds is only seen in low birth weight babies fed on cow's milk preparations but may occasionally be sufficiently severe to necessitate operation for removal of the curds.

Imperforate or ectopic anus

There is a great variety of different anomalies in this region (Plate 21). In the female, the commonest type is displacement forward of the anal opening so that it opens immediately behind the vulva, inside the vulva or, rarely, inside the vagina. In the male there may be no sign of an anus at all, a bulging membrane or triangular portion of skin at the anal site or a narrow subcutaneous channel leading forward from the true anus to a fistulous opening anteriorly (the 'covered anus'). Rectourethral fistulae also occur in males, but only rarely.

Even when there is simple anterior displacement of the anal opening it is usually a narrow one which allows some temporary passage of meconium but generally leads to partial obstruction sooner or later. It can be treated initially simply by dilatation, although further surgery is often needed later.

The assessment of the extent of the anomaly and the type of operation which is required is a matter for an experienced paediatric surgeon. In many cases, a simple cutting-back operation to enlarge the displaced opening is all that is necessary and does not interfere with sphincter control, but the more serious forms of the condition require operation via the abdomen in order to define the position, and a colostomy may be a necessary preliminary. Provided that use can be made of the puborectalis muscle sling, good results with faecal continence can be obtained.

Exomphalos

Exomphalos (Plate 22A) occurs once in every 5000 births. In this type of abdominal hernia, the protrusion occurs into the umbilical stalk itself so that the cord is inserted into part of the hernial sac consisting of amniotic membranes and peritoneum which may rupture during delivery, allowing the abdominal contents to spill out. Association with other congenital malformations, particularly of the alimentary tract, is common and exomphalos is one of the features of Beckwith's syndrome (p. 60).

Gastroschisis

In this condition (Plate 22B), the herniation occurs through a large defect in the abdominal wall adjacent to the umbilicus, so there is no covering sac. The protruding gut is usually inflamed from irritation by amniotic fluid and the baby often has peritonitis at birth. The bowel is oedematous, thickened and often appears blue due to interference with its blood supply.

Both conditions cause a rise in maternal alphafetoprotein levels in early pregnancy, but they can be distinguished from the more usual cause – an open spina bifida – by antenatal ultrasound scanning (p. 21).

Treatment

Immediate treatment of both exomphalos and gastroschisis is directed towards preventing drying out and infection of the protruding gut until the baby can be brought to neonatal paediatric surgery. One effective means of doing this is to wrap the whole abdomen, including the herniated intestine, loosely in clingfilm to prevent loss of fluid and to dress the baby with warm clothing to maintain her temperature.

Fluid and electrolyte losses from an exposed hernial sac or the protruding gut can be severe and an intravenous infusion of human albumin is essential if the baby is to be transferred to a distant hospital for surgery. Parenteral nutrition is often required postoperatively until the gut recovers its function.

The difficulty in surgical treatment is proportional to the amount and size of the viscera which have to be replaced. It is sometimes impossible to return all the abdominal contents and still close the abdominal muscles over them without compromising the baby's breathing, so in some cases a temporary cover with skin or a Dacron sheet is made and full repair is attempted later.

RESPIRATORY TRACT
Choanal atresia

This uncommon congenital obstruction to the posterior nasal airway shows itself as respiratory difficulty immediately after delivery if it is bilateral, since the baby at birth is dependent on the nose to breathe, but it can go unnoticed until later in childhood if it is only unilateral. It is occasionally associated with other congenital malformations and nerve deafness in a rare syndrome known as the CHARGE association.

Congenital laryngeal stridor

An inspiratory crowing noise noticeable in the first few days of life, louder at some times than others and especially with crying, is almost always due to a 'floppy larynx' or laryngomalacia. The noise is probably caused by a valvular closure of the glottis on inspiration due to softness of its supporting structures. Most cases recover spontaneously and gradually before the age of 2 years. It is alarming to the parents but appears to do no harm to the infant, and reassuring the parents is usually all the treatment that is needed.

Other abnormalities of the larynx, such as obstructing webs at different sites, are very much rarer causes of inspiratory stridor. Tracheal compression from a vascular ring, caused by abnormalities of the aortic arch, must be considered, especially if difficulty in swallowing and dyspnoea are also present. A barium swallow reveals the characteristic indentation in the oesophagus.

Congenital lung cysts

These rare malformations usually present at birth with respiratory difficulty although they occasionally remain symptomless until later childhood. They are often identifiable on examination of the fetal lungs on prenatal ultrasound, and after birth the chest X-ray may resemble a diaphragmatic hernia, but the condition can be distinguished from it by passing a nasogastric tube into a normally positioned stomach. The abnormal part of the lung should be removed surgically to prevent recurrent infection.

Sequestration of the lung

In this condition, the bronchi fail to communicate properly with a portion of lung tissue which remains unaerated after birth. It is often symptomless, but if it is identified on an X-ray surgical removal is indicated.

Diaphragmatic hernia

This abnormality occurs about once in 2000 births. Herniation of the stomach and other viscera into the chest is usually through a deficiency in the left leaf of the diaphragm. Before birth it is often associated with maternal polyhydramnios, and prenatal ultrasound examination can usually confirm the diagnosis. In some cases the pregnancy is uneventful and in these cases respiratory distress from birth is the presenting sign, due to shift of the mediastinum and reduced lung function which results from the associated hypoplasia of the lungs.

The main clinical features are a shift of the maximal heart sounds to the right side of the chest and apparent emptiness of the abdomen. X-ray of the chest in every baby with respiratory distress is the only sure way of not missing this abnormality, which constitutes a surgical emergency (Fig. 7.4, p. 101). Management in the early stages is described on page 100.

Hypoplasia

Hypoplasia of the lungs with diminished lung function and pulmonary hypertension may complicate several conditions including diaphragmatic hernia, oligohydramnios and the very rare bony abnormalities which restrict the growth of the chest wall. So long as the underlying problem is remediable, the lungs will usually develop improved function as the child grows.

THE HEART AND GREAT VESSELS

The true incidence of congenital malformations of the heart is uncertain because many, including some of the more serious lesions, are not detectable at birth by present methods of routine examination and some resolve completely without treatment, for instance the smaller ventricular septal defects. It is around 8 per 1000 births and about half of these will require medical and surgical treatment in the neonatal period. In about a quarter of cases, the cardiac malformation is only one of several congenital anomalies or is one feature of a syndrome associated with a chromosomal abnormality, such as Down's syndrome.

Surgical techniques have developed so rapidly that the number of completely inoperable abnormalities is now small. An increasing number of corrective procedures can now be undertaken in the newborn period and techniques to relieve cyanosis can reduce the morbidity of others considerably. It follows that early recognition of serious congenital heart disease is of great importance and it is this rather than detailed differential diagnosis of the numerous types of abnormality that will be described here.

For those who look after newborn babies, what matters is the ability to identify the infants whose problems are attributable to heart disease, to know how to select the ones who require early surgical treatment, and the means of maintaining the infant in the best condition to enable a safe transfer to a paediatric cardiology centre at the optimal time.

Congenital heart disease

Congenital heart disease can sometimes be diagnosed by ultrasound before birth, but in the newborn baby it is brought to notice in one or more of the following ways:

- Cardiac failure (p. 100) – tachypnoea, costal recession, tachycardia, enlargement of the liver and occasionally oedema are the main features. It is often difficult to be certain whether respiratory distress is due to pulmonary or cardiac disease.
- Central cyanosis, affecting the whole body and the mucous membranes of the mouth and conjunctiva, which is persistent and not confined to the extremities, in the absence of a pulmonary cause.
- A cardiac murmur or abnormality of the heart sounds themselves. It must be remembered, however, that moderately loud systolic murmurs may sometimes be heard in normal babies in the first few days; conversely, it should be remembered that the murmurs of certain types of congenital heart disease do not become audible for several days or weeks and that not all types of congenital heart disease cause a murmur.
- An arrhythmia (e.g. bradycardia with heart block, ectopic beats, supraventricular tachycardia).
- Lethargy, inactivity, poor feeding and later failure to thrive.

Investigations

The purpose of investigation of suspected congenital heart disease is to identify the type of defect present, to aid in the assessment of risk to the infant's immediate health and to monitor the need for, and the effects of, treatment. The investigations usually performed are:

- chest X-ray
- electrocardiogram (ECG)
- echocardiography
- blood gases
- pulse oximetry
- oxygen saturation test.

Interpretation of the chest X-ray at this age needs much experience; apparent enlargement is often misleading and may be due to a large thymic shadow amongst other possibilities.

Electrocardiograms are difficult to interpret during the first few days when big changes in the dynamics of the circulation are taking place (p. 47). However, findings that should alert suspicion include a superior axis, left axis deviation, left ventricular hypertrophy (tall R waves in V_6 and deep S waves in V_2), marked right ventricular hypertrophy (upright T wave after the fourth day, together with a tall R wave in chest lead V_1), or conduction abnormalities.

Echocardiography provides a non-invasive means of demonstrating the anatomical structure of the chambers, valves and vessels of the heart and the connections between them, together with measurement of pressure gradients across the valves if Doppler equipment is available. Colour flow mapping can also demonstrate abnormal patterns of blood flow in septal defects or in more complex anomalies. In some conditions, it provides enough information to plan surgical treatment, although cardiac catheterization is still required in a proportion of cases.

In a baby with significant cyanotic heart disease, transcutaneous pulse oximetry will demonstrate the degree of arterial oxygen desaturation. The oxygen saturation test can be used to distinguish cardiac from pulmonary cyanosis. An infant with cyanotic heart disease breathing 100% oxygen will fail to raise the arterial Po_2 above 13 kPa, whereas the Po_2 or oxygen saturation will rise significantly above this value in lung conditions.

Blood gases are particularly important in the cyanosed infant and will show whether the baby is becoming acidotic as a result of hypoxia. If much time is likely to elapse before the baby's arrival at the cardiac centre, the control of acidosis is crucial to the outlook for either survival or minimization of the risk of later neurological handicap. In some conditions, an infusion of prostaglandins is needed to keep the ductus arteriosus open during transfer (p. 208).

Common heart malformations

There are so many different types of possible cardiac malformation that only a very simplified account of those that most commonly occur will be given here. These will be classified according to their mode of presentation.

Malformations presenting mainly with cyanosis

Cyanotic congenital heart disease is usually complex and the physical signs vary greatly in the same basic condition from one infant to another; distinguishing the conditions clinically is often impossible and an accurate anatomical diagnosis can only be made with echocardiography or more complex investigations. All babies suspected of having a cyanotic heart malformation require urgent investigation and treatment to ensure adequate oxygenation of the blood.

Transposition of the great arteries. In this condition, the aorta arises from the right ventricle and the pulmonary artery from the left. Thus, unless a septal defect or open ductus arteriosus is also present, the two circulations are completely separate. Cyanosis from birth is usual, and typically the baby seems otherwise well in the first day or two until the ductus arteriosus begins to close. Thereafter, the progress depends upon how much oxygenated blood flows across any associated septal defect between the left and right sides. Cyanosis and respiratory difficulty usually become progressively worse within the first week. Murmurs and other signs – even the X-ray and ECG findings – are so variable at different stages that they prove to be of little diagnostic help. Echocardiography readily shows the pulmonary artery emanating from a narrow left ventricle and the aorta in an abnormally posterior position.

The development of balloon septostomy (Rashkind's procedure), which creates a large interatrial communication by the use of a balloon catheter alone and relieves cyanosis rapidly by allowing mixing of the saturated and unsaturated blood, means that early transfer to a cardiac centre on suspicion of the diagnosis is essential. Later a surgical procedure to create a cross-over of the circulations can be achieved at atrial level by Mustard's operation or, increasingly commonly, by an arterial switch procedure, and these are usually highly successful.

Pulmonary atresia. In this condition the pulmonary artery, pulmonary valve and the right ventricle are all hypoplastic and often cyanosis is the only abnormality on clinical examination. On the ECG there is usually left axis deviation, because of the diminished forces from the hypoplastic right ventricle, and the tall peaked P waves of right atrial hypertrophy. The X-ray shows gross cardiac enlargement with pulmonary arterial oligaemia but often obvious bronchial artery shadows. Immediate referral to a cardiac centre is essential since some cases may be helped by urgent pulmonary valvotomy or balloon valvuloplasty or by an arterial shunt operation, but the prognosis is often poor.

Tricuspid atresia. Atresia of the tricuspid valve is associated with a hypoplasia of the right ventricle, but a large ventricular septal defect often allows sufficient pulmonary blood flow to occur to maintain adequate oxygenation of the blood, and treatment can often be deferred until much later in childhood. It is often associated with the presence of marked left-sided dominance on ECG.

Total anomalous pulmonary venous drainage. This condition in which the pulmonary veins enter the right atrium instead of the left is usually associated with cyanosis and the early onset of cardiac failure. Murmurs may be absent. The lung fields on X-ray appear hazy due to pulmonary vascular congestion and the ECG shows right ventricular hypertrophy.

Persistent truncus arteriosus consists of a single artery leaving the heart which supplies both the aorta and pulmonary vessels. A systolic murmur and mild cyanosis are usually present, with breathlessness from increased pulmonary blood flow. Echocardiography shows the single arterial trunk emerging from the ventricles. A proportion of babies with this or other conotruncal abnormalities have a gene deletion on chromosome 22 (p. 194).

Single ventricle. A single ventricle, with or without other anomalies, is also likely to present with cyanosis.

Fallot's tetralogy. Later onset of cyanosis is seen in Fallot's tetralogy in which right ventricular hypertrophy occurs with pulmonary stenosis and an aorta which overrides a ventricular septal defect (Fig. 13.4). In the neonatal period the condition presents simply as a murmur at the left sternal edge, but a chest X-ray shows reduced pulmonary vascularity and the heart is usually of normal size.

Poor pulmonary perfusion. Occasionally cyanosis can result from poor pulmonary perfusion associated either with polycythaemia or with persistence of fetal pulmonary hypertension without a cardiac malformation. This latter problem requires treatment with oxygen and pulmonary vasodilator drugs, e.g. tolazoline, and sometimes the condition is sufficiently severe to need mechanical ventilation. It is often only diagnosed after full cardiac investigation has excluded any anatomical abnormality.

Management of the severely cyanosed infant

In transposition and pulmonary atresia, in particular, the baby's survival may depend on the

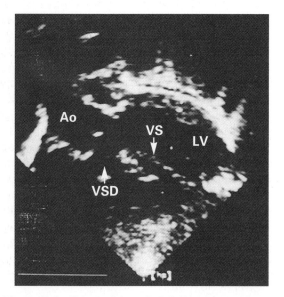

Figure 13.4 Echocardiogram in Fallot's tetralogy showing the ventricular septal defect (VSD, arrowed) and the aorta (Ao) overriding the interventricular septum (VS). (By kind permission of Dr Tony Salmon.)

small amount of oxygenated blood flowing through an open ductus arteriosus. Closure, which may occur at any time, results in the rapid onset of acidosis and severe hypoxia which can cause brain damage. In these infants, an intravenous infusion of prostaglandins E1 (or E2) at a rate of 0.01–0.05 µg/kg per minute may improve mixing of the circulations for long enough to enable the safe transfer of the infant to the cardiac centre.

Malformations presenting mainly with heart failure and respiratory distress

Hypoplastic left heart syndrome. This condition, consisting of aortic atresia and severe underdevelopment of the left ventricle, is the commonest fatal cardiac malformation in the newborn period and the only treatment available is heart transplantation, although results are currently very disappointing. Heart failure, which does not respond to medical treatment, appears within the first few days of life together with poor peripheral pulses and some degree of cyanosis. Occasionally a murmur may be present. The ECG usually shows gross right ventricular dominance and the diagnosis is readily confirmed on echocardiography. Death usually occurs within a week or two of birth.

Coarctation of the aorta (Fig. 13.5) is a localized narrowing of a small segment of the aortic arch which partially obstructs aortic blood flow. It is often associated with other anomalies, such as persistent ductus arteriosus or ventricular septal defect, and only presents at this age if it is severe. The femoral pulses are either not palpable or diminished and delayed, and the blood pressure is higher in the arms than in the legs. Cardiac failure usually occurs within the first 2 weeks. A murmur is often heard most easily between the scapulae. Unexpectedly, the ECG usually shows right dominance, probably because the ductus remains open. Urgent corrective surgery in the neonatal period is needed if the baby is in heart failure and is successful in most cases, although restenosis occurs in a minority of babies later in childhood.

Less severe coarctation without additional

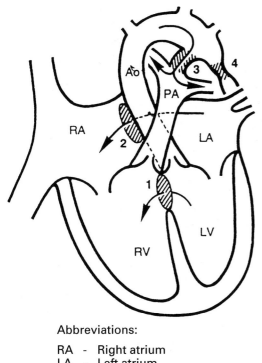

Abbreviations:

RA - Right atrium
LA - Left atrium
RV - Right ventricle
LV - Left ventricle
PA - Pulmonary artery
Ao - Aorta

Heart abnormalities illustrated:

1 - Ventricular septal defect
2 - Atrial septal defect
3 - Patent ductus arteriosus
4 - Coarctation of the aorta

Figure 13.5 Diagram of the position and direction of blood flow in the main acyanotic congenital heart lesions.

malformations, which is more common, can only be diagnosed at this age by the finding of absent or delayed femoral pulses and raised blood pressure in the arms.

Ventricular septal defect, persistent ductus arteriosus and atrial septal defect. In most cases of isolated ventricular septal defect or persistent ductus arteriosus (Figs 13.5 and 9.9), the baby remains well in the newborn period, there being no signs or symptoms until a murmur appears 2–6 weeks after birth. If the defects are large or associated with other cardiac anomalies, heart failure may ensue during the first week. In the case of a ventricular septal defect, a short systolic murmur appears in the first few weeks and only becomes pansystolic after a few weeks of age as the pressures in the right side of the heart fall naturally below the left, allowing blood to flow from left to right across the defect. The classical continuous or machinery murmur of the ductus arteriosus is not usually audible at this age for the same reason. Secundum atrial septal defects (Fig. 13.5) rarely present in the first few weeks of life, although infants with the more complex primum defects, which are often associated with defects of the mitral and tricuspid valves, often develop heart failure in the first few days of life.

Paroxysmal supraventricular tachycardia. In this condition, which is caused by an abnormality of the conducting tissues within the heart and is not uncommon, the rate of the heart suddenly rises, often reaching rates of well over 200 beats/min. Although the infant can often tolerate these rates and remain largely asymptomatic for many hours, eventually heart failure ensues. The diagnosis is made on the ECG which shows the very rapid rate (Fig. 13.6). The treatment consists of trying to reduce the rate to normal as quickly as possible. This can be achieved in an emergency by inducing a very strong vagal reflex by dipping the baby's face into ice-cold water momentarily, or by giving an injection of

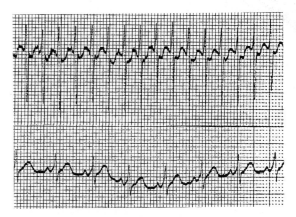

Figure 13.6 ECG traces showing supraventricular tachycardia (above) and the short P–R interval and slurred upstroke of the R wave in the baby's underlying Wolff–Parkinson–White syndrome (below).

intravenous adenosine 0.1–0.2 mg/kg, but in any case it is advisable to treat only in consultation with an experienced paediatric cardiologist. An ECG after the tachycardia has resolved often shows the Wolff–Parkinson–White anomaly (Fig. 13.6). The condition recurs in infancy in most, but not all, cases and may require treatment with other anti-arrhythmic drugs.

Other, rarer causes of heart failure. Fibrosis of the inner lining of the ventricles of unknown origin, which is known as subendocardial fibroelastosis, and myocardial infarction from anomalous origin of the coronary arteries are also rare causes of early heart failure. Myocarditis, sometimes due to Coxsackie virus infection, and mitochondrial disease can also rarely present in this way.

The medical management of heart failure

The infant is best nursed in a semi-erect posture and may be helped by raising the oxygen content of the inspired air to about 30%. Reduction of the venous pressure using a diuretic such as frusemide 1 mg/kg intravenously or intramuscularly is essential. Maintaining the diuresis can be achieved using oral frusemide or bendrofluazide with potassium supplements or spironolactone.

GENITOURINARY TRACT

Kidneys

Absence or severe dysgenesis of both kidneys gives rise to impaired fetal growth and oligohydramnios from lack of fetal urine production. Ultrasound examination of the fetus can identify the absence of the kidneys, and at birth there is a diagnostic frog-like appearance of the face (Potter's facies) with wide-set eyes, low-set ears, and a parrot-beaked nose.

Absence of one kidney may be suspected at routine neonatal examination if this is done carefully, since the lower poles of both are normally palpable in the newborn. Ultrasonography or isotope renography helps to confirm the diagnosis. A large mass in one or both renal regions is an occasional finding on prenatal ultrasound examination or at birth, and the differential diagnosis lies between Wilms' tumour (nephroblastoma), polycystic kidneys (usually bilateral) and severe hydronephrosis. Differentiation of the causes of the mass can be achieved using ultrasound, CT scanning or intravenous pyelography. If obstruction to the urinary tract or a tumour is suspected then early referral to a paediatric surgeon is essential to relieve the obstruction or remove the tumour.

Polycystic disease of the kidneys

Polycystic disease of the kidneys is usually classified into two main types. The 'infantile' variety is inherited as an autosomal recessive characteristic and the parents would therefore be expected to have normal kidneys. It presents as bilateral abdominal masses which can cause a marked abdominal distension and is often accompanied by cystic disease of the liver. It has a relatively poor prognosis owing to the deterioration of renal function or to the development of hypertension which ensues often within the first year. The 'adult' type is transmitted as a dominant condition from one or other parent and renal function is not usually impaired until adult life.

'Prune belly' syndrome

Congenital absence of part of the abdominal musculature in association with renal abnormalities – usually hydronephrosis and undescended testes – constitutes this rare condition.

Obstruction in the urinary tract

Congenital abnormalities resulting in obstruction to the flow of urine occur at the level of the pelviureteric junction, the lower ends of the ureters or at the outlet of the bladder, and many are identifiable on prenatal ultrasound examination of the fetal abdomen since they all result in dilatation of the renal tract. Since many cases of obstruction show no symptoms or abnormal physical signs in the neonatal period, but present later with pain, urinary tract infection or diminished renal function, the introduction of ultrasound screening has improved the outlook for these infants by allowing surgical correction, where necessary, before complications arise.

The most likely anomaly to present with symptoms in the newborn period is congenital valvular obstruction of the male posterior urethra. It may be possible to diagnose this condition in the first week if an observant mother or midwife notices a poor stream of urine or infrequent micturition. Delay in first passing urine beyond 24 hours is often reported but seldom has any serious significance, the apparent delay being caused by the fact that urine has passed unnoticed during delivery. If the urethral obstruction is anything more than slight, the bladder will probably be hypertrophied and palpable. Where such an obstruction is suspected, it is possible to confirm the presence of valves by radiography after introduction of radio-opaque material into the bladder. Surprisingly, little or no resistance to the passage of the catheter is encountered.

In female infants, an ectopic ureter, usually arising from one portion of a duplex kidney, may open into the vagina and cause continual dribbling of urine from birth.

Ectopia vesicae

A defect in the bladder and abdominal wall results in an everted bladder (and sometimes urethra), the ureteric orifices being visible on the surface. The symphysis pubis is often lacking and the pubic rami are widely separated. The condition is compatible with a long life span, but the disability of complete incontinence is such that an attempt at surgical treatment is always worthwhile. The type of procedure and the timing of it vary in the hands of different paediatric surgeons, but reconstruction operations are seldom done until after 6 months of age. Ureteric transplants into an isolated jejunal loop may be best if reconstitution of the bladder is impractical. Meanwhile, the exposed mucous membrane of the bladder is dressed with a non-stick application or moist padding until it becomes covered with thicker epithelium and the surrounding skin protected by a water-repellent ointment.

External genitalia

Hypospadias

In this malformation, the urethra fails to extend the whole length of the penis and opens on its ventral surface at varying points or sometimes in the perineum. The further down the shaft it opens, the more severe is the deformity and the more difficult is the surgical correction. In coronal hypospadias (Fig. 13.7), the urethral opening is situated at the junction of the glans and the shaft of the penis and the prepuce covers only the dorsal surface of the glans. Anchoring of the ventral surface of the penis by a fibrous structure (chordee), which results in a curvature of the penis on erection, may necessitate surgical correction, but otherwise treatment is not essential since it is compatible with normal micturition and sexual function. Where the urethral opening is placed further down the shaft or on the perineum, immediate surgery is only necessary if the urinary stream is poor or narrow, which suggests that there is some obstruction to the flow of urine. Otherwise surgery to move the urethral meatus as near to the tip of the penis as is possible is undertaken much later, usually between the age of 3 and 5 years. In the

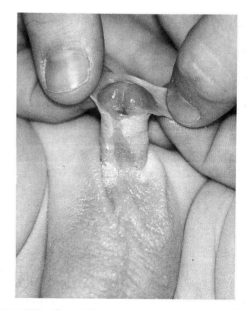

Figure 13.7   Coronal hypospadias.

most severe forms of the condition, especially where there is a bifid scrotum, the various causes of ambiguous genitalia must be borne in mind (p. 212).

Epispadias

Epispadias is much rarer than hypospadias, the urethral opening being on the dorsal surface of the penis.

Imperforate hymen

Imperforate hymen may be noticed in the newborn, attention being drawn to it by a cystic swelling between the labia minora and in the lower abdomen; this is due to the accumulation of mucus produced by the genital tract above the obstruction. It has to be distinguished clearly from a cyst of Gaertner's duct which arises from the wall of the vagina.

Adhesion of the labia minora

Adhesion of the labia minora is rarely seen at birth but is a fairly common disorder in the first 3 years; it is normally acquired rather than congenital. Separation can often be achieved after application of an oestrogen cream, and surgical separation is seldom necessary.

Ambiguous genitalia

The presence of external genitalia whose appearance is neither definitely male nor unequivocally female is distressing for both the parents of the child and the professionals involved in the delivery of the baby and results from a hormonal imbalance in early embryonic development. The strong temptation to declare the child male or female at once should be resisted as it is very important to establish the underlying cause from appropriate investigations so that the best ultimate decision about the sex of rearing can be made.

The investigations required include chromosome evaluation, ultrasound examination of the pelvic organs to demonstrate the presence of a uterus, endocrine studies of the several metabolic abnormalities known to cause this picture or even surgical exploration to identify the gonads. The main anomalies encountered are described in greatly simplified terms below.

Female pseudohermaphroditism

In this condition, the gonads are ovaries and ultrasound examination confirms the presence of a uterus in the pelvis. The external genitalia give the impression of being male with a hypertrophied clitoris, which resembles a penis, and sometimes wrinkling of the skin of the labia majora, which simulates that of a scrotum.

Smears from the buccal mucosa show that cell nuclei contain the chromatin body which indicates that there are two X chromosomes, and analysis of the chromosome complement in the white blood cells confirms the normal female pattern of 46XX. The great majority of these children have congenital adrenal hyperplasia, the clitoral hypertrophy resulting from overproduction of androgens. Occasionally a similar picture of rather lesser degree may result from administration of progesterone preparations to the mother in pregnancy. Even more rarely, the condition is found to have no hormonal basis and is of genetic origin.

Congenital adrenal hyperplasia

Congenital adrenal hyperplasia (Plate 23A) is inherited as an autosomal recessive condition so that the outwardly normal parents bear a 1 in 4 risk of having affected children. The gene mutation responsible for the condition is on chromosome 6 and can be identified in many cases by DNA analysis. It is due to the absence of an enzyme (most commonly 21-hydroxylase) concerned in the synthesis of cortisol by the adrenal gland. The lack of cortisol causes increased adrenocorticotrophic hormone (ACTH) production by the normal 'feedback' mechanism to the pituitary gland, which results in an overproduction of androgens. The condition can be diagnosed by finding a high level of 17-hydroxy progesterone in the blood. In nearly half the cases, a salt-losing adrenal crisis develops in the second or third week as a result of an accompanying lack of mineralocorticoid hormone secretion. The infant refuses feeds, fails to gain weight and vomits repeatedly, with resultant dehydration, electrolyte imbalance, hypotension and circulatory impairment. There is an elevation of the serum potassium level and usually a lowering of serum sodium. This requires immediate attention although it can be prevented if the diagnosis is suspected and the salt-losing state anticipated.

Intravenous normal saline and dextrose together with administration of fludrocortisone (0.05–0.1 mg daily) will be needed to correct the fluid and electrolyte disturbance, and hydrocortisone is also given on a long-term basis to suppress ACTH and thus reduce virilization. The dosage is about 2.5 mg twice daily, although greater amounts will be required if the baby is severely ill. Later surgical correction of the external genitalia may complete the functional cure.

Male pseudohermaphroditism

In male pseudohermaphroditism (Plate 23B), the gonads, if found, are testicles and the chromosome complement is 46XY, confirming that the child is genetically male. The external genitalia are feminized to a variable extent. The penis is hypoplastic and may resemble a clitoris, being bound down ventrally by a chordee. It usually results from either an inherited lack of sensitivity of the genitalia to the male hormone testosterone or the lack of an enzyme responsible for its production, some of which conditions are inherited in an autosomal recessive or X-linked fashion.

Full investigation of all male pseudohermaphrodite babies is essential in the first few days of life in order to establish a precise diagnosis, and therefore the prognosis, and to decide whether the infant should be reared as a boy or a girl.

True hermaphroditism

True hermaphroditism is extremely rare. Both testicular and ovarian tissue are present in the gonads and the external genitalia are variable in appearance, usually resembling one form of male pseudohermaphrodite as described above.

CENTRAL NERVOUS SYSTEM
Neural tube abnormalities

Anencephaly and spina bifida (p. 21) are examples of neural tube abnormalities. In the first weeks after fertilization, some cells form a groove along the length of the developing embryo which roll into a tube-like structure that eventually forms the fetal brain and spinal cord and its surrounding spine. A failure of complete closure of this tube is responsible for this group of disorders.

The incidence of this group of serious abnormalities has fallen substantially from the figure of approximately 4 per 1000 births, which applied in Britain some 20 years ago, to less than 0.3 per 1000 now. There are both genetic and environmental factors in the aetiology, the risk of the malformation being greatly increased when a previous child has been affected and being significantly greater in some parts of the country than in others. There used to be, for instance, twice as many anencephalic births in Wales as in East Anglia, although this difference has now substantially diminished. The incidence of live-born affected infants has fallen, partly as a result of the introduction of alpha-fetoprotein screening and ultrasound diagnosis followed by termination of affected fetuses, but it seems probable that improved maternal diet has had some effect, for the provision of preconceptional vitamin supplements with folic acid after an affected birth reduces the recurrence rate from 3.5 to 1% in a subsequent pregnancy (p. 21). A surviving affected girl who herself becomes pregnant has a 1 in 30 chance of bearing a child with a neural tube abnormality.

Anencephaly

This gross malformation, in which the forebrain is largely absent and the overlying skull and its coverings are missing, is usually identified at routine ultrasound screening and the pregnancy terminated, but if not the infant will be stillborn or will live only a few hours. Maternal polyhydramnios is often gross and may lead to suspicion of the disorder in pregnancy.

Encephalocele

Encephalocele, in which there is a large midline protrusion of brain substance through a skull defect either at the occiput or above the nose, is a severely disabling or lethal condition which is only rarely susceptible to successful surgical treatment.

Spina bifida with myelomeningocele or meningocele

A myelomeningocele (Plate 24) most commonly occurs in the lumbar region where there is a midline defect in the spine, with or without a swelling, covered only by a thin membrane of neuroepithelium and abnormal blood vessels. It contains either spinal cord or spinal nerve roots and almost always the surface oozes moisture, giving the appearance of a large ulcer. Less commonly it may be covered by true skin. Hydrocephalus of varying degree due to malformation of the cerebellum in the region of the foramen magnum (Arnold–Chiari malformation) is almost always present, although it may not always be severe enough to need immediate treatment.

The degree of disability which the child may be expected to suffer as she gets older depends upon the level and extent of the lesion and the severity of the hydrocephalus. In the majority of cases where the lumbar spine is involved, there is marked weakness or complete paralysis of the lower limbs, often with talipes deformity of the feet and congenital dislocation of the hips. With a small sacral lesion, there may be no loss of mobility, although because the nerve supply to the bladder and anal sphincter mechanism is impaired, urinary and faecal incontinence may occur. The bladder disturbance frequently leads to secondary disorders of the upper urinary tract, often with hydronephrosis and chronic urinary infection. In about 80% of cases, the hydrocephalus is associated with sufficiently raised intracranial pressure to require insertion of a ventriculoatrial or ventriculoperitoneal shunt to minimize the potential brain damage.

Follow-up studies of children with myelomeningocele have shown that the outlook for survival and the quality of life in the more severe cases after operation is so poor that many paediatricians and paediatric surgeons now recommend immediate surgical treatment in only about 25% of these infants. The selection is based upon a number of clearly demonstrable criteria, including the extent and level of the lesion, but each case must be carefully assessed in the light of all the available relevant facts. The situation requires a thorough discussion with both parents of the implications of the condition for the child and the family. This must be conducted by a paediatrician with experience and understanding to ensure that the facts are fully explained and the options made clear. In the selected cases, the myelomeningocele is repaired surgically within the first 24 hours of birth and thereafter, if hydrocephalus is present, its extent is monitored by repeated ultrasound measurements of the ventricles. Treatment of the hydrocephalus is by insertion of a shunt, using one of the variations of the Spitz–Holter valve and catheter which drains the cerebrospinal fluid from one lateral ventricle to the right atrium or into the peritoneum.

Thereafter, the treatment of these children must be a matter of well-organized teamwork by those with special experience in different fields, including neurosurgery for the hydrocephalus, orthopaedics for the hip and foot deformity, and genitourinary surgery for the later management of the bladder problems. Physiotherapists can encourage and facilitate the child's development, particularly her mobility, and advise about appropriate aids for walking or wheelchairs if needed. The social services will provide support for the family, and advice from the education authorities about special education will often be needed.

Occasionally spina bifida is accompanied by a meningocele only, the sac containing no spinal cord structures and being covered by skin, which may be considerably thinned. Hydrocephalus is much less common in these children and there are usually no neurological complications, so the outlook for normal mobility and cerebral function after operation is good.

Spinal dysraphism

In spinal dysraphism, the cord in the lumbar region is divided by a cartilaginous spur which gives rise to dysfunction of the nerves to the bladder and lower limbs in later childhood. Its presence should be suspected whenever there is a small midline defect of skin or a sinus above the sacrococcygeal region, especially when associated with a tuft of fine hair.

Congenital hydrocephalus

The great majority of cases of congenital hydrocephalus are associated with spina bifida and myelomeningocele.

Isolated hydrocephalus is most commonly due to obstruction of the cerebrospinal fluid pathways by adhesions somewhere in the subarachnoid space. More rarely it is due to a malformation of the ventricular system such as aqueduct stenosis, in which the narrowed channel between the third and fourth ventricles obstructs the flow of cerebrospinal fluid, or an intracranial cyst. Intracranial haemorrhage, particularly in pre-term infants, is another important cause and intrauterine infection with toxoplasmosis accounts for a few cases. In a small number of cases, it is familial and is inherited as an X-linked disorder (p. 192). Increasingly early detection by antenatal ultrasound may lead to termination of pregnancy in severe cases, so the incidence in liveborn infants is falling.

Undiagnosed isolated hydrocephalus is a rare cause of disproportion, giving rise to difficulties in labour. After birth it rarely causes immediate clinical disturbance in the baby, although exceptionally some drowsiness or vomiting may occur. Usually the enlarging head draws attention to the diagnosis and is confirmed by serial measurements of head circumference. An increase of more than 2.5 cm in the first 2 weeks justifies further investigation by ultrasound examination.

Clinical examination shows that the anterior fontanelle is wide and usually tense, with some separation of the sutures. (The normal size is extremely variable and a large fontanelle is by no means diagnostic.) As the pressure rises, the eyes are down-turned so that only the upper halves of the cornea can be seen (the 'setting sun' sign) and the scalp veins are dilated. The amount of neurological disturbance that results depends upon the cause of the hydrocephalus and the degree and duration of the raised intracranial pressure, but cerebral function is maintained surprisingly normally in some cases and treatment of advanced hydrocephalus can be compatible with normal intelligence. However, when the ventricular dilatation is identified in utero or occurs as a consequence of intraventricular haemorrhage, the prognosis is usually poor with severe developmental delay.

About 40% of cases progress for a time and then arrest spontaneously. Full investigation by ultrasound (Fig. 13.8) or CT scanning is necessary if early arrest does not take place, and surgical treatment with some form of bypass valve of the Spitz–Holter type is nearly always possible.

Hydranencephaly

In hydranencephaly the skull is intact and often of normal shape and size, but there is absence of most of the cerebral hemispheres, the space being filled by cerebrospinal fluid. Initially the condition may be hard to diagnose because the baby sucks without difficulty and abnormal neurological signs are not at first obvious. Transillumination of the head using a very bright light in a dark room is a simple and useful means of investigation for this at the bedside, but scanning by ultrasound is replacing it as it is now becoming a ward procedure.

Other abnormalities of head size and shape

Congenital microcephaly

The skull, particularly the frontal region, is small and the rest of the facial development relatively normal, producing a characteristic appearance. The outcome is severe learning difficulties. One

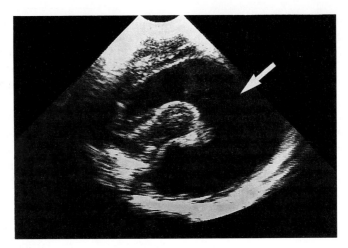

Figure 13.8 Cerebral ultrasound scan showing greatly dilated lateral ventricles (arrowed) in congenital hydrocephalus.

form of the disorder is inherited as an autosomal recessive characteristic occurring only in homozygotes (p. 194), but there are other causes, including intrauterine cytomegalovirus infection.

Craniosynostosis

Microcephaly must be distinguished clearly from the various forms of craniosynostosis in which early union of the cranial sutures forms a skull of reduced capacity and of deformed shape. For example, in turricephaly a tall narrow head results from fusion of the coronal sutures and in scaphocephaly a boat-shaped head with a prominent occiput is caused by closure of the saggital suture. In both these situations, the restriction of space interferes with brain growth and may cause increasing intracranial pressure, resulting in fits, learning difficulties and reduced sight from optic atrophy. Microcephaly and craniosynostosis can usually be differentiated on clinical findings, but X-rays of the skull are necessary for confirmation. If craniosynostosis is confirmed, early surgical excision of the fused sutures is required to allow more normal skull and brain growth.

EYES
Abnormalities of size

In the course of the neonatal examination the size of the eyes as well as other possible abnormalities should be noticed.

Microphthalmia

The abnormally small eye (microphthalmia), apart from being a feature of congenital toxoplasmosis, the rubella syndrome and cytomegalovirus infection, may occur as an isolated congenital defect or may be associated with colobomata and possibly with cerebral agenesis. No treatment is available and sight in the affected eye is usually very limited.

Macrophthalmia

More important from the point of view of early diagnosis is the abnormally large eye which may be due to congenital glaucoma (buphthalmos), in which case cloudiness of the cornea soon develops as the pressure of the fluid in the anterior chamber of the eye rises. The condition should be referred urgently to an ophthalmologist since the only hope of preserving vision lies in early surgical reduction of intraocular pressure.

Congenital cataracts

These are best seen when the eyes are examined with a light shining obliquely across them.

Although usually the sole abnormality and often hereditary, they may also point to the diagnosis of other disorders. These include the rubella syndrome, congenital toxoplasmosis, Down's syndrome, Lowe's oculorenal syndrome, congenital ectodermal dysplasia, and punctate epiphyseal dysplasia. They may develop later in congenital galactosaemia and neonatal hypocalcaemia.

Treatment is never urgent but early detection and referral to the ophthalmologist is advisable since early surgery can restore at least some vision and prevent a permanent amblyopia from developing.

LIMBS AND JOINTS
Congenital dislocation of the hip

Since early recognition and treatment of this condition from the newborn period is largely effective in preventing future disability from established dislocation, it is given special attention in the routine clinical examination and the manoeuvres for its detection are fully described on page 63.

Genetic factors must play a part in its causation since it is commoner in girls than in boys and in close relatives of affected children. Environmental factors are also involved since it is more common where the baby is of above average birth weight or, curiously, has suffered fetal growth retardation, and where there has been oligohydramnios, breech presentation or delivery by caesarean section. However, in 40% of cases, no predisposing factors are found. The incidence is variable in different parts of the world, but in Britain it is approximately 1–1.5 per 1000 births. Many more than this are found to have an unstable, but not actually dislocated, hip when examined within the first 2 days of life, the number varying from 3 to 20 per 1000 births according to the way in which the routine examination is carried out and interpreted. The shape of the acetabulum and the degree of instability of the joint can easily be demonstrated by ultrasound imaging (Fig. 13.9) and this should always be performed if instability is suspected. Among these unstable hips are some that would become

firmly dislocated if not treated, but some of them stabilize spontaneously leaving a normal hip joint without treatment within a week or so. There is therefore some difference of opinion about the correct approach to treatment by abduction splintage.

The unstable hip which can be easily relocated by gentle abduction should be kept in at least partial abduction and flexion by an abduction splint until it has stabilized. The hip which is in place at rest but can be displaced by testing may be treated in the same way, but it is equally reasonable to wait and review the hip with ultrasound evaluation to see whether it becomes stable within a few weeks.

If on first testing the hip shows limitation of abduction, suggesting that the joint is actually dislocated, no force should be used and abduction splinting should not be undertaken in view of the risk of damage to the femoral head. Treatment should be in the hands of an orthopaedic surgeon with neonatal experience, because early open surgical reduction or adductor tenotomy may in some cases be necessary.

Splintage

There are several accepted ways of keeping the hip joints in the flexed and abducted position. The von Rosen or Malmo splint is commonly used. It consists of a padded frame, the malleable metal arms of which bend to the position required for fixing the hips in relation to the trunk. It has the disadvantage of sometimes causing discomfort at first, which is also reflected in the baby's mother, who may feel that it impairs normal closeness and her confidence in handling her.

The 'Aberdeen' splint is simply a rigid cover for the napkin, the padded edges of which keep the thighs apart when it is strapped in place. It is less disturbing for both infant and mother but its weakness lies in the fact that it has to be taken off and reapplied each time the nappy is changed, which requires some practice to ensure that it is effective. The Pavlik harness (Fig. 13.10) is a more complicated device but has the advantage

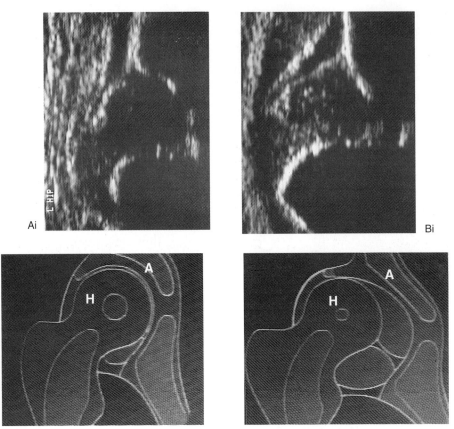

Figure 13.9 Ultrasound scans of the neonatal hip. A: The normal appearances. B: Lateral and upward displacement of the head of the femur in an infant with congenital dislocation of the hip. On the right, the diagrams show the relationship between the head of the femur (H) and the acetabulum (A). (By kind permission of Dr Sally Scott.)

of allowing the baby a little more freedom to move.

Whatever method is used, the apparatus must be put on very gently by someone experienced in its use, and the baby's progress must be followed carefully until she is walking satisfactorily. X-rays in the first month give limited information since the femoral head only becomes visible at around 4–6 months of age, but they are most helpful thereafter.

Ultrasound

Ultrasound examination of the hip joint shows its structure accurately in the first few weeks of life and can be used to follow its maturation for 6 months or more in babies with clinically unstable

hips to identify those hips which are likely to dislocate later or benefit from early surgery. Although it is used as a means of screening for the condition in some parts of Europe, it has not yet replaced the clinical indentification of the unstable hip in most areas of Britain.

Talipes equinovarus and calcaneovalgus

These deformities are partly genetic in origin and partly the result of malposition or abnormal pressures in utero. Certainly the baby can usually be 'folded' easily into the abnormal position which she occupied within the uterus, and reduction of the amount of amniotic fluid is commonly associated. The condition can be diag-

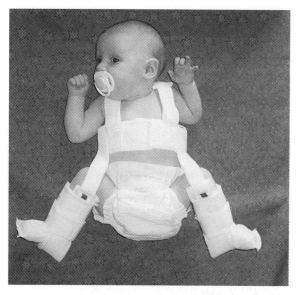

Figure 13.10   Infant fitted with a Pavlik harness to treat her unstable hips.

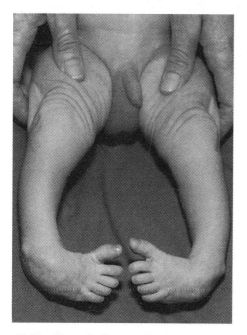

Figure 13.11   Bilateral talipes equinovarus.

nosed before birth in some cases by ultrasound scanning which shows the abnormal posture of the feet (Fig. 2.2).

Talipes equinovarus

The deformity (Fig. 13.11) consists of plantar-flexion at the ankle with varus deformity at the subtaloid joint and adduction of the forefoot producing an inward curve of the metatarsus. There is some degree of rigidity of the foot in this position and the deformity cannot be immediately corrected passively, thus distinguishing it from the temporary exaggerated postural inversion of the feet which is so common and which corrects itself.

Treatment should be started if possible in the first few days of life. The deformity is partially corrected by stretching and is then held in position either by the use of felt and adhesive strapping or by a splint. Frequent repetition of the procedure is necessary until overcorrection is achieved and the treatment must be followed up carefully until growth of the feet is complete. Occasionally an early operation to release the tight medial foot ligaments may be required and later lengthening of the Achilles tendon in severe cases. Night splints are worn to maintain a good foot posture until the child is about 3 years old and good foot function is usually obtained.

Talipes calcaneovalgus

Talipes calcaneovalgus is the opposite deformity, with the foot in extreme dorsiflexion and metatarsus valgus, so that the fifth toe approximates towards the outer border of the lower leg. There are all degrees of this deformity and in most cases the foot can easily be replaced passively into the normal position and no treatment is necessary. The more severe cases with much valgus deformity require firm manipulation of the foot towards the normal position and probably splints or strapping. It is worth noting that congenital dislocation of the hip is significantly more common in association with this type of talipes.

Scoliosis

This is infrequently recognized at birth unless it is due to structural abnormalities of the vertebrae when a relatively sharp angulation is present.

Infantile idiopathic scoliosis may, however, have its origin in intrauterine malposition, and if a lateral curve or an asymmetrical 'incurvation response' is noted at routine examination, the baby should certainly be examined again later. Most straighten spontaneously as the baby grows, but there may be a case for early postural treatment in selected instances.

Many other skeletal deformities, types of chondrodystrophy and soft tissue malformation are clearly recognizable in the newborn period. Major paediatric or orthopaedic textbooks describe them in full and they are not included here because of their individual rarity and because early recognition is not important for effective treatment.

LYMPHATIC SYSTEM

Lymphangiomas most commonly occur as cystic hygromas – soft multilocular cysts in the region of the neck or axilla. They are less common in other sites but may be associated with haemangiomas. The feasibility of surgical excision depends upon the extent and site of the lesion.

CONGENITAL ANOMALIES LEADING TO FAILURE OF NORMAL MENTAL DEVELOPMENT

Microcephaly

This abnormality has been discussed earlier in this chapter (p. 215).

Down's syndrome (trisomy 21)

Occurring as often as once in every 600 births, Down's syndrome is recognizable at or shortly after birth in nearly every case. It is due to the possession of extra chromosome material, either as a separate additional 21 chromosome (Fig. 13.12) or as a translocation of extra chromosome 21 material onto another chromosome. The incidence of the condition in different age groups and the ways in which it may be diagnosed antenatally so that termination of pregnancy becomes possible are fully discussed on page 19.

Recognition

Down's syndrome is usually recognized most

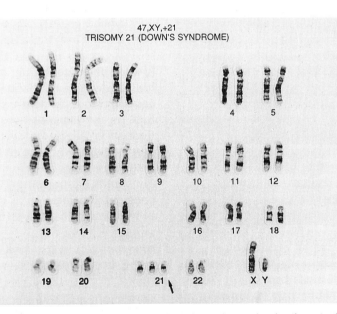

Figure 13.12 Chromosome pattern in Down's syndrome showing the extra 21 chromosome. (By kind permission of Prof. P. Jacobs.)

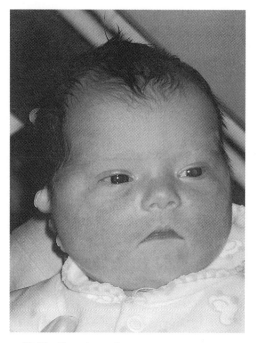

Figure 13.13 Down's syndrome.

easily from a general impression of the infant rather than by consciously taking note of the separate features (Fig. 13.13). Many abnormalities make up this clinical impression. The baby is often small. There is a general muscular hypotonia and laxity of joints. The head is rounded and relatively short from front to back. An extra fontanelle may be present in the sagittal suture line just above the posterior fontanelle. The features of the face are grouped more closely than normal and are in themselves generally smaller. The eyes show an oblique slant of the palpebral fissure outwards and upwards. The mouth is often turned downwards at the corners and the tongue frequently protrudes. The ears are small and simply formed. Small white flecks (Brushfield's spots) may be seen in a ring around the iris. The hands are short and wide, with stubby fingers, an incurved little finger and often a single transverse palmar crease. A congenital heart anomaly is present in nearly half of cases, although often it is not possible to recognize it on initial clinical examination. Cataracts, duodenal atresia and Hirschsprung's disease are also rela-

tively common. One of the most constant features is the abnormal pattern of dermal ridge (fingerprint markings) on the palms, but they are not easy to see on the small hand of the newborn child.

The diagnosis having been made, the parents must be informed. This difficult task ought only to be undertaken by a doctor who fully understands the effect it may have and who knows how to answer the many questions that will inevitably be put to her about the future. The subject is discussed in more detail in Chapter 14.

Other chromosome anomalies

'Fragile X' chromosomes

Recently the chromosomes of moderately mentally handicapped children have been examined and a number found to have fragments which appear to break off the end of the X chromosomes during chromosome culture in a folate-deficient medium. This appears to be a not uncommon finding and is associated with a number of physical features such as a long face and prominent jaw, large ears and a normal head circumference. After puberty, the testes are often unusually large. It is inherited as an X-linked condition, thus often affecting other male members of the family, and some 30% of the carrier mothers have some degree of learning difficulty. The location of the gene on the X chromosome has been identified by DNA analysis and this can now be used to confirm the diagnosis in the fetus or in the child after birth.

Other syndromes associated with chromosome anomalies are comparatively rare.

Trisomy 18

In trisomy 18, or Edward's syndrome, the multiple abnormalities include low-set ears, overlapping ulnar-deviated fingers, 'rocker' feet and congenital heart anomalies.

Trisomy 13

Trisomy 13 (Patau's syndrome) includes cleft

palate, brain defects, microphthalmia, absent testes and renal abnormalities.

Both these syndromes are almost always incompatible with survival.

Cri du chat

In the cri du chat syndrome there is deletion of part of chromosome 5. The mewing sound on crying gives rise to the name and the infant will usually be mentally handicapped.

Turner's syndrome

In this anomaly, one X chromosome is missing (chromosomes are 45 XO) and is associated with absence of the ovaries which results in infertility in adult life. The abnormal chromosome pattern may be found incidentally during the pregnancy whilst screening the fetal cells for other anomalies such as Down's syndrome. The disorder may be recognizable in the newborn by the presence of persistent oedema of the lower limbs or webbing of the neck, although most girls with the condition have no dysmorphic features and cannot be identified clinically on neonatal examination. Coarctation of the aorta is a common accompaniment. These girls often fail to thrive in infancy and grow slowly throughout childhood, ending up as short adults. The importance of early diagnosis rests in the hope of increased growth which may be achieved through giving low-dose oestrogen and growth hormone supplementation during childhood, but it is too early to know what increase in adult height can be achieved.

The dysmorphic syndromes

Many infants with chromosome anomalies will be noticed initially because of unusual physical features. Others with dysmorphic characteristics have normal chromosomes but may, because of the recognizable association of clinical features, be given a diagnosis as a specific named syndrome, although in some cases no diagnosis can be reached (Fig. 13.14). All of them are rare, but

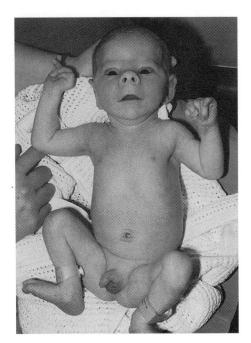

Figure 13.14 Dysmorphic facies, unusual posture of the fingers and bilateral undescended testes in a newborn baby. No diagnosis was reached in this case.

features which should suggest such a syndrome include:

- an odd facial appearance
- abnormalities of the limbs, particularly shortening
- malformations of the hands and digits
- abnormal genitalia
- unusual head shape
- abnormal position or structure of the eyes.

Since many of these babies will later become mentally handicapped and some are familial, the advice of a clinical geneticist should be sought if a syndrome cannot be easily diagnosed.

Congenital hypothyroidism

In about one baby in 3000, the thyroid gland fails to develop or is ectopic and produces inadequate amounts of thyroxine. The clinical signs of established hypothyroidism are only exceptionally recognizable in the newborn and usually only become apparent in the second or third month. Neonatal screening for the condition using estimation of thyroid-stimulating hormone (TSH) is now universal in Britain, making much earlier diagnosis possible and improving the prognosis for mental development (p. 68).

Without screening tests, hypothyroidism may be recognized in at least 50% of cases in the first 2 weeks if the physical signs are known, although at this stage they are often subtle. These are sluggish movements, slowness to cry, dryness of the skin, subnormal temperature and unexplained persistent mild jaundice. If X-ray of the long bones of the leg shows absence of the lower femoral epiphysis and the infant is not preterm, the diagnosis may be strongly suspected. Primary hypothyroidism may then be confirmed by finding a low serum thyroxine level with a high value of thyroid-stimulating hormone.

Treatment should start immediately the diagnosis is confirmed, with thyroxine 0.025 mg daily, subsequently increasing the dose as the child grows.

Hypothyroidism associated with congenital goitre is more easily recognizable at this age but is very rare. Endemic hypothyroidism from iodine deficiency is not a problem in Britain but families in which goitrous hypothyroidism occurs are described. More commonly, goitre in the newborn infant is due to drugs used in therapy for maternal thyrotoxicosis in pregnancy or to the administration of iodine. The signs of hypothyroidism do not always accompany the goitre, which gradually diminishes in size, but occasionally thyroxine administration is necessary in the first few weeks.

INBORN ERRORS OF METABOLISM

Biochemical techniques have brought to light a large number of different metabolic errors which are associated with impaired mental and physical development in childhood. Some are recognizable by means of screening tests in the neonatal period, but they are all rare and a few have been shown with certainty to be treatable by selective dietary restriction from the beginning, making early diagnosis essential (p. 67).

Galactosaemia

Galactosaemia is one condition in which treatment can be effective. Lack of an enzyme (galactose-l-phosphate uridyl-transferase) results in a failure of conversion of galactose to glucose and thus galactose accumulates, which results in damage to the liver and brain. Since the disease is inherited as a recessive condition, the parents are themselves unaffected clinically but the risk to each subsequent child is 1 in 4. Although rare, the condition should be suspected in any newborn infant who vomits, refuses feeds, fails to thrive and becomes jaundiced in the first week without any cause. Cataracts may be seen at an early stage. The diagnosis can be suspected if a reducing substance is identified in the urine using the Clinitest tablet method. A further test with Clinistix strips (which identify only glucose by the glucose oxidase method) confirms that the substance is not glucose, and specific laboratory testing identifies it as galactose. The diagnosis is confirmed by direct measurement of the red cell transferase enzyme content which is greatly reduced. Since galactose forms half of the disaccharide lactose, which is the sugar found in breast and most formula milks, treatment must be immediately started by withdrawing these completely and substituting a special low-lactose milk preparation, since if it is delayed, severe liver damage and learning difficulties may follow.

Phenylketonuria

Although occurring only once in 10 000–15 000 births, early recognition and treatment of the condition are essential if severe learning difficulties are to be prevented. It is inherited as a recessive characteristic, both parents are heterozygous carriers of the gene and each subsequent child has a 1 in 4 risk of having the disorder.

Congenital deficiency of the liver enzyme phenylalanine hydroxylase prevents the conversion of phenylalanine to tyrosine and increased amounts of phenylalanine accumulate in the blood and tissues while phenylpyruvic acid appears in the urine. The persistent high blood levels of phenylalanine in untreated cases are responsible for the progressive cerebral dysfunction and severe learning difficulties.

The diagnosis is suspected from the routine screening heel prick blood test as described on page 68. If positive, it must be urgently confirmed by more detailed biochemical investigation and a significantly high phenylalanine value found (above 725 μmol/L or 12 mg/100 ml) before starting dietary treatment using one of the low phenylalanine milk substitutes with the necessary vitamin and mineral supplements.

Regular blood phenylalanine checks are essential and the diet is subsequently regulated to maintain it near the minimal level required for normal growth and metabolism (120–240 μmol/L or 2–4 mg/100 ml) by means of calculated protein additions. Normal intellectual development can thus be achieved and no major deterioration results from relaxing the dietary restriction after 8–12 years of age. A woman with this disorder who wishes to become pregnant must, however, revert to a strict low phenylalanine diet before conception in order to reduce the risk of severe damage to the developing brain of her fetus (p. 26).

Other inborn errors of metabolism

There are many other recessively inherited conditions caused by a specific enzyme deficiency whose gene locations have been identified very recently, thus offering the chance of early prenatal diagnosis of the condition in an at-risk fetus by DNA analysis. In the majority of such conditions, there are no distinguishing features in the neonatal period to point to such a diagnosis. However, a very small number, including, for example, medium chain acyl coenzyme-A dehydrogenase deficiency (MCAD), may present in the early weeks of life with a serious metabolic disturbance, including acidosis, cerebral symptoms or even sudden unexpected death. It is clearly important to identify accurately which disorder is causing the problem as early as possible, since it is only feasible to test for it in a subsequent pregnancy if the enzyme defect has been characterized. In most cases an examination of the urine for amino acids and organic acids will identify the offending disease but more extensive discussion of the subject is beyond the scope of this book.

FURTHER READING

Baraitser M, Winter R 1996 Colour atlas of congenital malformations. Mosby Wolfe, UK

Boue A (ed) 1995 Fetal medicine – prenatal diagnosis and management. Oxford University Press, Oxford

Burns J 1994 Birth defects and their causes. Stress Books, Galway

Emery A E H, Rimoin D L 1990 Principles and practice of medical genetics. Churchill Livingstone, Edinburgh

Freeman N V, Burge D M, Griffiths M, Malone P (eds) 1994 Surgery of the newborn. Churchill Livingstone, Edinburgh

Hanna E J, Nevin N C, Nelson J 1994 Genetic study of congenital heart defects in Northern Ireland 1974–8. Journal of Medical Genetics 31: 858–863

Knox E, Lancashire R 1991 Epidemiology of congenital malformations. HMSO, London

Levene M, Liford R (eds) 1995 Fetal and neonatal neurology and neurosurgery. Churchill Livingstone, Edinburgh

Lloyd D A (ed) 1996 Seminars in neonatology: neonatal surgery. W B Saunders, London

Morrisey R 1990 Paediatric orthopaedics, 3rd edn. Lippincott, Philadelphia

Roberton N R C (ed) 1992 Textbook of neonatology. Churchill Livingstone, Edinburgh

Stevenson R E, Hall J G, Goodman R M 1995. Human malformations and related anomalies. Oxford University Press, Oxford

Weatherall D J 1991 New genetics and clinical practice. Oxford University Press, Oxford

Wiedemann H, Kunz J, Dibbern H 1992 An atlas of clinical syndromes. Wolfe, London

Young I D, Plaha D S 1992 The new genetics and its implications. In: David T J (ed) Recent advances in paediatrics 10. Churchill Livingstone, Edinburgh, ch 12

Yu V Y H (ed) 1995 Clinical paediatrics: pulmonary problems in the perinatal period and their sequelae. Baillière Tindall, London

14

Helping the parents

The birth of a healthy and contented infant who feeds and sleeps well is a fulfilling experience for both parents, especially if this has been achieved with the minimum of professional assistance. Preparation for parenthood classes are a most valuable training for the birth and care of the infant, but the reality of having a real baby to nurture is not always as smooth as anticipated. The emotions of the delivery, the blues in the first few days and the demands from the infant all affect the parents' confidence, and if they have had little prior experience of baby care they have to learn quickly how to understand, anticipate and respond to the baby's needs. No two babies are alike, yet the majority of newborns slip easily into a regular pattern of activity, feeding and sleep and present few problems to new parents. However, if the baby does not conform to the expected pattern of behaviour, anxiety easily arises. Successful breast feeding, for instance, does not necessarily come naturally to a new mother nor is it easily achieved. The baby may have an irregular sleep pattern or may simply be unsettled and such features can result in one or both parents becoming very tired. In such instances, understanding and informed nursing support are invaluable.

As many as one baby in 12 will require medical attention for a problem of some sort in the first few weeks. In such cases, the added anxiety will greatly affect the parents' confidence in the future and this will need considerable understanding from all medical and nursing staff concerned. It is essential that, as well as having knowledge of the conditions affecting the newborn infant, those caring for the family must be aware of their likely emotional reactions when faced with caring for an unhealthy or malformed child and know how best to support them. They should also know about the services available to assist in providing care and support to the family on their return home.

PREPARATION FOR THE BIRTH OF THE BABY

During the pregnancy, the information given in the 'education for parenthood' classes will concentrate largely on the care of the healthy baby. This will cover such aspects of care as breast (or artificial) feeding, the variation of feeding patterns from one baby to another, the different sleep rhythms which may be experienced, the normal pattern of weight gain and some information on how the baby will develop. The programme of care in the community for healthy infants from the midwife, health visitor and family doctor should also be described, together with the schedule of immunizations against infectious diseases in infancy which the baby should receive.

The best medical support that can be given to parents during a pregnancy is to assure them that all is well with mother and fetus. However, it is also important to identify any increased risk to the infant before birth so that plans for the future can be made. A past history of many miscarriages, a stillbirth or neonatal death, a malformed infant or a family history suggesting a genetic disorder may increase the parents' anxieties about their anticipated infant and it is wise to notify the paediatric team of such situations so that they can be prepared for it. In many areas, a special programme of support is introduced in the antenatal period to parents who have previously lost a baby from the sudden infant death syndrome. This provides a package of care for the baby after birth involving frequent assessment of his progress by the health visitor, weekly plotting of the infant's weight on special charts designed to identify those babies whose weight is suboptimal, accelerated access to medical or paediatric examination when needed and the provision of an apnoea alarm or weighing scales for use at home. After the baby's birth, the parents are also taught how to resuscitate him should he be found to be seriously ill.

If a congenital abnormality is found on prenatal examination (p. 19) of the baby, it is often appropriate to involve a paediatric specialist to discuss its significance and to describe any treatment which may be available. Since about 8% of all infants born have some condition needing paediatric attention and may need admission to the neonatal unit, a case can be made for discussing this possibility with the parents during the antenatal period. However, those advising the parents must also take into account how much anxiety this might create for them and judge accordingly what to tell them and when. It must be remembered that, because of religious or cultural beliefs, prenatal intervention may not be acceptable to some parents and such views must colour the discussion about the management of the baby's condition. On the whole, it is best to tell the couple something of the range of possibilities since they are then less likely to be shocked if mother and baby do have to be separated at birth.

The antenatal period also affords the opportunity to identify any social problems or disadvantages which might affect the mother's ability to cope with the baby after delivery. These may include lone parenthood, housing problems, social isolation, unemployment, language difficulties and poverty. Parental physical or psychiatric illness or the presence in the family of other children with illness or disability may affect parenting ability. In a small number of cases there may be more serious social concern, such as another child in the family whose name is on the child protection register for child abuse or a person in the home who has a conviction for offences against children. In such circumstances, social services, or occasionally legal, action may be required during the pregnancy to protect the baby after birth. Support from the social worker may be needed in such cases and this will become more important if the baby is found to have medical problems after birth.

There may also be cultural matters about

which those caring for the mother and baby should know. Such things as dietary taboos, religious customs, mothers who find it unacceptable to be examined by a male doctor and which family member will make the decisions about the care of the baby may be of great importance, particularly for a family from a minority group in society. Religious circumcision requirements may also need to be discussed. Blood transfusion may be unacceptable to some groups. Each of these should be discussed, and an acceptable way found of accommodating the parents' requirements.

THE ILL OR ABNORMAL INFANT

It is when a sick, malformed or immature infant is born that the greatest understanding of the emotional and psychological needs of the parents is required. They will experience emotions which have features in common with the grief reaction following bereavement, and each parent will react individually, influenced by their beliefs, their past experiences and how responsible they feel for what has happened.

Parental reaction to the birth of a sick or malformed infant

The parents' initial reaction on realizing or being told that their baby is malformed, handicapped or ill is one of shock, emotional disorganization and confusion. Soon afterwards, these feelings may turn into a period of denial in which they cannot believe the facts they have heard and they may even become hostile to the paediatrician who gave them the news. Feelings of rejection and even malice towards the child may follow, sometimes subsequently being replaced by feelings of guilt at having such thoughts. Each parent may react in different ways at different times and in varying order, and they may become bewildered in their attempts to support each other.

Such questions as 'why did it happen?'; 'why did it happen to our baby?'; 'did we do something wrong?'; or 'did we fail to do something we should have?'; 'could it have been caused by . . .?'

are all common and indicate that the parents are experiencing a feeling of guilt that they are in some way at fault for having a baby who is not perfect. This may be particularly poignant in cultures which believe malformations to be an act of God. 'There is nothing like this on my side of the family' is another frequent statement in which a parent tries to absolve him or herself from responsibility for the baby's condition. This fear of 'blame' becomes particularly acute when the baby's condition has a genetic origin. When it is X-linked, the fact that the condition is passed to a male child by an asymptomatic mother who carries the abnormal gene can cause particularly acute tension.

Gradually, as the condition of the infant becomes clearer or the diagnosis is confirmed, the parents' reactions may become less acute and other, more considered reactions emerge. These also vary enormously, ranging from complete acceptance of the situation, through resignation to their plight and denial that anything is wrong, to outright rejection of the child. Many parents find solace and help in adapting to their unexpected situation by joining with other parents in self-help groups and fundraising organizations for the condition concerned, supporting the professionals already involved or learning about the condition so that they can themselves counsel others who find themselves in the same position. Health professionals should be aware of these groups and of how to obtain addresses, books and other information should it be needed. Such groups are now catalogued and their details are available in most paediatric departments.

Breaking the bad news

The way in which the parents are first told that their baby has a serious abnormality has an important bearing upon how they come to terms with it. It is essential that they should be given every possible help to accept the child, and that trust in those responsible for the medical care should be firmly established from the beginning.

The timing must depend on circumstances but, if the abnormality is obvious at birth, the first explanation of what the parents can expect is best given as soon as the condition has been clinically assessed. Even when a full diagnosis cannot be made without further investigation, a preliminary discussion at the earliest possible time is necessary. If the birth is in hospital, all staff should be aware of who is to take on this responsibility and should themselves avoid impulsive, well-intentioned but often misleading advice or reassurance based upon their own feelings rather than on sound knowledge of all the circumstances. The parents may have to take difficult decisions about their child and it is important that whoever gives them guidance must be thoroughly informed about the family so that they can feel comfortable about those decisions.

The explanation should in general be given by a senior paediatrician, preferably by the one who will be responsible for the baby's ongoing care, and certainly by one who understands the background culture of the family. If the first language of the clinician is not that of the parents, a skilled interpreter with some understanding of the medical problems and insight into the religious, cultural and family issues is invaluable. It is wise to arrange to see both parents together to hear the news and to provide support for each other. It is often helpful to explain the situation while the mother is holding the baby in her arms. Sometimes it may be thought best just to sow the seeds of doubt in the parents' minds, but there is seldom justification for withholding the truth in so far as it is known, for parents are very perceptive and will often deduce from the actions and manner of the care givers that they are worried about the infant. It is not enough simply to restrict the explanation to answering questions from the parents – the most important ones are often not asked. The parents may have recognized the problem for themselves when, for instance, the infant has Down's syndrome, and in these circumstances it is best to confirm their suspicions and begin to explain the significance of the abnormality at once.

If the concern about the infant is that he will have significant learning difficulties as a result of a serious cerebral insult or a complication occurring during intensive care in a pre-term infant, the same principles apply. Giving both parents together an honest appraisal of the situation, including its uncertainties, is almost always the best policy in the long term. Great patience, an unhurried approach and a real concern for the family are some of the qualities that help to establish trust, and opportunities must be found at agreed dates for further interviews to expand upon aspects which may not previously have been dealt with. Often the parents will take in only a small amount of what is said and they are frequently confused about the significance of the abnormality. It may be necessary to repeat almost everything at subsequent interviews. There should also be close liaison with those asked to give support, including the family doctor and health visitor, and some agreement should be reached about who should be the person to whom the family turns first for advice when they are uncertain about the infant's care.

Bringing up a child with a handicap, whatever its nature, is a difficult task and it can be most helpful for parents to meet at an early stage the therapists and social workers available to treat the child and support the family. They can then introduce them to the local and national voluntary organizations from which they can obtain additional help. Although the best place for any baby is at home with the natural parents, there are occasions when they cannot provide the necessary care for the child, in which case the paediatric social worker will help in advising about the financial benefits available and assist the family in discussing the available alternatives to care at home should this become necessary.

Counselling the distraught parent

Although doctors, nurses and midwives have their own skills in understanding and counselling people in distress, there are some attitudes which are known to be helpful and others which can be destructive. The empathic person is one who can feel for the parents and get alongside them in their distress, and it is this type of care giver who will be most supportive to them. Such a person will respect the parents' feelings and help them to understand that their emotions are natural and acceptable, however uncomfortable for others. They will share in the parents' sorrow and encourage them to know that they will grow through the experience, that they do have the strength to cope and will have the support they need to enable them to do so. They will also allow the parents the space and time they need and will respect those times when they need privacy. By contrast, additional burdens can be placed on the parents by a person who fails to get alongside them, being obviously in a hurry, offering quick and slick solutions rather than listening to what they are really saying, or worst of all implying disapproval and giving the impression that the parents are behaving unreasonably.

DYING BABIES

Approximately eight babies in every 1000 are stillborn or die in the first month of life in the UK despite the best available attention, but in places where experienced antenatal and neonatal care is not well developed, the rate is much higher. Thus, the death of a newborn infant is not an uncommon event and every midwife, neonatal nurse and doctor caring for newborn infants should know how to care well for the dying baby and help the parents.

The types of condition which result in the death of a newborn baby nowadays are discussed in Chapter 1, but many of them relate to incomplete antenatal care, premature birth, maternal illness associated with the pregnancy or unexpected malformation of the baby. In some cases, such as stillbirth or overwhelming sepsis, death may be sudden and unexpected but in the rest it is possible to anticipate at least briefly that the baby's life is ending, though there is often little time for the parents to prepare themselves for the event. Whatever the cause, it must be remembered that, however small and immature, every dying baby deserves all the dignity and respect which is afforded to a grown child. Many dying neonates will be undergoing some form of intensive care with all its associated equipment but this should not blind the care givers to the human needs of both the baby and the parents. It is often possible to involve the parents in their baby's physical care, however intensive it is, and if it is clear that the baby is dying, their contribution can be increased if they so wish. They should also be encouraged to express their wishes about the care to be given and the religious or cultural customs they wish to be observed, and those caring for the baby should adapt the treatment to accommodate them appropriately. It can be helpful to parents if some of the carers are involved in such ceremonies to demonstrate that they too share in the family's feelings.

Although it is entirely proper to strive to maintain the life of an infant, a time may come when it is more important for the parents to have and hold their baby without the apparatus and accompaniments of intensive care, so that his last moments may be peaceful and the parents' later recollections more personal. If this can occur in a private place away from clinical activity, it gives a greater opportunity for the parents' grief to be expressed more naturally. Sometimes the presence of medical, nursing or other staff is helpful in this process, but all carers should be sensitive to the wishes and feelings of the family and as far as possible they should be allowed to choose those they wish to support them at that time. The parents often value a photograph of themselves with the baby, even one taken after he has died.

Helping parents after a perinatal death

The support of parents after the death of their newborn baby is complex and requires particular understanding and empathy. They will require comfort in their initial sorrow, advice about arranging the funeral and information on how to register both the birth and the death of their infant. Each person who has provided care to the mother during the pregnancy should be informed of the baby's death. All available information relating to the cause of the death must be sought and collated, so that later on the family can be given the opportunity to discuss it with the paediatrician in order to help them understand more fully what happened and why.

Whatever the cause of death, the parents will

be deeply affected by their loss after the great hopes and expectation raised during the pregnancy. The grief of such a loss afffects people in different ways and at different rates. Sometimes this can confuse a couple who are at different stages of the process and can lead to additional tension between them. Simply explaining to such parents that this is a natural and normal situation can often be very supportive. The emotional reactions experienced during the initial grieving include bitterness, anger, helplessness, fear, disbelief and sometimes a guilt that they may have contributed to the death of the baby. If the parents' anger is turned towards one or more of the carers, perhaps focused on a decision made or a perceived delay in an action being taken, it can be hurtful to the person concerned but it is not helpful to the family to discuss the substance of the complaint at this stage. It is also out of place to offer casual words of sympathy to the parents or a hollow reassurance that they will be able to have a replacement for the dead infant. The opportunity must be found for an unhurried listening to the parents' natural desire to unburden their sorrow and their concerns about the circumstances of the death.

In most cases the parents are present when the baby dies, but if not they can be gently encouraged to see and hold their dead infant as this can help them overcome their sense of disbelief. Even when there is a severe congenital malformation, ways can be found to present the baby with much of the affected area covered to enable them to see and hold the infant without causing undue shock if this is what the parents wish. For others, it is important that they see the abnormalities for themselves to help them understand what has happened and why the baby has died. The caring staff themselves often feel deeply for the family and sharing their grief can provide comfort to them.

Most maternity departments have a checklist of all those professional carers who need to be informed of a baby's death so that they can continue to provide appropriate advice and help. In the UK it is the parents' responsibility to register the birth and death of the infant, a task which can accentuate the confused emotions of the situation. If the death was expected and its cause beyond doubt the doctor caring for the baby will complete and sign a death certificate which the registrar will need in order to complete the necessary registrations. After this, the baby's body can be released for the funeral. The parents may need advice on how to arrange the funeral and will wish to do it themselves, although many hospitals will make the arrangements for them if they so wish. Occasionally the death may be of uncertain cause or unexpected. In these situations the local coroner should be consulted and he will often require a postmortem examination to be carried out to establish the cause of death before he allows the death to be registered and the body released for the funeral.

Postmortem examination of the baby

Confirmation of the clinical diagnosis by postmortem examination has traditionally been thought to help the clinician without providing the parents with much useful information. Developments in autopsy techniques have now added cytogenetic analysis and X-rays of the bones to the traditional direct inspection of the internal organs, microscopical analysis of relevant tissues and microbiological culture of fluids and organ surfaces. Recent research into the value of such extended postmortem examination on stillbirths and neonatal deaths has shown that, where there was uncertainty about why the baby died, either the cause of death or important information of relevance in future pregnancies was found at autopsy in about a quarter of cases. Unexpected congenital abnormalities, cytogenetic abnormalities and infections were found particularly frequently. Clinicians have been reticent about suggesting such examinations in the past, but since their value is now clear, an autopsy should be offered to parents in most cases.

Some groups, such as Muslims, will not normally allow postmortem examination for religious reasons, except where the law requires one to be done. Other people may refuse permission for cultural or emotional reasons and this should usually be respected. Some will allow very limited examination such as an organ biopsy, blood sampling or X-ray imaging and these can provide valuable information in some cases.

Although there is a need to inform the parents at the time of death of what is known about its cause, detailed discussions including the result of the autopsy and any subsequent tests are best left until the initial shock has receded. This explanation should wait until both parents can be present and must be given by a senior paediatrician who is well informed of all the facts and understands the implications for the parents' decisions about having further children.

Stillbirth

Until a few years ago, there was a tendency to treat the misfortune of a stillbirth somewhat differently from that of a neonatal death, but it is now better understood that the needs of these parents are much the same and their expressions of grief very similar. Counselling as described for neonatal death is equally appropriate and the parents should be offered the benefit of a postmortem examination of the baby. A dignified disposal of the baby's body should be arranged according to the parents' wishes and customs. It may assist the parents' grieving to realize that they can give the baby a personal name.

Whether the baby was stillborn or died in the first few days, some parents find comfort from having a tangible reminder of the infant such as a photograph, a hand or foot print or a lock of hair and these should be offered if they so wish.

Continuing care for the parents

Grieving will continue long after the parents return home and will involve the other members of the family so it is important that those providing care in the community should have all possible information to enable them to help the family through the process of adjustment. Other children in the family will also grieve for the lost baby and their understanding of what has happened will vary according to their ages. Their needs should also be taken into account as part of the support given to the family.

The continuing flow of lochia and secretion of milk serve as frequent reminders of the bereavement and may accentuate the depression that often ensues as part of the normal grieving process.

To assist parents to grieve the loss of their baby many hospitals provide a 'book of remembrance' in which parents may record a personal memory and the name of their infant. Some families may wish to turn their tragedy into a positive contribution and can be advised about charitable organizations and self-help groups relevant to their experience which they may join. For others, the sense of loss may be so great that more formal treatment may be needed, but fortunately only a small number are affected to this extent.

If the baby's death was due to a congenital abnormality, referral to a clinical geneticist is advisable since it is being increasingly recognized that genetic factors are involved in the origin of many such abnormalities and information gained may be important in the management of subsequent pregnancies.

FURTHER READING

Henley A, Kohner N 1995 When a baby dies: the experience of late miscarriage, stillbirth and neonatal death. Pandora, London
Kimpton D 1990 Special child in the family. Sheldon Press, London
Kohner N 1995 Pregnancy loss and the death of a baby: guidelines for the professional. Stillbirth and Neonatal Death Society, London

Murphy S 1990 Coping with cot death. Sheldon Press, London
Prince J, Adams E 1987 The psychology of childbirth. Churchill Livingstone, Edinburgh
Qureshi B 1989 Transcultural medicine. Kluwer, Dordrecht
Schaffer R 1977 Mothering. Fontana, London
Sinclair J, Bracken M 1992 Effective care of the newborn infant. Oxford University Press, Oxford

15

Neonatal pharmacopoeia

Prescribing drugs for the newborn infant is more complex than for the older child. Drug doses are almost all related to the weight of the infant, which can at times mean greatly different doses of the same drug for two babies in the same unit. The rate at which the infant metabolizes or excretes drugs is often slower, so doses must be given at less frequent intervals to avoid side-effects from accumulation of the substance. A relatively lower blood albumin level may mean that less of the drug is bound and more is in a free, active state in the circulation. Some drugs interact with others and alter their effectiveness or increase the risk of toxicity. It is advisable to avoid using such drugs together. Important interactions are noted in the comments section of the pharmacopoeia. Great care must be taken in prescribing and administration of drugs at this time, and the doses given in this pharmacopoeia (Table 15.1) are a guide to the amount a baby requires rather than a firmly fixed dose. Published doses of drugs for use in the newborn baby vary considerably from one text to another. In this section the doses given correspond closely to those most commonly encountered in other recent books and journals.

Table 15.1

Drug	Route	Single dose	Frequency*	Comments
Adenosine	i.v.	100 µg/kg	1	Flush in with 1 ml of 0.9% saline; use only with ECG monitoring
Aminophylline	i.v.	5 mg/kg	1	Loading dose
	i.v.	2.5 mg/kg	2	Infuse over 30 minutes
	Rectal	5 mg/kg	3	Blood level monitoring needed
Bendrofluazide	Oral	1.25 mg/kg	1	Measure electrolytes; potassium supplements usually required
Caffeine citrate	Oral	20 mg/kg	1	Loading dose
	Oral	5 mg/kg	1	Daily maintenance; keep blood level 25–35 µmol/L
Calciferol (Vit. D$_2$)	Oral	10–25 µg	1	Daily requirements
Calcium chloride	Oral	33 mg/kg	4	With milk feeds
Calcium gluconate	i.v.	0.25 mmol/kg (2 ml/kg of 10% solution)	1	Slow infusion in 0.9% sodium chloride solution under ECG monitoring
	Oral	0.25 mmol/kg	4	With milk feeds
Chloral hydrate	Oral	30 mg/kg	up to 4	
		45 mg/kg	1	Single hypnotic dose
Chlorothiazide	Oral	10 mg/kg	1–2	Give spironolactone 1 mg/kg twice daily also to counteract potassium loss
Chlorpromazine	Oral	500 µg/kg	4	Reduce only slowly in babies of drug-addicted mothers
Cisapride	Oral	0.2 mg/kg	3–4	15 minutes before feeds; do not give with erythromycin or miconazole
Dexamethasone	i.v./oral	200–500 µg/kg	1	Infuse over 5 minutes. For treatment of BPD (p. 139)
Diamorphine	s.c.	50 µg/kg	6	
	i.v.	10–15 µg/kg	Up to hourly	Respiratory depression can be reversed by nalorphine
Diazepam	i.v.	0.2 mg/kg	1–3	Bolus injection over 3 minutes
	Rectal	0.3 mg/kg		Repeat after 10 minutes if fitting persists
Digoxin	i.v.	10 µg/kg	1–3	Loading dose
	Oral	5–10 µg/kg	1	Daily maintenance
Dobutamine	i.v.	5 µg/kg/min	Continuous infusion	Adjust infusion rate according to response
Dopamine	i.v.	2–5 µg/kg per min	Continuous infusion	Adjust infusion rate according to response
Edrophonium	i.m.	100–200 µg/kg	1	Diagnostic test dose
Erythropoietin	s.c.	250 units/kg		3 times per week for 4–6 weeks
Ethamsylate	i.v./i.m.	12.5 mg/kg	4	For 4–6 days
Folic acid	Oral	1 mg	Weekly	
Frusemide	Oral	1 mg/kg	1	
	i.v.	0.5–1.0 mg/kg	1	
Heparin	i.v.	2 units/hour	Continuous infusion	Infuse as a solution of 2 units/ml
Hepatitis B vaccine	i.m.	0.01 mg (0.5 ml)	Single dose	Single dose; repeat at 6 and 12 months of age
Hepatitis B immunoglobulin	i.m.	200 U	Single dose	Give with hepatitis B vaccine
Indomethacin	i.v./oral	0.1–0.3 mg/kg	1	Give for up to 6 days as bolus injections over 10 seconds

Table 15.1 (*cont'd*)

Drug	Route	Single dose	Frequency*	Comments
Insulin	i.v.	0.1 U/kg	Continuous infusion	Dose adjusted according to response
Magnesium sulphate 50%	i.m.	0.2 ml/kg	1–2	Maximum of 3 doses
Mannitol 20% solution	i.v.	0.5–1.0 g/kg	1	Infuse over 30 minutes
Midazolam	i.v.	150 μg/kg	1	For sedation for painful procedures; effect may be reversed by flumazenil 20 mg/kg i.v.
Naloxone	i.v./i.m.	30 μg/kg	1	For immediate reversal of opiate effect
	i.m.	70 μg/kg	1	For continued effect over 24 hours
Pancuronium	i.v.	50–80 μg/kg	Up to hourly	Repeat 1–4 hourly as needed
Paraldehyde	i.m.	0.1 ml/kg	Up to 6	Inject deep into muscles
Pethidine	i.m./i.v.	0.5–2.0 mg/kg	4	Lower doses by the i.v. route
Phenobarbitone	i.v./i.m.	20 mg/kg	1	Loading dose
	Oral	2.5 mg/kg	1–2	Maintenance dose
Phenytoin	i.v.	8 mg/kg	1	No faster than 1 mg/kg per minute; may be repeated after 1 hour
	Oral	2.5–4 mg/kg	2	Keep blood level in target range 40–80 μmol/L
Phytomenadione	i.m./oral	1 mg		Single dose as prophylaxis or to correct deficiency
Prostaglandin E$_2$	i.v.	0.6 μg/kg per hour	Continuous infusion	
Sodium valproate	i.v.	10 mg/kg	1	Loading dose; infuse over 5 minutes
	Oral	10 mg/kg	1–3	Maintenance dose
Spironolactone	Oral	0.5–1.5 mg/kg	2	
Theophylline	Oral	5 mg/kg	1	Loading dose
	Oral	2–3 mg/kg	4	Maintenance dose
Tolazoline	i.v.	1.0 mg/kg	1	Infuse over 10 minutes
	i.v.	0.1–1.0 mg/kg	Hourly	Maintenance infusion
Vitamin E	i.m.	25 mg/kg		3 daily doses
	Oral	10 mg		Daily requirement

*Number of doses per day, or as stated.

FURTHER READING

British National Formulary. Current edition. British Medical Association and Royal Pharmaceutical Association of Great Britain, London

Fleming P, Speidel B, Marlow N, Dunn P 1991 A neonatal vade mecum. Edward Arnold, London

Schott J, Henley A 1996 Culture, religion and childbearing in a multicultural society. Butterworth Heinemann, Oxford

The Northern Neonatal Network 1996 Neonatal formulary. BMJ Publishing Group, London

Index